BRAIN DYSFUNCTION IN INFANTILE FEBRILE CONVULSIONS

International Brain Research Organization
Monograph Series
Volume 2

INTERNATIONAL BRAIN RESEARCH ORGANIZATION MONOGRAPH SERIES

SERIES EDITOR: MARY A. B. BRAZIER

INTERNATIONAL BRAIN RESEARCH
ORGANIZATION MONOGRAPH SERIES
Volume 2

Brain Dysfunction
in Infantile Febrile Convulsions

Edited by

Mary A. B. Brazier

Brain Research Institute
University of California, Los Angeles
Los Angeles, California

Flavio Coceani

The Research Institute
The Hospital for Sick Children
Toronto, Ontario, Canada

Raven Press ▪ New York

Raven Press, 1140 Avenue of the Americas, New York, New York 10036

Made in the United States of America

International Standard Book Number 0–89004–068–0
Library of Congress Catalog Card Number 75–14564

The IBRO Monograph Series

The International Brain Research Organization (IBRO) was founded in 1961 with the goal of fostering, in all countries, fundamental research leading to knowledge of the brain, both normal and abnormal. IBRO is represented by several hundred members drawn from 45 countries. Membership carries no dues and is based only on the contribution that the individual is making to brain science.

Eight categories of membership (the panels) subdivide the membership according to major interests, namely neuroanatomy, neurochemistry, neuroendocrinology, neuropharmacology, neurophysiology, behavioral sciences, neurocommunications and biophysics, and brain pathology.

In order to effect its major goal, IBRO, among its several activities, designs and runs educational workshops in brain science in less scientifically developed countries and, additionally, as evidenced by this volume, organizes major symposia, usually one a year on some special topic, to which members gather from many countries.

The first volume of the series was published in 1975 and contains the proceedings of a symposium held in New Delhi as a satellite to the XXVIth International Congress of Physiology: The subject was *Growth and Development of the Brain: Nutritional, Genetic, and Environmental Factors.*

In October of 1975, an invited symposium was held in Toronto ancillary to the 1st International Congress of Child Neurology. The subject was *Brain Dysfunction in Infantile Febrile Convulsions* and the proceedings form this volume, the second in the IBRO Monograph Series.

Mary A. B. Brazier

Preface

This volume, the second in the Monograph Series of the International Brain Research Organization, contains the proceedings of an IBRO Symposium held in Toronto, Canada in October 1975 as a satellite to the 1st International Congress of Child Neurology with speakers from 12 different countries.

The approach was international and multidisciplinary, and the goal was to achieve a better understanding of the etiology and pathogenesis of this condition and to indicate procedures for prevention and treatment.

Febrile convulsions occur in about 5% of children and complications are a very significant cause of irreversible brain damage leading to mental retardation and temporal lobe epilepsy.

The program was therefore planned to develop knowledge in the field from basic studies of the electrophysiological and morphological features of the maturing brain together with the neurochemical correlates of maturation of the central nervous system. Reports concerning the ontogenesis of thermoregulation and sensitivity to pyrogens led into the subject of pyrexia and the mechanism of action of antipyretic drugs.

The program of the third day of the symposium, held in conjunction with the Congress of Child Neurology, brought these fundamental studies into the consideration of the clinical problem. Susceptibility to febrile convulsions was examined from the point of view of inheritance factors, as well as nutritional deficits, and the neurological sequelae were described. These reports led up to the important subject of acute and prophylactic treatment, the ultimate goal.

This monograph takes its place as an outlet of the activities of the International Brain Research Organization, which was founded in 1961 with the goal of fostering, in all countries, fundamental research leading to knowledge of the brain, normal and abnormal.

IBRO is indebted to Dr. John Stobo Prichard, President of this International Congress of Child Neurology, for his enthusiastic support and to our editorial assistants, Denise Campbell and Gwen Garvin.

Mary A. B. Brazier
Flavio Coceani

Contents

Contributors

J. Aicardi
Clinique de Pediatrie et Puericulture
Hôpital Saint-Vincent de Paul
74, Avenue Denfert-Rochereau
75674 Paris Cedex 14, France

K. P. Bhargava
Department of Pharmacology and Thera-
    peutics
King George's Medical College
Lucknow-2260003, India

Mary A. B. Brazier
Brain Research Institute
University of California Los Angeles
Los Angeles, California 90024

N. A. Buchwald
Mental Retardation Research Center
University of California Los Angeles
Los Angeles, California 90024

D. L. Cheney
Laboratory of Preclinical Pharmacology
National Institute of Mental Health
Saint Elizabeths Hospital
Washington, D.C. 20032

Jean-Jacques Chevrie
Clinique de Pediatrie et Puericulture
Hôpital Saint-Vincent de Paul
74, Avenue Denfert-Rochereau
75674 Paris Cedex 14, France

Flavio Coceani
The Research Institute
The Hospital for Sick Children
555 University Avenue
Toronto M5G 1X8, Ontario, Canada

K. E. Cooper
Division of Medical Physiology
Faculty of Medicine
The University of Calgary
2920 24th Avenue N.W.
Calgary T2N 1N4, Alberta, Canada

E. Costa
Laboratory of Preclinical Pharmacology
National Institute of Mental Health
Saint Elizabeths Hospital
Washington, D.C. 20032

J. T. Coyle
Department of Pharmacology and Experi-
    mental Therapeutics
The Johns Hopkins University
School of Medicine
725 North Wolfe Street
Baltimore, Maryland 21205

C. A. Dinarello
Laboratory of Clinical Investigation
National Institute of Allergy and Infectious
    Diseases
Department of Health Service
National Institutes of Health
Bethesda, Maryland 20014

Murray A. Falconer
Neurological Unit
The Maudsley Hospital
DeCrespigny Park
London SE5 8AZ, England

J. H. French
Department of Pediatrics
Albert Einstein College of Medicine
1300 Morris Park Avenue
Bronx, New York 10461

N. Hashem
Medical Genetics and Pediatrics Division
Faculty of Medicine
Ain-Shams University
5 El-Goumhouria Street
Cairo, Egypt

James N. Hayward
Department of Neurology
Reed Neurological Research Center
University of California Los Angeles
Los Angeles, California 90024

C. D. Hull
Mental Retardation Research Center
University of California Los Angeles
Los Angeles, California 90024

P. Krupp
Research Department
Pharmaceuticals Division
Ciba-Geigy Limited
Basel CH-4002, Switzerland

Margaret A. Lennox-Buchthal
Institute of Neurophysiology
University of Copenhagen
Juliane Mariesvej 36
2100 Copenhagen, Denmark

M. S. Levine
Mental Retardation Research Center
University of California Los Angeles
Los Angeles, California 90024

Peter Lomax
Department of Pharmacology
University of California Los Angeles
School of Medicine
Los Angeles, California 90024

Brian S. Meldrum
Department of Neurology
Institute of Psychiatry
DeCrespigny Park
Denmark Hill
London SE5 8AF, England

A. S. Milton
Department of Pharmacology
University of Aberdeen
University Medical Building
Forester Hill
Aberdeen AB9 22D, Scotland

Nisha Misra
Department of Pharmacology and Thera-
peutics
King George's Medical College
Lucknow-2260003, India

Christopher Ounsted
Human Development Research Unit
The Park Hospital for Children
Old Road
Headington
Oxford OX3 7LQ, England

Q. J. Pittman
Division of Medical Physiology
The University of Calgary
2920 24th Avenue N.W.
Calgary T2N 1N4, Alberta, Canada

E. Preston
Pharmacological Research and Develop-
ment Laboratory
Scientific Development Group
Organon International B.V.
Oss, The Netherlands

J. S. Prichard
Division of Neurology
Hospital for Sick Children
555 University Avenue
Toronto M5G 1X8, Ontario, Canada

David A. Prince
Department of Neurology
Stanford University School of Medicine
Stanford, California 94305

Dominick P. Purpura
Department of Neuroscience
Rose F. Kennedy Center for Research in
Mental Retardation and Human De-
velopment
Albert Einstein College of Medicine
1300 Morris Park Avenue
Bronx, New York 10461

Th. Rabinowicz
Division of Neuropathology
University Hospital, Lausanne
Lausanne 1011, Switzerland

G. Racagni
Laboratory of Preclinical Pharmacology
National Institute of Mental Health
Saint Elizabeths Hospital
Washington, D.C. 20032

E. Schönbaum
Pharmacological Research and Develop-
ment Laboratory
Scientific Development Group
Organon International B.V.
Oss, The Netherlands

K. K. Tangri
Department of Clinical Pharmacology
Royal Postgraduate Medical School
Ducane Road
London W12, England

W. L. Veale
Division of Medical Physiology
The University of Calgary
2920 24th Avenue N.W.
Calgary T2N 1N4, Alberta, Canada

J. R. Villablanca
Mental Retardation Research Center
University of California Los Angeles
Los Angeles, California 90024

Sheila J. Wallace
Department of Child Health
The Welsh National School of Medicine
University Hospital of Wales
Heath Park
Cardiff CF4 4XW, Wales

S. M. Wolff
Laboratory of Clinical Investigation
National Institute of Allergy and Infectious
* Diseases*
National Institutes of Health
Bethesda, Maryland 20014

R. Ziel
Research Department
Pharmaceuticals Division
Ciba-Geigy Limited
Basel CH-4002, Switzerland

G. Zsilla
Laboratory of Preclinical Pharmacology
National Institute of Mental Health
Saint Elizabeths Hospital
Washington, D.C. 20032

Brain Dysfunction in Infantile Febrile
Convulsions, edited by M. A. B. Brazier and
F. Coceani. Raven Press, New York © 1976.

Morphological Features of the Developing Brain

Th. Rabinowicz

Division of Neuropathology, University Hospital,
Lausanne 1011, Switzerland

The neural plate of the human embryo at a gestational age of 1 month shows both an up- and a downward movement of closure. At this stage the central part of the neural tube is closed earlier than the caudal and cephalic regions. Thus already in the first month of our development some quite important topographic differences exist in the maturation of the nervous system, the central part of the neural tube which later will command the musculature of the trunk being the earliest to be developed. Later the caudal part of the neural tube closes also, thus being more mature than the cephalic part, so that we can consider that the neural tube at the level commanding the movements of the legs develops earlier than the cephalic part, which commands the movements of the arms and hands. Using quantitative methods that same sequence of maturation can be observed later, in the 8-month-old premature, in the precentral gyrus of the frontal lobe (Fig. 1). On the other hand, the development progresses much more slowly for the cephalic part of the neural tube: the rhombencephalon and the mesencephalon mature earlier than the prosencephalon.

As for the cerebral cortex, at a gestational age of 4.5 months the hippocampus is already developed and quite clearly recognizable while the rest of the cortex is still at an embryonic stage of development. Even in that embryonic brain, however, some regions are more advanced than others. Not only is Ammon's horn fairly well elaborated but most of the basal ganglia present a well-recognizable structure. At the same time, in the cerebral cortex only the area which will correspond to the precentral gyrus is beginning to take shape.

One of the most important features during that time is represented by the migration of the neuroblasts from their germinal centers up to the future cerebral cortex. However, there are important differences in the speed of maturation of the cerebral cortex, which are quite clear if one studies the histological parameters quantitatively, point by point, at different ages during the entire period of maturation.

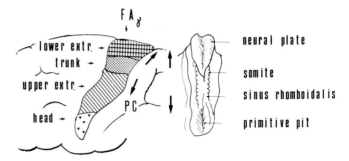

FIG. 1. Right: Period of closure of the neural plate (1 month gestational age). The central part of the plate is now closed, forming the neural tube. The closure is progressing both in caudal and cephalic directions. The closed part later commands the musculature of the trunk. The caudad movement is slightly more rapid than the cephalad movement. **Left:** Premature of the 8th month. Degrees of maturation (number of differentiated nerve cells/ number of neuroblasts, see Rabinowicz, 12). Precentral gyrus, area FA$_\gamma$ (4). The first to mature is the cortical area commanding the movements of the trunk, then that for the legs and feet. The cortex controlling the lower extremity matures earlier than that for the upper extremity, which in turn matures earlier than that for the head. Thus the same spread of maturation (both up- and downward) is realized in the motor cortex as it was 7 months earlier in the neural tube.

TECHNIQUES

Quantitative studies on the number of nerve cells, their sizes, and the thickness of the cerebral cortex and of each of its layers have been performed and were published in 1925 on adults by Economo and Koskinas (3). More recently, between 1936 and 1967, Conel (1) published quantitative data from the full-term newborn and from children 1, 3, 6, and 15 months of age and 2, 4, and 6 years of age. We completed this work with the same methods in the same areas in prematures of 6, 7, and 8 calendar months, two 8-year-old children, and one patient each of 10 and 22 years of age. Some of this work is still ongoing and some is now completed (the 8-month-old premature and the 8-year-old child).

Quantitative information on the cerebral cortex is obtained by counting neurons and glial cells in a 100-μm-side square on sections 25 μm thick after cresyl violet staining on paraffin-embedded material. In the premature the number of well-differentiated neurons is compared to that of the neuroblasts. This gives a ratio which yields information on the degree of maturation of each area. The thickness of the whole cortex and of each layer is also measured. More information on methodology is given elsewhere (11).

Some Morphological and Quantitative Data Related to Neuronal Growth

Evolution of Betz Cells

Stained with cresyl violet, no Nissl substance can be found in Betz cells in the 6-month-old premature. A month later one can find sometimes a few dusty points of cresyl violet-positive substance in the protoplasm of Betz cells in the fifth layer of the precentral gyrus. At the eighth month almost all the protoplasm is filled with a fine dust of cresyl violet-positive substance, but no build-up Nissl bodies are seen like those which will be visible later. These appear first at birth, as described by Conel (1). At 8 years of age (Fig. 2) medium-sized Nissl bodies can be seen at the outer part of the cytoplasm, while the rest of the cytoplasm contains less-well-stained Nissl bodies. These are not present in the same amount in all the Betz cells. In the adult (a 41-year-old patient) the Nissl substance is well developed, heavily stained at the periphery, and clearer around the nucleus. Some Nissl bodies are also quite visible at the beginning of the dendrites.

Neurofibrils

The modified Cajal silver impregnation method reported by Conel and by out laboratory (11) showed that some powdery argentophilic substance was present in a few Betz cells from a 6-month-old premature. An 8-month-old premature showed much more developed Betz cells still containing a powdery argentophilic substance with a few short, but clearly recognizable fibrils. At age 6 years, argentophilic fibrils were quite numerous but seem to be a little shorter than at age 8 years when these fibrils were quite easily demonstrated. At 35 years argentophilic fibrils were quite obvious, but one must note also the presence of a fair amount of lipofuchsin on one side of the protoplasm, a sign of aging.

The *development of the dendrites* goes also through a considerable evolution: The apical dendrite early has a quite remarkable increase in length. A 6-month-old premature shows Betz cells of the fifth layer in which the apical dendrite is approximately five to six times shorter than in the 8-month-old premature. Moreover, not only does the apical dendrite grow fairly rapidly, it appears in the second layer at birth but the basal dendrites are developing as well. While the thorns and bulbs are present as early as in the 6-month-old premature, their number is much higher in the 8-month-old premature and increases considerably throughout the development. We do not yet have quantitative data on the number of these thorns and pedunculated bulbs, but we are working on it. Another important feature is the remarkably good development of the horizontal fibers, mainly in the fourth and fifth layers. Some vertical fibers are also present in the fifth and sixth layers in the subjacent white matter in the precentral gyrus.

As for the *axonal growth,* Rabinowicz (10) noted that at the eighth month there are few collaterals (usually one). They were described by Conel as being more numerous from the fourth year on.

The evolution of the *length and width of the cell body of Betz cells* (Fig. 3) measured at the level of the precentral gyrus commanding the movements of the trunk shows quite interesting features. The thick dotted lines in Fig. 3 give minimum and maximum values of the width of the cells measured be-

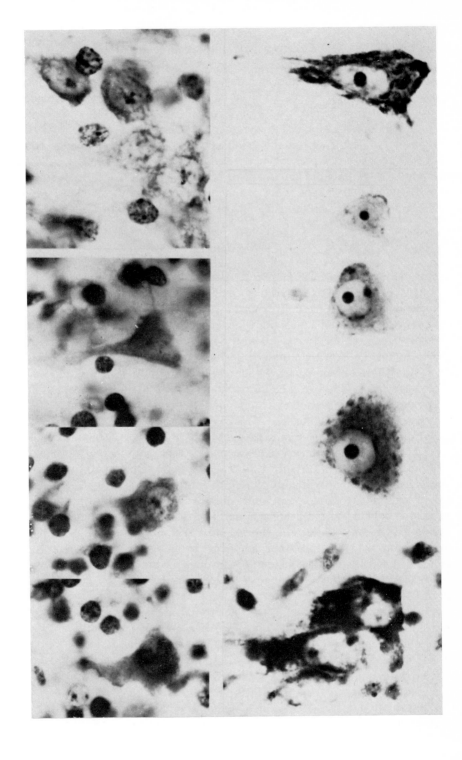

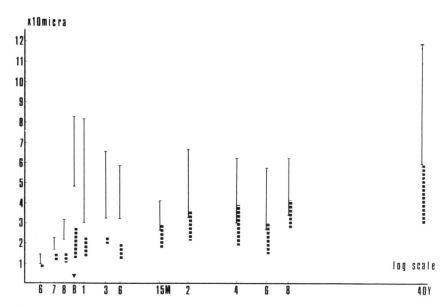

FIG. 3. Evolution of the length and width of the cell body of Betz cells (FA$_\gamma$ trunk) in human brains. Thin lines represent the maximal and minimal values of cell body length. Dotted lines are the maximal and minimal values of cell body width. Note the elongated cells both around birth and in the adult. Between 4 and 8 years most Betz cells are as wide as they are long. Note also the two periods of decreased size of the Betz cells: at approximately 15 months and 6 years.

tween the emergence of the basal dendrites at the largest part of the cells in cresyl violet-stained sections. The thin lines give minimum and maximum values of the length of the cell body measured between the base of the cell and the beginning of the apical dendrite (Fig. 3). The length and width of the cell-body increase rather sharply from the 6-month-old premature until birth. From the moment of birth on, the length of the cell body no longer increases but clearly decreases, while the width is also smaller than at birth, giving the Betz cell-body a rather elongated shape between birth and age 6 months. The minimum length after birth is seen at age 15 months, at which

---

←

FIG. 2. Area FA$_\gamma$ (4). **Top row** (from left to right): First and second frames: Betz cells of a 6-month-old premature. Small cells with no Nissl bodies and a pale nucleus with one or more nucleoli. Third frame: Betz cell from a 7-month-old premature. The cell is triangular and small, with no Nissl bodies. Fourth frame: Betz cell from an 8-month-old premature, with a slightly larger nucleus with one nucleolus. There is some chromophil substance but no Nissl bodies. **Bottom row** (from left to right): First frame: Betz cells with much chromophil substance, a slightly larger nucleus, and some small Nissl bodies. Note the elongated shape of the cell (compare with Fig. 3). Frames 2–4: Three Betz cells from an 8-year-old child. Note the broadly triangular shape of the cells (Fig. 3). Easily recognizable Nissl bodies are present, the darkest along the outer limits of the cytoplasm. The nucleus has a large nucleolus. Frame 5: Betz cell from a 41-year-old man. Note the elongated shape of the cell body, with much Nissl substance (compare with Fig. 3). Cresyl violet staining after paraffin embedding. ×850.

time the cells are almost as wide as they are long. This will last till age 8 years, maybe later, and gives the Betz cell a broadly triangular shape (Fig. 3). In adults the width is less than the length according to measurements established by Economo and Koskinas (3) using the same methods. We do not at present understand the variability in the size of Betz cells nor do we understand their reduction in size around age 1.5 years. Later, at 6 years, there is again a slight reduction, but of much lesser degree than that at 15 months. It is remarkable that the evolution of the thickness of the whole cortex also shows some reduction at approximately the same ages (see below).

Morphological Features of the Development of the Cerebral Cortex and of Its Layers

Generally, in the 6-month-old premature the definition of the layers is very poor, and the cell density is extremely high. Moreover, the layers are much less even than in the 7-month-old premature. The thickness of the layers is also much less in the 6-month-old than in the 7-month-old premature, and much less in the 7-month-old than in the 8-month-old. Our data show the differences of speed of growth measured as an increase in thickness of the layers.

In the 6-month-old premature, except for the first layer, which is always quite easy to recognize, the second layer is extremely irregular in shape everywhere, mostly rather thick and poorly defined towards the third layer. The latter is sometimes indistinguishable from the fourth layer. The fifth layer is somewhat clearer but still sometimes hard to locate. The sixth layer is rather easy to recognize while being still poorly defined toward the fifth layer and the white matter. This description is referred to most of the isocortical areas, whereas areas like the hippocampus behave differently, as we will see. Generally the fifth and sixth layers develop earlier than the others. Some of their features, like columns, begin to be recognizable in the 7-month-old premature. One month before birth the layers are quite similar to the structure seen in older children, but all the layers and particularly the second layer still show a high cellular density and the layers are not as well defined as later.

One may also notice (Fig. 4) that the columnar structures, when present, are built much more densely, and the columns are much narrower. This gives a good representation of the relatively slow growth of the horizontal

———————————————————→

FIG. 4. FA$_y$ trunk. Top left: Six month-old premature. Lower left: Seven-month-old premature. Middle: Eight-month-old premature. Right: Eight-year-old child. The first clear differentiation of the layers is shown at 7 months. Betz cells are in clusters and well recognizable at 8 months. In the 8-year-old child the structure is a rather adult one, and Betz cells are disposed slightly one over the other. Note also the slow increase in thickness of the whole cortex between the 6th and 8th months compared to the thickness in the 8-year-old child. Cresyl violet staining after paraffin embedding. ×39.

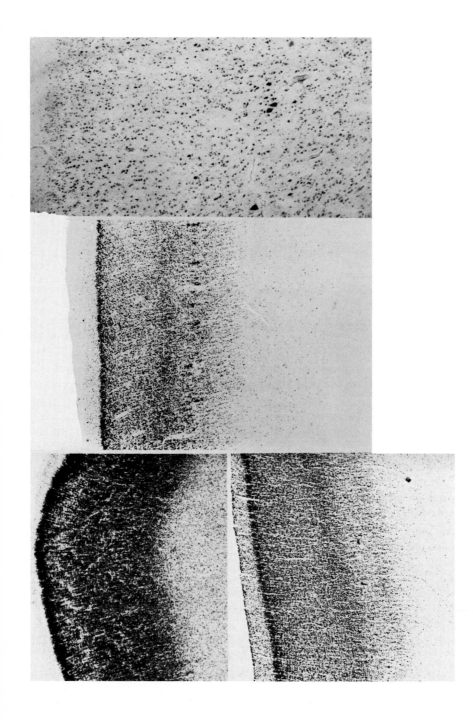

dendrites, which increases the distance between cells of the same layers; apical dendrites grow much faster but with much less branching. Progressively with age and the basal dendrites' growth, the columnar structures are less close and the neuronal density decreases.

It is remarkable that many neurons are displaced from their proper layer, and one can easily find large pyramidal cells in the fourth and sometimes even in the third layer, while their definitive location is in the fifth layer (13).

Another frequently seen feature is the presence of poorly oriented and sometimes even inverted neurons. The large pyramidal cells and Betz cells are mostly agglutinated in the 6- and 7-month-old prematures, while they begin to separate in the 8-month-old premature (Fig. 4) and continue to do so.

Cell Density

One other general feature of the developing cerebral cortex is the rapidly decreasing number of cells per unit of volume. As has been shown (12), the higher the neuronal density the less mature is the tissue. In area FA_γ, at the level commanding the movements of the trunk (precentral gyrus area 4) more than 5,000 cells have been counted by unit of volume in the 6-month-old premature in the second layer and more than 900 cells have been found in the fifth layer (Fig. 5A). At the seventh month the number decreases to 3,100 for the second layer and to approximately 700 for the fifth layer. In the 8-month-old premature the second layer shows approximately 2,200 cells. At birth there is still a decrease in the cell density of the second layer — a phenomenon which lasts until approximately age 15 months — while the fifth layer in a full-term newborn has almost attained a density similar to the one found in adults.

Remarkably enough, the same dynamics of development may be seen in experimental material (Swiss albino mice) (Fig. 5A), the second layer of area 4 having a slower speed of maturation than the fifth layer. Of course there are still some important differences between the cerebral cortex of mice, which is lissencephalic, and that of humans. Moreover, cell densities were studied in our laboratories during the postnatal stages of mice whereas our study in humans is partly prenatal.

Considering our data on cell densities, it would be more accurate to compare the development of the mice brain at 5 days postnatally to the one of the 8-month-old human prematures. In 1918 Sugita (14) admitted that at 5 days postnatally the development of the mice brain corresponded approximately to the development of the human at birth. Recently Dobbing (2) mentioned a period of rapid growth called "brain growth spurt" and insisted on the importance of comparing the same stages of development rather than the same ages between different animals. (The brain growth spurt has been based mainly on biochemical data, including measurements

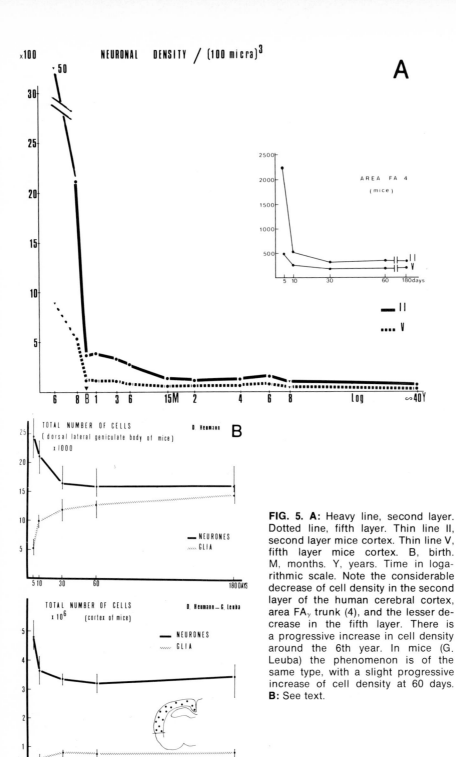

FIG. 5. A: Heavy line, second layer. Dotted line, fifth layer. Thin line II, second layer mice cortex. Thin line V, fifth layer mice cortex. B, birth. M, months. Y, years. Time in logarithmic scale. Note the considerable decrease of cell density in the second layer of the human cerebral cortex, area FA$_\gamma$ trunk (4), and the lesser decrease in the fifth layer. There is a progressive increase in cell density around the 6th year. In mice (G. Leuba) the phenomenon is of the same type, with a slight progressive increase of cell density at 60 days. **B:** See text.

of the amounts of DNA, RNA, proteins, and cholesterol.) This period is mostly postnatal in rats and mice, and pre- and postnatal in humans. At 5 days in mice, the cell density is still very high and decreases rapidly until 10 days; this leads us to presume that we are probably still in the brain growth spurt much before 5 days. Moreover, the growth spurt in mice is much more prominent for the second than for the fifth layer, the latter maturing earlier. As already stated, our data on cell densities reflect the same dynamics in the human brain, the fifth layer also developing earlier. According to Dobbing (2), the brain growth spurt in man seems to begin around the fourth gestational month, the maximum being around birth with a period of decrease extending up to the first postnatal year; we can confirm this grossly on a histoquantitative basis. Nevertheless, our data suggest that the brain growth spurt in man shows a maximum much before birth, probably around the sixth gestational month if not earlier. While Dobbing (2) established the brain growth spurt according to biochemical criteria, the quantitative histological data show that in humans there are actually different growth spurts, not only for the whole brain but also for each area and even for each layer.

As we have seen, cell densities are extremely high in 6-month-old prematures, decreasing rather rapidly during the prenatal period. One may wonder where all these cells go. One of the main reasons for the decreasing number of neurons in our 100-μm unit cube is the growth and development of dendrites, separating the cells from each other. Even so, if the decreased cell density is compared with the increased thickness of the cerebral cortex at the same place, these curves do not quite correspond. It may thus be suspected that a certain number of nerve cells disappear, as has been described by Hamburger (4) and others.

As it is extremely difficult to isolate a part of the cerebral cortex in the human brain in order to follow its development, we tried to investigate this phenomenon in mice: In our laboratory, Heumann (5) and Leuba (9) established by serial sections the volume of a given group of areas [17–18–18a–41–20–2–3–4–10, according to Krieg (7,8)] of the cerebral cortex in mice. The volume was chosen between natural limits established anteriorly by the fornix, laterally by the entorhinal fissure, medially by the pericallous fissure, and posteriorly and inferiorly by the well-recognizable subiculum. The volume was determined at 5, 10, 30, 60, and 180 days postnatally, and the total number of cells was established in this total volume for each age. To control our cortical data, the evolution of the volume of the dorsal lateral geniculate body of mice was also established by Heumann (5) in the same animals, and the total number of cells counted in it at the same ages. Our curves (Fig. 5B) show a very good correspondence between the values of the cerebral cortex and those of the geniculate body. They strongly suggest that there is indeed a decrease in the number of neurons in these volumes (amounting to approximately 30%), most of the decrease occurring between the fifth and tenth postnatal days. Moreover, the total numbers of glial cells increase in both the dorsal lateral geniculate body and the given cerebral areas.

Nevertheless, there are some differences between the geniculate body and the cerebral cortex of mice. The number of neurons in the geniculate body decreases a bit more slowly and the cell density stabilizes slightly faster than in the cerebral cortex. In the latter, the number of glial cells does not increase as rapidly as in the dorsal lateral geniculate body. Our results do not indicate whether the glial cells replace, cell by cell, the disappearing nerve cells. We assume that the slower increase of glial cells in the cerebral cortex compared to that of the geniculate body may reflect a better development of the dendritic system in the cerebral cortex, provided the vascular net does not also absorb a rather important part of the volume. As anatomically and histologically it is much easier and more precise to establish the volume of the dorsal lateral geniculate body, one can assume that the decrease in the number of nerve cells in such a well-defined nucleus can confirm the same phenomenon in a slightly less-well-definable volume of the cerebral cortex. Such a loss of nerve cells has already been shown by Zilles and Wingert (15) in the oculomotor nucleus of mice.

Quantitative and Morphological Study of Some Areas

Hippocampal areas

It is well known that the region of the hippocampus is one of the earliest to develop. As most areas of this region do not have six layers, but four or three—which comprises a more primitive type of cortex—these regions are called allocortical areas. Quantitative data have not been obtained from all of them because it is extremely difficult to count nerve cells irregularly distributed or scattered in small groups or layers not well delineated.

Nevertheless, we tried to establish the evolution of the thickness of the cerebral cortex in *area HE 1β* (according to Economo and Koskinas), which is a pyramidal cortex of three recognizable layers containing medium-sized pyramidal cells in the second layer. It constitutes a portion of the subiculum, which is continued into area HE 1α. Part of area HE 1β, as well as part of area HE 2, constitutes the Sommer sector, which is frequently involved in epileptic seizures. The evolution of the thickness of the HE 1β area shows (Fig. 6) that in the 8-month-old premature and at birth the thickness is slightly less than in the 6- or 7-month-old premature or in the 1-month-old child. Between 3 and 15 months the thickness is greater than that at 2 years up to around 6 years. From 10 years on, the thickness is mostly increased, approximately to what it was around the first year of life. The values from adult brains (3) show quite clearly that the heterogeneity of the cases was so great that two average values had to be given (Fig. 6): One group of cases increased in thickness while the other showed a thinner cortex with age.

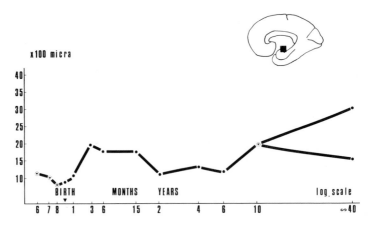

FIG. 6. Evolution of the thickness of the cortex (human) in area HE 1β of the hippocampus. Thickness is measured on cresyl violet-stained sections after paraffin embedding. See text for further details.

In *area HE 1α*, the second layer, which is a pyramidal one whose cells are mostly grouped in glomerules, has approximately the same structure as the adjacent area HE 1β, except that in the latter the glomerular layer is almost continuous. Figure 7A shows the evolution of area HE 1α with the densely packed glomerules or groups of pyramidal cells. The section from the 6-month-old premature shows also the great number of migrating neuroblasts present in the "white matter." At age 8 years the glomerular layer has a well-defined shape and an adult appearance. Comparing the drawings from Golgi-Cox impregnations (Fig. 7B) from the 8-month-old premature with those of the 8-year-old shows the importance of the increased length of the apical dendrites and of the development of the horizontal dendrites. However, in the 8-month-old premature all the different cell types are already clearly recognizable. They are small, with a relatively well-developed cell body, while the dendrites are scarce, the whole structure of that area is already built up, and the different types of cells are at their proper places.

The most internal part of the hippocampus is called Ammon's horn and is shown in Figs. 8A and B in 6- and 8-month-old prematures and an 8-year-old child. The most internal part of Ammon's horn is constituted by a vaguely triangular area defined as *field HF* or *area dentata*. The latter is almost completely surrounded by a layer of granular cells which constitutes "Giacomini's strip" (stratum granulosum). In the 6-month-old premature the entire structure is clearly developed, except that the cell density is extremely high. Two months later, in the 8-month-old premature, the cell density is much less, the molecular layer is rather broad, and the granular layer is thin with neurons already showing well-developed dendrites. Compared with the 8-year-old child, the emphasis in the development is mainly on the dendrites.

Part of *area HE 2* adjacent to area HE 1β represents, together with field HF, a region that is mostly resistant to seizures or hypoxemia and has therefore been called the "resistant stripe."

The longitudinal study of the thickness of area HE 1β (Fig. 6) evokes some questions. There seem to be two periods in our life during which this area is thinner: one period before the age of 1 month and the other between 2 and 6 years. One may wonder if the diminution in thickness in some adult brains is related to the diminution of the functions in that area. (If the ammonic and hippocampal areas are related to some functions in memory, these two groups of thicknesses could have some meaning.)

Frontal area FA_γ (4)

The frontal area FA_γ (4) was studied at all its levels, which on the precentral gyrus allows a separate study of the areas commanding the movements of the head, the arms, the trunk, and the legs, as well as the area commanding the movements of the feet, which is the paracentral lobule. These areas have been studied together with the postcentral gyrus. As we showed (12) in the 8-month-old premature, the most advanced area in the precentral gyrus is the one commanding the movements of the trunk muscles; maturation of the precentral gyrus develops in two directions, both up and down from the more or less central part of the gyrus. Thus maturation of the motor cortex corresponds almost exactly to the closing of the neural tube 6–7 months earlier.

Different general features of the developing cortex are illustrated here using the level of the trunk as an example. As shown in Fig. 4 in the 6-month-old premature, layers 1, 2, and 3 are recognizable, while layer 4 is extraordinarily thick and dense, layer 5 appears clear, and layer 6 is still densely packed. At that time clusters of rather thick pyramidal Betz cells are found mainly in the fifth layer, although some are seen rather frequently in the fourth layer, sometimes even at the base of the third layer, and occasionally in the sixth layer. One month later only the second layer is extremely dense. In the 8-month-old premature, some Betz cells begin to be clearly in a staircase disposition, as they will be later. In the 8-year-old child the cell density is considerably lower and the second layer no longer has a granular appearance but is constituted only of small pyramidal cells.

We have already seen the longitudinal study of the nerve cell density in layers 2 and 5 of FA_γ trunk. Corresponding to the decrease in thickness at around the sixth year, the cell density increases slightly at the same time. If you remember how these data are obtained (in a 100-μm-side cube), it is clear that this does not necessarily mean a real reduction in the number of nerve cells; it could also be interpreted as being the same number of

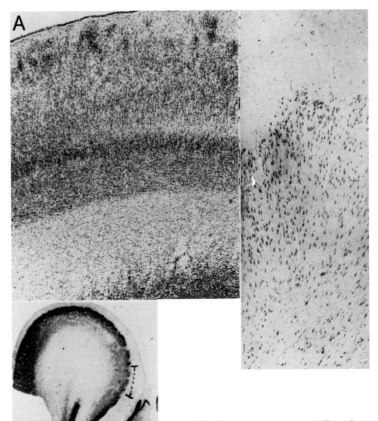

FIG. 7A. Area hippocampi HE 1α. **Lower left:** Dotted line shows the site of area HE 1α. **Top left:** Six-month-old premature. **Right:** Eight-year-old child. See text for further details. Top left and at right: Cresyl violet staining. ×35.

cells but in a thinner cortex. Consequently the cell population seems more or less stable in the second layer from approximately 2 years on, and in the fifth layer from approximately 6 months on—illustrating the differences in the speed of growth between these two layers and the fact that the same area may simultaneously show quite differently matured layers as we have already shown in mice.

The evolution of the thickness of FA_γ area 4 at the level commanding the muscles of the trunk (Fig. 9A) is more or less progressive, with a rather rapid growth period until the sixth postnatal month except during the perinatal period. Growth in that area seems to be rather stable between the ages of 6 months and 8 years. (Data concerning the thickness at 8 and 10 years must still be confirmed, the number of cases being insufficient.) The inter-

K_t for GABA does not change significantly between birth and adulthood, a result similar to that obtained with norepinephrine (10). However, the V_{max} of uptake first increases from birth to 15 days postpartum and then decreases toward adult values, a pattern which coincides with findings in the striatum. These changes in V_{max} are unlikely to be due simply to homo-exchange because the amount of endogenous GABA in the synaptosomal fraction remains relatively constant throughout the developmental period (13). A similar finding has been reported with slices of chick brain (33). Thus it is unlikely that the increased GABA uptake at an early stage of development represents an artifact of the homogenization procedure.

The reason for this unique fluctuation in the V_{max} of GABA uptake during development is unknown at present. It is possible that transport sites are particularly abundant in the immature neuron and then decrease as the neuron differentiates after 2 weeks postpartum. An alternative hypothesis originates from the assumption that the magnitude of GABA uptake, as in the case of dopamine and norepinephrine, is a reflection of the density of specific nerve terminals. If so, one may speculate that GABAnergic neurons yield a rich innervation by 2 weeks postpartum, and that nerve terminals later undergo atrophy or are dispersed among other neuronal and non-neuronal constituents of the brain. Whatever the explanation, there is in the immature brain a marked disparity between the endogenous GABA levels and the activity of the uptake process, which is responsible for the inactivation of synaptically released GABA.

DEVELOPMENT OF CHOLINERGIC NEURONS IN THE STRIATUM

Since choline acetyltransferase levels in the striatum are little affected by lesions to the major afferent pathways (38), cholinergic neurons, like GABAnergic neurons, are thought to be intrinsic to the striatum. Based on ultramicroscopic characteristics, it has been surmised that certain small interneurons are cholinergic (1,38). Autoradiographic studies of the incorporation of ^{3}H-thymidine demonstrate that cell division in the rat striatum peaks during the final days of gestation and continues for several days after birth, particularly in the case of small interneurons (16,17,49). Thus cholinergic neurons are probably still in the process of multiplication or in the early stage of differentiation by the time dopaminergic processes begin to provide a significant innervation to the striatum.

Unlike acetylcholinesterase, which occurs in both neuronal and non-neuronal elements of the CNS, choline acetyltransferase is specific to cholinergic neurons and thus is a reliable marker for these cells (38). The specific activity of choline acetyltransferase in the neonatal striatum is only 2% that of the adult, and it rises to 4% during the first 7 days after brith (Fig. 4). Afterwards, choline acetyltransferase levels increase linearly and

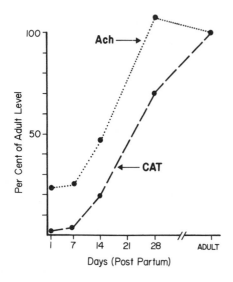

Days (Post Partum)

FIG. 4. Development of cholinergic neurons in the rat striatum. Activity of choline acetyltransferase (CAT) was measured by the method of Bull and Oderfeld-Nowak (4). For determination of endogenous acetylcholine, rats were killed by microwave irradiation focused on their skulls to preclude postdecapitation changes in the levels of the neurotransmitter; Ach was measured by the enzymatic-radiometric method of Goldberg and McCaman (19). Results are presented in terms of percent of adult specific activity or concentration. Values for the adult striatum per milligram wet weight are: CAT, 32 nmoles-hr^{-1}; Ach, 65 pmoles. Each point is the mean of five or more separate preparations; SEMs are $\leq$ 10%.

reach 70% of adult values by 28 days. Similar to findings with GABA, the concentration of acetylcholine in the neonatal striatum is quite high, being 23% that of the adult. Thus there is a 10-fold difference between acetylcholine content and choline acetyltransferase activity in the neonate relative to the adult. Like choline acetyltransferase activity, acetylcholine content increases only 2% during the first week after birth. However, the concentration of the neurotransmitter increases linearly from 7 days onwards and attains adult levels by 28 days. Notably, the rise in tissue acetylcholine precedes the increase in specific activity of choline acetyltransferase throughout ontogenesis; however, the two processes develop in parallel.

DEVELOPMENT OF THE DOPAMINE RECEPTOR
IN THE STRIATUM

A dopamine-sensitive adenylate cyclase has been demonstrated in the corpus striatum and other regions of the CNS that are innervated by dopaminergic neurons (5,29,41). This adenylate cyclase demonstrates many properties that are expected for the "dopamine receptor" from pharmacologic and physiologic findings. It is responsive to low concentrations of dopamine with a K_m of 4 μM. It is inhibited by neuroleptic drugs including phenothiazines, butyrophenones, and thiozanthines; but β-agonists and β-blockers have negligible effects on its activity. Little is known about the development of the dopamine-sensitive adenylate cyclase except for reports by Lolley et al. (37) on its ontogenesis in the mouse retina and by Von Hungen et al. (54) on its presence in subcortical regions of the immature rat brain.

Activity of the dopamine-sensitive adenylate cyclase was measured in cell-free homogenates of the striatum at different stages of development according to the method of Kebabian et al. (29). Synthesis of adenosine-3′, 5′-cyclic monophosphate (cyclic AMP) was determined for homogenates incubated in the presence of 50 μM dopamine or in the presence of 50 μM dopamine plus 5 μM fluphenazine, a potent blocker of the dopamine receptor (5,41). Dopamine stimulated significantly the formation of cyclic AMP in both the mature and immature striatal preparation, and the effect was completely reversed by the presence of fluphenazine. At birth the dopamine-sensitive cyclase activity in the striatum is 20% that of the adult (Table 2). It increases rapidly and linearly during the early postnatal period and attains adult values by 28 days. Notably, adenylate cyclase and the presynaptic markers for the dopaminergic neuron (i.e., tyrosine hydroxylase, endogenous dopamine, dopamine uptake) develop in parallel; however, adenylate cyclase matures first. Thus in dopaminergic synapses the maturation of the postsynaptic receptor precedes that of the presynaptic mechanisms.

Most neurons in the striatum are depressed by iontophoretically applied dopamine (6,40). Interestingly, cyclic AMP is a depressor agent on the same neurons (51), which accords with the concept that adenylate cyclase is the postsynaptic receptor in dopaminergic synapses. Conversely, blockade of dopamine receptors by treatment with neuroleptics results in increased rates of neuronal firing (6). Further, there is strong evidence that dopaminergic neurons impinge on cholinergic neurons in the striatum. Systemic administration of dopamine receptor blockers results in lower levels of acetylcholine in the tissue, whereas an opposite effect follows treatment with dopamine receptor agonists (22,50). A possible explanation for these findings is that the nigral dopaminergic pathway exerts a tonic inhibitory influence on cholinergic neurons in the striatum.

TABLE 2. *Development of dopamine-sensitive adenylate cyclase in the striatum*

Age	Dopamine + fluphenazine	Dopamine	Δ	% Stimulation
Newborn (3)	1.0 ± 0.4	3.0 ± 0.3	2.0 ± 0.2	200
8 days (3)	2.0 ± 0.2	6.4 ± 0.8	4.4 ± 0.8	220
15 days (3)	3.8 ± 0.2	8.6 ± 0.2	5.7 ± 0.9	126
21 days (1)	4.5	14.1	9.6	213
28 days (3)	6.6 ± 0.6	18.8 ± 1.2	12.2 ± 0.6	185
Adult (3)	10.2 ± 1.9	20.2 ± 2.3	10.0 ± 1.1	98

Corpora striata were dissected from brain of rats at 3°C immediately after killing and were homogenized in 25 or 50 volumes of tris acetate buffer. Adenylate cyclase activity of homogenates was measured according to the method of Kebabian et al. (29). Measurements were done in triplicate in control tissues and in tissues treated with dopamine (50 μM) or dopamine (50 μM) plus fluphenazine (5 μM). Results (mean ± SEM) are expressed in terms of picomoles of cyclic AMP formed per milligram tissue during a 150-sec incubation. Number of separate preparations assayed is in parentheses.

To determine when the dopaminergic pathway acquires the postulated functional control over striatal cholinergic neurons, we examined the effects of the potent neuroleptic fluphenazine on the levels of acetylcholine in the striatum of rats of various ages. Rats were administered fluphenazine (5 mg/kg) subcutaneously and were decapitated 30 min after treatment. The concentration of acetylcholine in the striatum of fluphenazine-treated animals was compared to that of vehicle-treated controls (Table 3). Fluphenazine treatment results in a 38% decrement in the concentration of acetylcholine in adults, but has no significant effect on acetylcholine levels in the striatum of newborn or 5-day-old rats. A response to fluphenazine appears at 8 days after birth and consists of a 26% decrease in acetylcholine levels. A comparable response is obtained in the 17-day-old or adult animals. The present findings are in agreement with recently published results of Guyenet et al. (21).

These studies indicate that the dopamine-sensitive adenylate cyclase and the responsiveness of cholinergic neurons to dopamine receptor blockade do not develop concurrently in the striatum. The lack of response to fluphenazine until 8 days after birth does not appear to be due to hypoactivity of the dopaminergic mechanism: Keller et al. (30) have shown that the turnover of dopamine is quite high in the neonatal striatum, and that dopamine receptor stimulation or blockade results in appropriate responses. Possibly the dopamine-sensitive cyclase measured in the striatum during the first week after birth is localized to noncholinergic neurons and nonneuronal cells. Cholinergic neurons would acquire adenylate cyclase only at 8 days postpartum, when they cease dividing and undergo differentiation. In this

TABLE 3. *Effect of fluphenazine on acetylcholine levels in the striatum*

| | Acetylcholine (% of mean control value) | |
Age	Control	Fluphenazine
Newborn (5)	100 ± 9	101 ± 14
5 days (10)	100 ± 6	119 ± 9
8 days (5)	100 ± 4	74 ± 3^a
17 days (5)	100 ± 9	64 ± 6^a
Adult (5)	100 ± 8	62 ± 7^a

Rats of various ages were administered fluphenazine (5 mg/kg) or the equivalent volume of vehicle by subcutaneous injection. Immature rats were maintained at 35°C to preclude hypothermia. The rats were decapitated 30 min after treatment and the corpora striata rapidly dissected at 3°C and frozen on solid CO_2. The concentration of acetylcholine in the tissue was measured by the radiometric-enzymatic assay of Goldberg and McCaman (19). Results are expressed in terms of percent of control values. Number of rats in each experimental group is given in parentheses.
  [a] $p \leq 0.01$.

regard it is noteworthy that the choline acetyltransferase activity exhibits a sharp rise at 8 days postpartum, when the pharmacologic effects of fluphenazine first appear. Alternatively, there may be in cholinergic neurons a delay between the time of appearance of dopamine-sensitive adenylate cyclase and the time when the enzyme becomes functional.

DISCUSSION

Our previous studies on the ontogenesis of noradrenergic neurons in whole rat brain demonstrated a remarkably close correlation in the development of several presynaptic mechanisms. The present investigation focused on the dopaminergic innervation to the striatum and proved that several presynaptic components of the dopaminergic system (i.e., tyrosine hydroxylase, uptake of dopamine, dopamine content) develop concurrently. Each component has a separate cytologic location. The high-affinity transport mechanism is located in the neuronal membrane (15); tyrosine hydroxylase is a soluble enzyme in the neuroplasm (8); and levels of dopamine probably reflect the density of storage vesicles derived from the agranular reticulum (27). Since presumably each component is under distinct genetic control, differentiation of dopaminergic neurons appears to be a well-coordinated process. This coordination is even more remarkable if one considers findings with GABAnergic and cholinergic neurons of the striatum. In the latter neurons, biosynthetic enzyme, level of neurotransmitter, and (if present) the uptake mechanism do not develop concurrently.

From the foregoing it follows that immature GABAnergic and cholinergic neurons differ from adult neurons in that they lack an appropriate balance in the activity of presynaptic mechanisms. These mechanisms condition the availability of the neurotransmitter in the synaptic cleft. If one uses the activity of glutamic acid decarboxylase as the norm in GABAnergic neurons, GABA levels and the activity of the synaptosomal uptake mechanism are, respectively, 6- and 12-fold higher in neonatal than in adult striatum. Similarly, there is a 10-fold disparity between acetylcholine concentration and choline acetyltransferase activity in the neonatal striatum. In the adult pharmacologic interference with processes responsible for the synthesis, storage, or inactivation of a neurotransmitter can have considerable effects on the function of neurons. Therefore the occurrence of a different ratio of these three parameters in the immature versus the mature brain suggests that developing neurons are functionally quite different from fully differentiated neurons. For example, in the 2-week-old rat the postsynaptic action of GABA may be severely curtailed by the presence of a remarkably avid presynaptic uptake mechanism.

An additional feature of the developing striatum is the occurrence of a varying functional relationship among neuronal pathways. If it is assumed that the steady-state ratio among levels of the three neurotransmitters is optimal in the adult striatum, there are considerable deviations from such a ratio early in development. With levels of dopamine as the norm, levels of acetylcholine and GABA are, respectively, two- and fourfold higher in the neonatal than in the adult striatum. Furthermore, synapses may become functional long after the development of the appropriate receptor site. Thus striatal cholinergic neurons become receptive to the inhibitory action of dopaminergic afferents only several days after dopaminergic terminals and dopamine-sensitive adenylate cyclase can be demonstrated in the tissue.

These studies clearly demonstrate the heterogeneous nature of neuronal differentiation in a well-defined region of the CNS. First, the presynaptic mechanisms that regulate the availability of neurotransmitter show different rates of development in a particular neuronal type; the varying balance among these mechanisms would affect the function of the neuronal pathway. Second, neuronal pathways differ substantially with regard to the time of their appearance in the developing nervous tissue. The combined effect of these *intra-* and *inter*neuronal developmental changes results in an immature nervous system that is not merely quantitatively but also qualitatively different from that of the adult. These factors may explain in part the unusual manifestation of neurologic disorders, the paradoxical action of pharmacologic agents, and the lower seizure threshold during childhood.

ACKNOWLEDGMENTS

Portions of this work were done in collaboration with S. J. Enna and P. Campochiaro. The author wishes to thank Robert Zaczek for his excellent technical assistance and Nancy Hiatt and Vickie Rhodes for their secretarial assistance. This research was supported by USPHS Grant DA 00266.

REFERENCES

1. Bak, I. J., Choi, W. B., Hassler, R., Usunoff, K. G., and Wagner, A. (1975): Fine structural synaptic organization of the corpus striatum and substantia nigra in rat and cat. *Adv. Neurol.*, 9:25–41.
2. Bernheimer, H., Birkmayer, W., Hornykiewicz, O., Jellinger, K., and Seitelberger, F. (1973): Brain dopamine and the syndromes of Parkinson and Huntington: Clinical, morphological and neurochemical correlations. *J. Neurol. Sci.*, 20:415–455.
3. Bird, E. D., Mackay, A. V. P., Rayner, C. N., and Iversen, L. L. (1973): Reduced glutamic acid decarboxylase activity of post-mortem brain in Huntington's chorea. *Lancet*, 1:1090–1092.
4. Bull, G., and Oderfeld-Nowak, B. (1971): Standardization of a radiochemical assay of choline acetyltransferase and a study of the activation of the enzyme in rabbit brain. *J. Neurochem.*, 19:935–947.
5. Clement-Cormier, Y. C., Parrish, R. G., Petzold, G. L., Kebabian, J. W., and Greengard, P. (1975): Characterization of a dopamine-sensitive adenylate cyclase in rat caudate nucleus. *J. Neurochem.*, 25:143–150.
6. Connor, J. D. (1970): Caudate nucleus neurones: Correlation of the effects of substantia nigra stimulation with iontophoretic dopamine. *J. Physiol. (Lond.)*, 208:691–703.

7. Cotzias, G. C., Papavasilion, P. S., and Gellene, R. (1969): Modification of parkinsonism— chronic treatment with L-DOPA. *N. Engl. J. Med.*, 280:337–345.
8. Coyle, J. T. (1972): Tyrosine hydroxylase in rat brain—cofactor requirements; regional and subcellular distribution. *Biochem. Pharmacol.*, 21:1935–1944.
9. Coyle, J. T. (1974): Biochemical aspects of the catecholaminergic neurons in the brain of the fetal and neonatal rat. In: *Dynamics of Degeneration and Growth in Neurons*, edited by K. Fuxe, L. Olson, and Y. Zotterman, pp. 425–434. Pergamon Press, New York.
10. Coyle, J. T., and Axelrod, J. (1971): Development of the uptake and storage of L-[^{3}H]nor-epinephrine in the rat brain. *J. Neurochem.*, 18:2061–2075.
11. Coyle, J. T., and Axelrod, J. (1972): Dopamine-β-hydroxylase in the rat brain: Developmental characteristics. *J. Neurochem.*, 19:449–459.
12. Coyle, J. T., and Axelrod, J. (1972): Tyrosine hydroxylase in rat brain: Developmental characteristics. *J. Neurochem.*, 19:1117–1123.
13. Coyle, J. T., and Enna, S. J. (1975): Ontogenesis of GABAnergic neurons in the rat brain. *Brain Res. (in press)*.
14. Coyle, J. T., and Henry, D. (1973): Catecholamines in fetal and newborn rat brain. *J. Neurochem.*, 21:61–67.
15. Coyle, J. T., and Snyder, S. H. (1969): Catecholamine uptake by synaptosomes in homogenates of rat brain: Stereospecificity in different areas. *J. Pharmacol. Exp. Ther.*, 170:221–231.
16. Creeps, E. S. (1974): Time of neuron origin in preoptic and septal areas of the mouse: An autoradiographic study. *J. Comp. Neurol.*, 157:161–244.
17. Das, G. D., and Altman, J. (1970): Postnatal neurogenesis in caudate nucleus and nucleus accumbens septi in the rat. *Brain Res.*, 21:122–127.
18. Ellenberger, C., Hanaway, J., and Netsky, M. G. (1969): Embryogenesis of the inferior olivary nucleus in the rat: A radioautographic study and a re-evaluation of the rhombic lip. *J. Comp. Neurol.*, 137:71–83.
19. Goldberg, A. M., and McCaman, R. E. (1973): The determination of picomole amounts of acetylcholine in mammalian brain. *J. Neurochem.*, 20:1–8.
20. Graham, L. T., and Aprison, M. H. (1966): Fluorometric determination of aspartate, glutamate and γ-aminobutyric acid in nerve tissue using enzymatic methods. *Anal. Biochem.*, 15:487–497.
21. Guyenet, P. G., Beaujouan, J. C., and Glowinski, J. (1975): Ontogenesis of neostriatal cholinergic neurons in the rat and development of their sensitivity to neuroleptic drugs. *Naunyn Schmiedebergs Arch. Pharmacol.*, 288:329–334.
22. Guyenet, P. G., Javoy, F., Agid, Y., Beaujouan, J. C., and Glowinski, J. (1975): Dopamine receptors and cholinergic neurons in rat neostriatum. *Adv. Neurol.*, 9:43–51.
23. Hammill, J., and Carter, S. (1966): Febrile convulsions. *N. Engl. J. Med.*, 274:563–565.
24. Hattori, T., McGeer, P. L., Fibiger, H. C., and McGeer, E. G. (1973): On the source of GABA-containing terminals in the substantia nigra: Electron microscopic autoradiographic and biochemical studies. *Brain Res.*, 54:103–114.
25. Hokfelt, T., Fuxe, K., and Goldstein, M. (1973): Immunohistochemical studies on monoamine-containing cell systems. *Brain Res.*, 62:461–469.
26. Hokfelt, T., Jonsson, G., and Lidbrink, P. (1970): Electron microscopic identification of monoamine nerve ending particles in rat brain homogenates. *Brain Res.*, 22:147–151.
27. Holtzman, E., Teichberg, S., Abrahams, S. J., Citkowitz, E., Crain, S. M., Kawai, N., and Peterson, E. R. (1973): Notes on synaptic vesicles and related structures, endoplasmic reticulum, lysosomes and peroxisomes in nervous tissue and the adrenal medulla. *J. Histochem. Cytochem.*, 21:349–385.
28. Iversen, L. L., and Bloom, F. E. (1972): Studies of the uptake of [^{3}H]-GABA and [^{3}H]-glycine in slices of homogenates of rat brain and spinal cord by electron microscope autoradiography. *Brain Res.*, 41:131–143.
29. Kebabian, J. W., Petzold, G. L., and Greengard, P. (1972): Dopamine-sensitive adenylate cyclase in caudate nucleus of rat brain and its similarity to the "dopamine receptor." *Proc. Natl. Acad. Sci. USA*, 69:2145–2149.
30. Keller, H. H., Bartholini, G., and Pletscher, A. (1973): Spontaneous and drug-induced changes of cerebral dopamine turnover during post natal development of rats. *Brain Res.*, 64:371–378.

31. Klawans, H. L. (1970): A pharmacologic analysis of Huntington's chorea. *Eur. Neurol.,* 4:148–163.
32. Lamprecht, F., and Coyle, J. T. (1972): DOPA decarboxylase in the developing rat brain. *Brain Res.,* 41:503–506.
33. Levi, G. (1972): Transport systems for GABA and for other amino acids in incubated chick brain tissue during development. *Arch. Biochem. Biophys.,* 151:8–21.
34. Levi, G., and Raiteri, M. (1973): Detectability of high and low affinity uptake systems for GABA and glutamate in rat brain slices and synaptosomes. *Life Sci.,* 12:81–88.
35. Loizou, L. (1971): Effect of inhibition of catecholamine synthesis on central catecholamine-containing neurones in the developing albino rat. *Br. J. Pharmacol.,* 41:41–48.
36. Loizou, L. A. (1972): The postnatal ontogeny of monoamine-containing neurones in the central nervous system of the albino rat. *Brain Res.,* 40:395–418.
37. Lolley, R. N., Schmidt, S. Y., and Farber, D. B. (1974): Alterations in cyclic AMP metabolism associated with photoreceptor cell degeneration in C3ZH mouse. *J. Neurochem.,* 22:701–708.
38. Markham, C. H., and Knox, J. W. (1965): Observations on Huntington's chorea in childhood. *J. Pediatr.,* 67:46–57.
39. McGeer, P. L., McGeer, E. G., Fibiger, H. C., and Wickson, V. (1971): Neostriatal choline acetylase and cholinesterase following selective brain lesions. *Brain Res.,* 35:308–314.
40. McLennan, H., and York, D. H. (1967): The action of dopamine on neurons of the caudate nucleus. *J. Physiol. (Lond.),* 189:393–402.
41. Miller, R. J., Horn, A. S., and Iversen, L. L. (1974): The action of neuroleptic drugs on dopamine stimulated adenosine-3'5'-monophosphate production in rat neostriatum and limbic forebrain. *Mol. Pharmacol.,* 10:759–766.
42. Nicholson, J. L., and Bloom, F. E. (1973): Cell differentiation and synaptogenesis in the locus coeruleus, raphe nuclei and substantia nigra of the rat. *Anat. Rec.,* 175:398–399.
43. Olson, L., and Seiger, A. (1972): Early prenatal ontogeny of central monoamine neurons in the rat: Fluorescence histochemical observations. *Z. Anat. Entwicklungsgesch.,* 137:301–316.
44. Olson, L., Seiger, A., and Fuxe, K. (1972): Heterogeneity of striatal and limbic dopamine fluorescent islands in developing and adult rats. *Brain Res.,* 44:283–288.
45. Perry, T. L., Hansen, S., and Kloster, M. (1973): Huntington's chorea: Deficiency of γ-aminobutyric acid in brain. *N. Engl. J. Med.,* 288:337–342.
46. Pickel, V. M., Joh, T. H., Field, P. M., Becker, C. G., and Reis, D. J. (1975): Cellular localization of tyrosine hydroxylase by immunohistochemistry. *J. Histol. Cytochem.,* 23:1–12.
47. Roberts, E., Harman, P. J., and Frankel, S. (1951): γ-Aminobutyric acid content and glutamic decarboxylase activity in developing mouse brain. *Proc. Soc. Exp. Biol.,* 78:799–803.
48. Sachs, Ch., De Champlain, J., Malmfors, T., and Olson, L. (1970): The postnatal development of noradrenaline uptake in adrenergic nerves of different tissues from the rat. *Eur. J. Pharmacol.,* 9:67–79.
49. Schultze, B., Nowak, B., and Maurer, W. (1974): Cycle times of neural epithelial cells of various types of neurons in the rat: An autoradiographic study. *J. Comp. Neurol.,* 158:207–218.
50. Sethy, V. H., and Van Woert, M. H. (1974): Modification of striatal acetylcholine concentration by dopamine receptor agonists and antagonists. *Res. Commun. Chem. Pathol. Pharmacol.,* 8:13–28.
51. Siggins, G. R., Hoffer, B. J., and Ungerstedt, U. (1975): Electrophysiologic evidence for involvement of cyclic adenosine monophosphate in dopamine responses of caudate neurons. *Life Sci.,* 15:779–792.
52. Van den Berg, C. J., Van Kempen, G. M. J., Schade, J. P., and Veldstra, H. (1965): Levels and intracellular localization of glutamate decarboxylase and other enzymes during the development of the brain. *J. Neurochem.,* 12:863–869.
53. Vernadakis, A., and Woodbury, D. M. (1962): Electrolyte and amino acid changes in rat brain during maturation. *Am. J. Physiol.,* 203:748–752.
54. Von Hungen, K., Roberts, S., and Hill, D. F. (1974): Development and regional variations

in neurotransmitter sensitive adenylate cyclase systems in cell free preparations from rat brain. *J. Neurochem.*, 22:811–819.

55. Wender, P. H. (1972): The minimal brain dysfunction syndrome in children. *J. Nerv. Ment. Dis.*, 155:55–64.
56. Whittaker, V. P. (1965): The application of subcellular fractionation techniques to the study of brain function. *Prog. Biophys. Mol. Biol.*, 15:41–96.
57. Wilson, S. H., Schrier, B. K., Farber, J. L., Thompson, E. J., Rosenberg, R. N., Blume, A. J., and Nirenberg, M. W. (1972): Markers for gene expression in cultured cells from the nervous system. *J. Biol. Chem.*, 247:3159–3169.

Brain Dysfunction in Infantile Febrile
Convulsions, edited by M. A. B. Brazier and
F. Coceani. Raven Press, New York © 1976.

Cholinergic and Adenylate Cyclase Systems in Rat Brain Nuclei During Development

D. L. Cheney, E. Costa, G. Racagni, and G. Zsilla

Laboratory of Preclinical Pharmacology, National Institute of Mental Health, Saint Elizabeths Hospital, Washington, D.C. 20032

Available studies of cholinergic mechanisms in the central nervous system indicate that the highest concentration of acetylcholine and the highest activity of choline acetyltransferase occur in the nuclei accumbens, caudatus, and interpeduncularis (8,61). In evaluating the synaptic interactions in these nuclei it must be considered that while nuclei accumbens and caudatus contain important dopaminergic afferents, nucleus interpeduncularis is devoid of such afferents. Although little is known about the functional neuroanatomical relationships of cholinergic and dopaminergic neurons within the nucleus accumbens, the choline acetyltransferase activity of the striatum has been located in small interneurons with bifurcating axons which exclusively synapse with striatal cells (6,30,35). Several lines of indirect neurochemical evidence suggest that dopaminergic nerve terminals of the nigrostriatal pathway regulate the metabolism of striatal acetylcholine (2,34,45,51,54,55). It is possible, however, that the dopaminergic afferents to the nucleus accumbens may not exactly replicate the type of control on cholinergic activity as has been described for the nucleus caudatus.

The ontogenesis of cholinergic and dopaminergic neurons in the striatum and the development of interrelationships between these two systems has been the objective of several studies (21,40). These studies have shown that a dopaminergic system is functional in the striatum of 1-day-old rats while a functional cholinergic system cannot be demonstrated even in 10-day-old rats. The mechanisms which initiate the maturation of the cholinergic system in the striatum are unknown. However, evidence has been presented that the striatum contains a dopamine-sensitive adenylate cyclase (28) whose maturation (23,24,58) parallels that of choline acetyltransferase (32,40). Whether adenylate cyclase or the cyclic nucleotides are causally related to the maturation process of the striatal cholinergic system has not been studied. In fact, the exact role of the cyclic nucleotides in the development and function of the striatum is currently unknown (23). However, the cyclic nucleotides have been shown to participate in the function of postsynaptic receptors for catecholamines (14,15,22,29,59). Cyclic adenosine 3',5'-monophosphate (c-AMP) has been implicated in the dopaminergic hyperpolarization of ganglion cell neurons (27,38,39), while cyclic guanosine 3',5'-monophosphate (c-GMP) appears to be involved in the depolarization of these neurons following transsynaptic activation of muscarinic receptors (29). The *in vivo* synthesis of c-AMP has been shown to be increased by transsynaptic activation of noradrenergic neurons (12) and by agonists of dopamine receptors (7,9). The striatal concentrations of c-GMP are increased by several analgesics (46) and to a smaller extent by drugs which inhibit γ-aminobutyric acid (GABA) synthesis (5). Moreover, in the cerebellum the c-GMP content of the molecular and Purkinje cell layers can be increased by activation of the climbing fibers (10,37), which probably are not cholinergic neurons. In adrenal medulla the chromaffin cells are innervated by cholinergic neurons impinging on nicotinic and muscarinic receptors (16). Nicotinic receptors control the adenylate cyclase activity and the concentration of c-AMP, while muscarinic receptors control guanylate cyclase activity and the concentration of c-GMP (18). In this tissue a sustained increase of c-AMP content promotes a delayed increased synthesis of tyrosine hydroxylase. This is mediated by the activation and translocation of a protein kinase from the cytosol to the nucleus. These considerations suggest that postsynaptically a given receptor may include either guanylate cyclase or adenylate cyclase. Moreover, c-AMP has been shown to play a role in the transsynaptic control of protein synthesis (18).

Most studies on the development of either cholinergic neurons or the enzymes that control synthesis and/or metabolism of the cyclic nucleotides have been concerned with whole brain or have been limited to a single brain region which includes various anatomical subsystems. Consideration of the variety of receptor functions regulating c-AMP or c-GMP synthesis spells out the inherent difficulties in interpreting ontogenesis of the cyclases in relation to neuronal systems. In the present study we have attempted to minimize these difficulties by measuring the concentrations of acetylcholine, choline, and c-AMP as well as the activity of choline acetyltransferase and adenylate cyclase at selected times after parturition in various stereomicroscopically isolated nuclei of the rat brain. The nuclei we selected do not contain a homogenous population of postsynaptic receptors, but they do contain some biochemically identified neuronal systems.

METHODS

Pregnant rats which had all been artificially inseminated on the same day (Zivic-Miller, Allison Park, Pa.) were housed for at least 2 weeks prior to parturition in separate cages at 22°C with a 12-hr light-dark cycle. Following parturition neonatal rats of either sex were killed by decapitation for the enzyme studies or by focused microwave radiation (2.4 kW; 2.45 GHz; 75 W/cm^2; 1–1.5 sec) (17) for measurement of tissue concentrations of choline, acetylcholine, and c-AMP. Irrespective of the manner in which the neonates were killed, the brains were quickly removed from the skull and frozen in powdered dry ice.

For some experiments the frozen brains were mounted on a microtome stage (8), and a series of successive coronal sections (400 μm thick) were cut (0°–2°C). The sections were collected and kept frozen on glass slides. Various brain nuclei were localized and punched out with stainless steel tubing (1.2 mm i.d.), transferred to 1.5-ml micro test tubes (Brinkman Instruments, Westbury, N.Y.), and kept frozen at −70°C until assayed.

Choline acetyltransferase activity was assayed according to the procedure described by Schrier and Schuster (50) and modified by Trabucchi et al. (56). Acetylcholine and choline concentrations were determined by gas chromatography-mass spectrometry (Finnigan 3000, Finnigan Inc., Palo Alto, Calif.) using the method of Jenden and Hanin (25) as modified by Cheney et al. (8) for small tissue samples. Adenylate cyclase activity was measured by the method of Kebabian et al. (28) modified by Zivkovic et al. (62). Cyclic AMP was isolated, purified (19,20,36), and assayed by the activation of a purified c-AMP-dependent protein kinase isolated from beef heart (31).

RESULTS

Choline Acetyltransferase

Rats were decapitated at various times after parturition and the activity of choline acetyltransferase determined in several brain nuclei (Fig. 1).

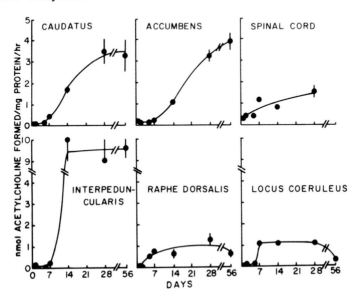

FIG. 1. Choline acetyltransferase activity in rat brain nuclei at various times following parturition. Values represent the mean ± SE of five determinations.

The choline acetyltransferase activity was very low between 1 and 7 days after birth in the nuclei caudatus, accumbens, and interpeduncularis. Adult activity was reached at 14 days in the nucleus interpeduncularis. There was a significant increase in activity in the nucleus accumbens and nucleus caudatus at 14 days, but the adult activity level was reached only by 28 days. In the spinal cord, nucleus raphe dorsalis, and nucleus locus coeruleus, there was a much smaller total increase in choline acetyltransferase with age. An increment over that of 1-day-old rats was evident at 7 days in the spinal cord and the nucleus locus coeruleus, and at 5 days in the nucleus raphe dorsalis. In the nuclei included in Fig. 1 the choline acetyltransferase activity at 28 and 56 days was essentially comparable.

Acetylcholine and Choline

The concentrations of acetylcholine and choline in brain nuclei at 1–60 days are shown in Figs. 2 and 3. On day 1 the acetylcholine concentration in the nuclei accumbens, caudatus, and interpeduncularis was approximately 25% of adult levels. Between 7 and 14 days these values increased significantly over the values at birth, the adult concentrations being reached by 28 days. In the spinal cord there was a significant increase in acetylcholine content by 14 days. Unfortunately, older animals could not be studied be-

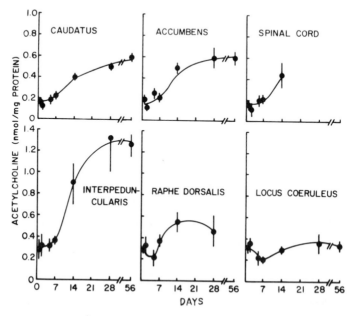

FIG. 2. Acetylcholine content of rat brain nuclei at various times following parturition. Values represent the mean ± SE of five determinations.

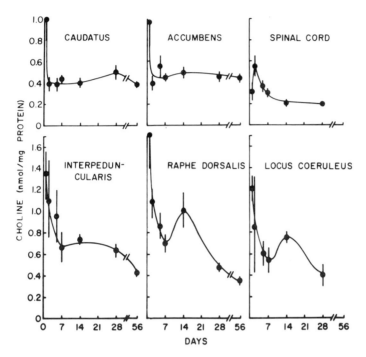

FIG. 3. Choline content of rat brain nuclei at various times following parturition. Values represent the mean ± SE of five determinations.

cause our microwave apparatus does not allow us to fix the whole spinal cord of rats when their age exceeds 28 days. The acetylcholine content of the nucleus raphe dorsalis doubled between birth and 14 days of age. No significant change in acetylcholine content occurred in the nucleus locus coeruleus at any time after birth.

In the nuclei caudatus and accumbens the choline content decreased dramatically between 1 and 2 days following parturition, to a level that remained constant throughout the time interval we studied. In the nuclei interpeduncularis, raphe dorsalis, and locus coeruleus the adult level was reached somewhat more gradually. The decline was rapid from 1 day to 7 days and then more gradual from 14 days until adult values were reached at 56 days. To test whether the dramatic decline of choline content was due to a change in choline permeability, 1- and 28-day-old rats were injected subcutaneously with choline-D_4 (200 μmole/kg) and killed by microwave radiation 1, 2, and 5 min later. Choline-D_4 was measured in whole brain (Fig. 4). In 28-day-old rats the choline-D_4 content failed to change at various times after injection, whereas in the whole brain of 1-day-old rats the choline-D_4 content increased gradually with time.

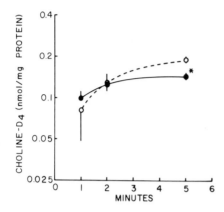

FIG. 4. Incorporation of choline-D₄ (200 μmole/kg s.c.) into rat brain as a function of time. One day (*open circles*) and 28 days (*closed circles*) after parturition. Values represent the mean ± SE of five determinations. Asterisk indicates a statistically significant difference.

Adenylate Cyclase

Figure 5 compares the activities of choline acetyltransferase and adenylate cyclase in rat nucleus caudatus at various times following parturition. The increment of the adenylate cyclase activity with time paralleled that of the choline acetyltransferase activity. The activities of both enzymes were low during the first few days after birth. Only after 15 days did the activities of the two enzymes reach 40–50% of the 28-day values.

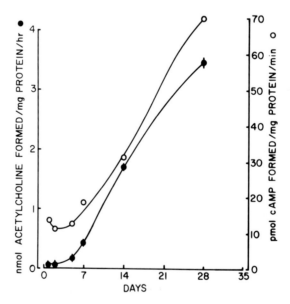

FIG. 5. Adenylate cyclase (*open circles*) and choline acetyltransferase (*closed circles*) activities in rat nucleus caudatus at various times after parturition. For adenylate cyclase activity each value represents the average of two determinations which did not differ from each other by more than 10%. For choline acetyltransferase activity each value represents the mean ± SE of five determinations.

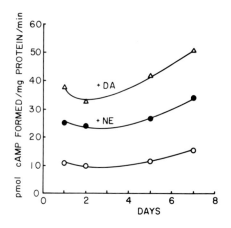

FIG. 6. Catecholamine-stimulated adenyl-ate cyclase activity at various times following parturition. Open circles, control values. Closed circles, norepinephrine (NE) (10^{-5} M) stimulation. Open triangles, dopamine (DA) (10^{-5} M) stimulation. Values for control and norepinephrine stimulation represent the average of two determinations which did not differ from each other by more than 10%. Values for dopamine stimulation represent the mean ± SE of three determinations.

The adenylate cyclase activity in homogenates of the nucleus caudatus from rats killed at various times after parturition was measured in the presence and absence of low concentrations of norepinephrine (10^{-5} M) and dopamine (10^{-5} M) (Fig. 6). At birth dopamine stimulated adenylate cyclase

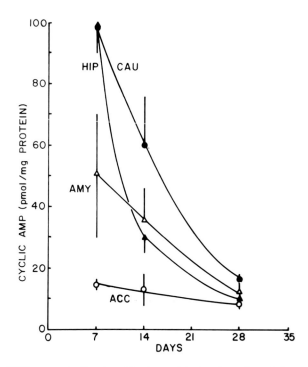

FIG. 7. Cyclic AMP concentration in rat brain nuclei at various times following parturition. Closed circles, nucleus caudatus (CAU). Closed triangles, hippocampus (HIP). Open triangles, nucleus amygdaloideus (AMY). Open circles, nucleus accumbens (ACC). Values represent the mean ± SE of five determinations.

by 3.6-fold, whereas norepinephrine stimulated the enzyme by 2.4-fold. The extent of adenylate cyclase activation remained stationary for the first 5 days but increased significantly at 7 days after parturition. During the entire time period, the activity was always greater in the presence of dopamine than in the presence of norepinephrine.

Cyclic AMP

Concentrations of c-AMP were determined in the nuclei caudatus, accumbens, amygdaloideus, and hippocampus (Fig. 7). In all regions the c-AMP content was highest at birth and decreased between 7 and 10 days postnatally. The largest decrease occurred in the nucleus caudatus and the hippocampus, while in the nucleus accumbens the decrease was slight.

DISCUSSION

In the rat brain many enzyme systems involved in the regulation of neurotransmitter mechanisms begin to develop during the second postnatal week (3,44). This developmental pattern was described for choline acetyltransferase (32,40) and adenylate cyclase (23,24,58). Developmental studies of the concentration of the substrate for choline acetyltransferase and the product of adenylate cyclase have been complicated by the rapid postmortem changes which occur in the brain content of these two compounds. Studies have shown that c-AMP levels in the central nervous system increase rapidly postmortem (11,17,52,57). It is therefore mandatory that the brain content of c-AMP or choline during ontogenesis is measured after almost instantaneous inactivation of metabolic enzymes. When this was done it was found that both choline and c-AMP concentrations decline after birth. While the phenomenon is apparently similar, the cause for the decline of these two compounds is probably different. We have shown that there is a greater permeability of the blood-brain barrier to choline-D_4 immediately after birth than at 28 days. This finding suggests, but does not prove, that developmental changes in the permeability to quaternary compounds may be operative in causing the abrupt decline of brain choline content. Permeability changes are less important in controlling the brain content of c-AMP because this nucleotide is synthesized in brain. Since available evidence suggests that a number of cholinergic neurons in the striatum contain dopamine-dependent adenylate cyclase, it became of interest to study whether a dopamine-dependent adenylate cyclase was present at birth. The experiments reported in Fig. 6 show that as early as 1 day after parturition there is a substantial amount of enzyme which is susceptible to dopamine stimulation.

The neonatal development of cholinergic interneurons in striatum was investigated by measuring the tissue content of choline and acetylcholine and the tissue activity of choline acetyltransferase and adenylate cyclase as a function of time after parturition. The activity of choline acetyltransferase was very low in the nuclei caudatus, accumbens, and interpeduncularis from day 1 until approximately day 7. Then the activity increased rapidly, reaching adult values between 14 and 28 days after birth. These results are in agreement with previous observations in the striatum (21,40) and whole brain (32). Thus one might infer that the nuclei accumbens and interpeduncularis also contain small cholinergic interneurons. Such dramatic increases in enzyme activity were not seen with the nuclei raphe dorsalis, locus coeruleus, or spinal cord. In these tissues comparatively smaller increases were seen between 7 and 28 days after birth. The very high increase of choline acetyltransferase activity occurring in the nucleus caudatus during development may be due to formation of axons and dendritic processes in the small cholinergic interneurons (6,33). This view is in keeping with the parallel increase of choline acetyltransferase and adenylate cyclase activity shown in Fig. 5. In the nuclei raphe dorsalis and locus coeruleus—which contain either the cholinergic nerve terminals (8,43) impinging on serotonergic (raphe dorsalis) (4) and noradrenergic (locus coeruleus) (26,41,42) cell bodies or cholinérgic axons *en passant*—the increase in choline acetyltransferase activity and acetylcholine content during development is much less evident.

Although the rise in acetylcholine levels in the various brain nuclei is not as marked as that of the choline acetyltransferase activity, the two processes appear to develop in a time-related fashion. Presumably this relationship is possible because acetylcholinesterase activity is present at birth in all brain areas and increases by only two- to threefold from birth to adulthood (1,40). Thus the enzyme that degrades acetylcholine does not appear to be the limiting factor for the tissue concentration of acetylcholine.

Adenylate cyclase activity in the nucleus caudatus was low for several days after birth (Fig. 5). A significant increase was seen in 7-day-old rats; in 14-day-old rats the activity was 50% of that at 28 days. Studies by others have demonstrated an increase in adenylate cyclase activity (which reaches a maximum at approximately 30 days after birth) in whole brain (23) and cerebrum (58). Phosphodiesterase activity has been shown to increase to a maximum approximately 25–30 days after parturition in the cerebrum (58) and in soluble and particulate fractions of whole brain (48). It is rather difficult to explain on the basis of available data why the c-AMP content decreases so markedly after birth. Since this decrease is not associated with a change of adenylate cyclase activity, we must assume that the regulation of c-AMP content depends to a large extent on other factors. Perhaps changes in phosphodiesterase activity and the possible influence of a phosphodiesterase activator (53) account for this finding.

Earlier studies, performed without rapid fixation of brain tissues with microwave radiation, showed that either the c-AMP content of whole brain increases during development (47,48) or that no change occurs from birth to 63 days of age (60). Following decapitation the c-AMP content of brain increases at a very fast rate (17,57). It is therefore impossible to compare these data on the c-AMP content with those obtained after instantaneous inactivation of brain enzymes (16,49).

The observation that the striatum contains a catecholamine-sensitive adenylate cyclase at birth (24,28,49) indicates that the mechanisms for postsynaptic receptor function of dopaminergic synapses are already present. Moreover, the intensity of dopamine stimulation increases with time after birth in parallel with the increase of choline acetyltransferase and adenylate cyclase activities. These observations raise the possibility that at birth a portion of the adenylate cyclase of the nucleus caudatus is located in small cholinergic interneurons. Moreover, it appears that following the functional innervation of the receptors after birth the interneurons acquire the capability of controlling the c-AMP content, and this may result in lower c-AMP levels. Conversely, it is possible that the decrease in c-AMP content after birth reflects the development of another cell system which exerts an inhibitory influence on the adenylate cyclase. Some lines of evidence have suggested that GABA-containing cells may be present in the striatum (13). These cells may express their synaptic function by inhibiting adenylate cyclase either directly or through suppression of the dopaminergic stimulation.

REFERENCES

1. Abdel-Latif, A. A., Smith, J. P., and Ellington, E. P. (1970): Subcellular distribution of sodium-potassium adenosine triphosphate, acetylcholine and acetylcholinesterase in developing rat brain. *Brain Res.*, 18:441–450.
2. Anden, N-E., and Bedard, P. (1971): Influences of cholinergic mechanisms on the function and turnover rate of brain dopamine. *J. Pharm. Pharmacol.*, 23:460–462.
3. Baker, P. C., and Quay, W. B. (1969): 5-Hydroxytryptamine metabolism in early embryogenesis and the development of brain and retinal tissues: A review. *Brain Res.*, 12:273–295.
4. Bertilsson, L. M. (1975): Effect of p-chloroamphetamine on the concentration of 5-hydroxytryptamine in rat raphe nuclei measured by mass fragmentography. *Fed. Proc.*, 34:800.
5. Biggio, G., and Guidotti, A. (1976): Climbing fiber activation and 3',5'-cyclic guanosine monophosphate (cGMP) content in cortex and deep nuclei of cerebellum. *Brain Res.*, 107:365–374.
6. Butcher, S. G., and Butcher, L. L. (1974): Origin and modulation of acetylcholine activity in the neostriatum. *Brain Res.*, 71:167–171.
7. Carenzi, A., Guidotti, A., Revuelta, A., and Costa, E. (1975): Molecular mechanisms in the action of morphine and viminol (R_2) on rat striatum. *J. Pharmacol. Exp. Ther.*, 194:311–318.
8. Cheney, D. L., LeFevre, H. F., and Racagni, G. (1975): Choline acetyltransferase activity and mass fragmentographic measurement of acetylcholine in specific nuclei and tracts of rat brain. *Neuropharmacology*, 14:801–809.
9. Costa, E., Carenzi, A., Guidotti, A., and Revuelta, A. (1973): Narcotic analgesics and the regulation of neuronal catecholamine stores. In: *Frontiers in Catecholamine Research*, edited by E. Usdin and S. Snyder, pp. 1003–1010. Pergamon Press, New York.

10. Costa, E., Guidotti, A., Mao, C. C., and Suria, A. (1975): New concepts on the mechanism of action of benzodiazepines. *Life Sci.,* 17:167–186.
11. Dross, K., and Kewitz, H. (1972): Concentration and origin of choline in rat brain. *Naunyn Schmiedebergs Arch. Pharmacol.,* 274:91–106.
12. Ebadi, M. S., Weiss, B., and Costa, E. (1970): Adenosine 3'-5'monophosphate in rat pineal gland: Increase induced by light. *Science,* 170:188–190.
13. Fonnum, F., Grofova, I., Rinvik, E., Storm-Mathisen, J., and Walberg, F. (1974): Origin and distribution of glutamate decarboxylase in the substantia nigra of the cat. *Brain Res.,* 71:77–82.
14. Greengard, P., and Kebabian, J. W. (1974): Role of cyclic AMP in synaptic transmission in the mammalian peripheral nervous system. *Fed. Proc.,* 33:1059–1067.
15. Greengard, P., McAfee, D. A., and Kebabian, J. W. (1972): On the mechanism of action of cyclic AMP and its role in synaptic transmission. *Adv. Cyclic Nucleotide Res.,* 1:337–355.
16. Guidotti, A., and Costa, E. (1974): A role for nicotinic receptors in the regulation of the adenylate cyclase of adrenal medulla. *J. Pharmacol. Exp. Ther.,* 189:665–675.
17. Guidotti, A., Cheney, D. L., Trabucchi, M., Doteuchi, M., Wang, C., and Hawkins, R. A. (1974): Focussed microwave radiation: A technique to minimize post mortem changes of cyclic nucleotides, DOPA and choline and to preserve brain morphology. *Neuropharmacology,* 13:1115–1122.
18. Guidotti, A., Hanbauer, I., and Costa, E. (1974): Role of cyclic nucleotides in the induction of tyrosine hydroxylase. *Adv. Cyclic Nucleotide Res.,* 5:619–639.
19. Guidotti, A., Weiss, B., and Costa, E. (1972): Adenosine 3',5'-monophosphate concentrations and isoproterenol-induced synthesis of deoxyribonucleic acid in mouse parotid gland. *Mol. Pharmacol.,* 8:521–530.
20. Guidotti, A., Zivkovic, B., Pfeiffer, R., and Costa, E. (1973): Involvement of 3',5'-cyclic adenosine monophosphate in the increase of tyrosine hydroxylase activity elicited by cold exposure. *Naunyn Schmiedebergs Arch. Pharmacol.,* 278:195–206.
21. Guyenet, P. G., Beaujouan, J. C., and Glowinski, J. (1975): Ontogenesis of neostriatal cholinergic neurones in the rat and development of their sensitivity to neuroleptic drugs. *Naunyn Schmiedebergs Arch. Pharmacol.,* 288:329–334.
22. Hoffer, B. J., Siggins, G. R., Oliver, A. P., and Bloom, F. E. (1972): Cyclic AMP-mediated adrenergic synapses to cerebellar Purkinje cells. *Adv. Cyclic Nucleotide Res.,* 1:411–423.
23. Hommes, F. A., and Beere, A. (1971): The development of adenyl cyclase in rat liver, kidney, brain and skeletal muscle. *Biochim. Biophys. Acta,* 237:296–300.
24. Hungen, K. Von, Roberts, S., and Hill, D. F. (1974): Developmental and regional variations in neurotransmitter-sensitive adenylate cyclase systems in cell-free preparations from rat brain. *J. Neurochem.,* 22:811–819.
25. Jenden, D. J., and Hanin, I. (1973): Gas chromatographic microestimation of choline and acetylcholine after n-demethylation by sodium-benzene-thiolate. In: *Choline and Acetylcholine: Handbook of Chemical Methods for Quantitative Microassay in Tissue Extracts,* edited by I. Hanin, pp. 135–155. Raven Press, New York.
26. Jones, B. E., and Moore, R. T. (1974): Catecholamine-containing neurons of the nucleus locus coeruleus in the cat. *J. Comp. Neurol.,* 157:43–51.
27. Kebabian, J. M., and Greengard, P. (1971): Dopamine-sensitive adenyl cyclase: Possible role in synaptic transmission. *Science,* 174:1346–1349.
28. Kebabian, J. W., Petzold, G. L., and Greengard, P. (1972): Dopamine-sensitive adenylate cyclase in caudate nucleus of rat brain, and its similarity to the "dopamine receptor." *Proc. Natl. Acad. Sci. USA,* 69:2145–2149.
29. Kebabian, J. W., Steiner, A. L., and Greengard, P. (1975): Muscarinic cholinergic regulation of cyclic guanosine 3',5'-monophosphate in autonomic ganglia: Possible role in synaptic transmission. *J. Pharmacol. Exp. Ther.,* 193:474–489.
30. Kemp, J. M., and Powell, T. P. S. (1971): The structure of the caudate nucleus of the cat: Light and electron microscopy. *Philos. Trans. R. Soc. Lond. [Biol.],* 262:383–390.
31. Kuo, J. F., and Greengard, P. (1972): An assay method for cyclic AMP and cyclic GMP based upon their abilities to activate cyclic AMP dependent and cyclic GMP dependent protein kinase. *Adv. Cyclic Nucleotide Res.,* 2:41–50.
32. Ladinsky, H., Consolo, S., Peri, G., and Garattini, S. (1972): Acetylcholine, choline and

choline acetyltransferase activity in the developing brain of normal and hypothyroid rats. *J. Neurochem.*, 19:1947–1952.

33. Lake, N. (1973): Studies on the habenulo-interpeduncular pathway in cats. *Exp. Neurol.*, 41:113–132.

34. Lloyd, K. G., and Bartholini, G. (1974): The effect of methiothepin on cerebral monoamine neurons. *Adv. Biochem. Psychopharmacol.*, 10:305–309.

35. Lynch, G. S., Lucas, P. A., and Deadwyler, S. A. (1972): The demonstration of acetylcholinesterase containing neurons within the caudate nucleus of the rat. *Brain Res.*, 45:617–621.

36. Mao, C. C., and Guidotti, A. (1974): Simultaneous isolation of adenosine 3′,5′-cyclic monophosphate (cAMP) and guanosine 3′,5′-cyclic monophosphate (cGMP) in small tissue samples. *Anal. Biochem.*, 59:63–68.

37. Mao, C. C., Guidotti, A., and Costa, E. (1975): Inhibition by diazepam of the tremor and the increase of cerebellar cGMP content elicited by harmaline. *Brain Res.*, 83:516–519.

38. McAfee, D. A., and Greengard, P. (1972): Adenosine 3′,5′-monophosphate: Electrophysiological evidence for a role in synaptic transmission. *Science*, 178:310–312.

39. McAfee, D. A., Schorderet, M., and Greengard, P. (1971): Adenosine 3′,5′-monophosphate: Increase associated with synaptic transmission. *Science*, 171:1156–1158.

40. McGeer, E. G., Fibiger, A. C., and Wickson, V. (1971): Differential development of caudate enzymes in the neonatal rat. *Brain Res.*, 32:433–440.

41. Olsen, L., and Fuxe, K. (1971): On the projections from the locus coeruleus noradrenaline neurons: The cerebellar innervation. *Brain Res.*, 28:165–171.

42. Olsen, L., and Fuxe, K. (1972): Further mapping out of central noradrenaline neuron systems: Projections of the "subcoeruleus" area. *Brain Res.*, 43:289–295.

43. Palkovits, M., and Jacobowitz, P. M. (1974): Topographic atlas of catecholamine and acetylcholinesterase containing neurons in the rat brain. II. Hindbrain (mesencephalon, rhombencephalon). *J. Comp. Neurol.*, 157:29–42.

44. Pitts, F. N., Jr., and Quick, C. (1967): Brain succinate semialdehyde dehydroxygenase-II. *J. Neurochem.*, 14:561–570.

45. Racagni, G., Cheney, D. L., Trabucchi, M., and Costa, E. (1976): In vivo actions of clozapine and haloperidol on the turnover rate of acetylcholine in rat striatum. *J. Pharmacol. Exp. Ther.*, 196:323–332.

46. Racagni, G., Zsilla, G., Guidotti, A., and Costa, E. (1975): Accumulation of cGMP in striatum of rats injected with narcotic analgesics: Antagonism by naltrexone. *J. Pharm. Pharmacol.*, 28:258–260.

47. Schmidt, M. J., and Robison, G. A. (1972): The effect of neonatal thyroidectomy on the development of the adenosine 3′,5′-monophosphate system in the rat brain. *J. Neurochem.*, 19:937–947.

48. Schmidt, M. J., Palmer, E. C., Dettbarn, W-D., and Robison, G. A. (1970): Cyclic AMP and adenyl cyclase in the developing rat brain. *Dev. Psychobiol.*, 3:53–67.

49. Schmidt, M. J., Schmidt, D. E., and Robison, G. A. (1971): Cyclic adenosine monophosphate in brain areas: Microwave irradiation as a means of tissue fixation. *Science*, 173:1142–1143.

50. Schrier, B. K., and Schuster, L. (1967): A simplified radiochemical assay for choline acetyltransferase. *J. Neurochem.*, 14:977–985.

51. Stadler, H., Lloyd, K. G., Gadea-Cira, M., and Bartholini, G. (1973): Enhanced striatal acetylcholine release by chlorpromazine and its reversal by apomorphine. *Brain Res.*, 55:476–480.

52. Stavinoha, W. B., and Weintraub, S. T. (1974): Choline content of rat brain. *Science*, 183:964–965.

53. Strada, S. J., Uzunov, P., and Weiss, B. (1974): Ontogenetic development of a phosphodiesterase activator and the multiple forms of cyclic AMP phosphodiesterase of rat brain. *J. Neurochem.*, 23:1097–1103.

54. Trabucchi, M., Cheney, D. L., Racagni, G., and Costa, E. (1974): Involvement of brain cholinergic mechanisms in the action of chlorpromazine. *Nature (Lond.)*, 249:664–666.

55. Trabucchi, M., Cheney, D. L., Racagni, G., and Costa, E. (1975): In vivo inhibition of striatal acetylcholine turnover by L-dopa, apomorphine and (+)-amphetamine. *Brain Res.*, 85:130–134.

56. Trabucchi, M., Cheney, D. L., Susheela, A. K., and Costa, E. (1975): Possible defect in cholinergic neurons of muscular dystrophic mice. *J. Neurochem.,* 24:417–423.
57. Uzunov, P., and Weiss, B. (1971): Effect of phenothiazine tranquillizers on the cyclic 3′,5′-adenosine monophosphate system of the rat brain. *Neuropharmacology,* 10:697–708.
58. Weiss, B. (1971): Ontogenetic development of adenyl cyclase and phosphodiesterase in rat brain. *J. Neurochem.,* 18:469–477.
59. Weiss, B., and Costa, E. (1968): Selective stimulation of adenyl cyclase of rat pineal gland by pharmacologically active catecholamines. *J. Pharmacol. Exp. Ther.,* 161:310–319.
60. Weiss, B., and Strada, S. J. (1973): Adenosine 3′,5′-monophosphate during fetal and postnatal development. In: *Fetal Pharmacology,* edited by L. Boreus, pp. 205–235. Raven Press, New York.
61. Yamamura, H. I., Kuhar, M. J., Greenberg, D., and Snyder, S. H. (1974): Muscarinic cholinergic receptor binding: Regional distribution in monkey brain. *Brain Res.,* 66:541–546.
62. Zivkovic, B., Guidotti, A., Revuelta, A., and Costa, E. (1975): Effect of thioridazine, clozapine and other antipsychotics on the kinetic state of tyrosine hydroxylase and on the turnover rate of dopamine in striatum and nucleus accumbens. *J. Pharmacol. Exp. Ther.,* 194:37–46.

Brain Dysfunction in Infantile Febrile
Convulsions, edited by M. A. B. Brazier and
F. Coceani. Raven Press, New York © 1976.

Prostaglandin System in Developing and Mature Central Nervous Tissue

Flavio Coceani

The Research Institute, The Hospital for Sick Children, Toronto M5G 1X8, Canada

It is now well established that the prostaglandins (PGs) are ubiquitous compounds capable of varied and potent actions on a wide range of cellular processes. My object here is to review the present state of knowledge about the PGs in the central nervous system (CNS), dwelling specifically on topics that seem relevant to the theme of this volume. The reason for referring to the "PG system" in the title is twofold; first, it implies that I am concerned not only with the PGs and their possible function in the CNS but also with the organization of synthetic and degradative pathways; and second, it underlines the fact that PG biosynthesis generates, besides the PGs proper, several other compounds of biological interest.

PROSTAGLANDIN BIOSYNTHESIS

Since the pioneer work in Bergström's and van Dorp's laboratories (reviewed in ref. 49), it has been known that the PGs are formed from essential fatty acids. Arachidonic acid is the most common precursor, at least in mammals. For many years the biosynthetic process was visualized as a sequence of reactions yielding first an oxygenated intermediate, the cyclic endoperoxide, and then the various PG types. Implicitly, it was assumed that only fatty acid derivatives possessing the prostanoate structure are biologically active and that E- and F-type PGs are, functionally speaking, the major endproducts of the reaction. Recent advances in the field (i.e., the characterization of an active non-PG metabolite of arachidonic acid—thromboxane A_2[1]—and the demonstration of biological actions of the intermediates in PG biosynthesis) modified that "classic" scheme and afforded new concepts on the organization of the biosynthetic enzyme system and on the function of the PGs (21; see also 49). Since PG biosynthesis has been studied primarily in nonneural tissues (e.g., the sheep vesicular gland), it is convenient first to integrate all experimental data into a comprehensive scheme and then examine how such a scheme is applicable to the CNS. The

---

[1] Thromboxane A_2 is thought to be identical with the "rabbit aorta contracting substance" of Piper and Vane (46).

biosynthetic process (Fig. 1) is initiated by the enzymic cleavage of arachidonic acid from a membrane lipid that is likely a phospholipid (31). This
step is considered rate-limiting for the subsequent reactions (31,34). Free
arachidonic acid may then be metabolized to several products via three
pathways. In pathway 1 the fatty acid is converted to a nonprostanoate
product—12L-hydroxy-5,8,10,14-eicosatetraenoic acid (HETE)—by an
oxygenase-catalyzed reaction (17,18). No data are available on the function
of this pathway except for a recent report (55) proving that HETE is a
chemotactic agent for neutrophils. Pathways 2 and 3 generate several active
compounds. They are thromboxane A_2, the endoperoxide intermediates
PGG_2 and PGH_2, and the PGs proper. Several enzymes, known collec-
tively as the PG synthetase complex, catalyze these reactions (17,18,21,
22,42; reviewed in ref. 49).

According to this novel scheme, the biosynthetic process is potentially

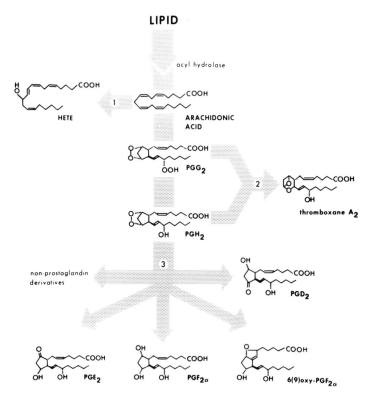

FIG. 1. Pathways in the metabolism of arachidonic acid. The initial step of the reaction
(*interrupted arrow*) is rate-limiting. Note that all biologically active products, with the
exception of thromboxane A_2, possess the prostanoate structure, i.e., the structure of a
20-carbon monocarboxylic acid with a cyclopentane ring. See text for details.

very flexible and may yield a variable mixture of active and inactive products depending on the tissue, the functional state, or both. Several observations are consistent with this possibility:

1. PGs are distributed unevenly in the body (reviewed in ref. 29); and in some organs the pattern of PG release changes on stimulation (50). Incubation experiments with the endoperoxide intermediates demonstrate organ differences in the activity of PG-forming enzymes (39,41,42).

2. Arachidonic acid is metabolized to nonprostanoate products, rather than to PGE_2 and $PGF_{2\alpha}$, in platelets (20) and lung tissue (18). One of such products is the hemiacetal derivative of 8-(1-hydroxy-3-oxopropyl)-9,12L-dihydroxy-5,10-heptadienoic acid (thromboxane B_2), the inactive metabolite of thromboxane A_2 (21).

3. PG endoperoxides are more potent smooth muscle stimulants than PGs proper on the respiratory tract (19) and on certain vessels (19,56). Further, biological actions of the endoperoxides differ qualitatively from those of the PGs in two cell systems, i.e., platelets (34) and adipocytes (14).

While these data substantiate the original postulate of an organ-specific pattern for arachidonic acid metabolism, they also suggest that the PG endoperoxides and thromboxane A_2, rather than the PGs proper, function as the active species of the PG system at some sites.

Relatively little is known of the sequence and pathways of arachidonic acid metabolism in the CNS. Several workers (38,40,57) have demonstrated that the mammalian brain is a site of active PGE_2 and $PGF_{2\alpha}$ biosynthesis. PGD_2 is also synthesized in the tissue (L. S. Wolfe, *personal communication*), but no information is available on its rate of synthesis. Brain lacks the enzyme(s) catalyzing the conversion of PGH_2 to 6(9)oxy-$PGF_{2\alpha}$ (42). Both absolute and relative amounts of PGE_2 and $PGF_{2\alpha}$ formed vary with the species, the brain region, and the experimental condition (Table 1). Among the brain regions examined, the cerebellum stands out for its greater capacity to synthesize PGE_2 than $PGF_{2\alpha}$, and this unique condition may have functional implications (see below). Interestingly, PG biosynthesis in the late foetal or neonatal brain, whether from an immature (rat) or a mature (lamb) species at birth, is similar to that of the adult brain. This suggests that the biosynthetic enzyme system, or at least the component of the system concerned with synthesis of the PGs proper, becomes functional at an early stage of neurogenesis. Consistent with this concept is the finding that undifferentiated, proliferating neuroblastoma cells produce PGEs (23). The CNS therefore has the main pathway—i.e., pathway 3 (Fig. 1)—for arachidonic acid metabolism. A major question remains whether nervous tissue can synthesize thromboxane A_2. Further, it is not known how much arachidonic acid is converted to non-PG, nonthromboxane derivatives.

TABLE 1. *Biosynthesis of PGE₂ and PGF₂α in mammalian brain*

Age	Preparation		PG formed (μg/g tissue)	
	Tissue slice[a]	Homogenate[b]	E_2	$F_{2\alpha}$
Man				
Adult	Cerebral cortex		0.05	0.37
Cat				
Adult	Cerebral cortex		0.85	2.03
Adult	Cerebellum		0.84	0.73
Adult	Caudate nucleus		0.38	0.77
Adult	Hypothalamus		0.31	0.74
Rat				
Adult	Cerebral cortex		0.17[c]	0.60[c]
Adult		Whole brain	1.75	0.42
One day		Whole brain	1.90	0.23
Lamb				
Foetus at term		Whole brain	0.50	0.10
Two days		Whole brain	0.53	0.13

Note that the PG levels reported here are several-fold higher than those found in the quickly frozen tissue (57). Hence these findings are an overestimate of the condition *in vivo* (for more details see ref. 8).

[a] Wolfe et al. (57). Slices were incubated (60 min, 37°C) without added arachidonic acid.

[b] Pace-Asciak (40; see also ref. 8). Homogenates were incubated (10 min, 37°C) in the presence of arachidonic acid (100 μg/g tissue).

[c] Nicosia and Galli (38) reported identical results.

Activation and Inhibition of PG Biosynthesis

Several factors stimulate PG biosynthesis in the CNS (for review see ref. 8). Pyrogens, for example, accelerate formation of a PG compound tentatively identified with PGE₂ (Milton, *this volume*). Conversely, substances of diverse chemical structure, including aspirin and other antipyretics, are potent blockers of PG biosynthesis (12; see also Ziel and Krupp, *this volume*). The above findings form the basis for the theory implicating PGs in the pathogenesis of fever (Cooper et al., *this volume*).

It is generally assumed that stimulatory agents exert their action on the rate-limiting step (i.e., the acyl hydrolase reaction) in the biosynthetic process. Consistent with this concept is the finding that phospholipase A₂, a major hydrolytic enzyme in the CNS (10,11), is activated by neurohormones such as norepinephrine and 5-hydroxytryptamine (16). These compounds are known stimulators of PG biosynthesis in the CNS (28,48) and other organs (47). However, the greater formation of one or more PGs under stimulation could also result from a shift in the direction of arachidonic acid metabolism. For example, PGE₂ could be formed at the expense of other endoperoxide by-products. No conclusion on this point is possible until all metabolites of arachidonic acid are identified and measured.

While the site of the action of stimulatory agents remains undefined, there is good evidence that most inhibitory agents (13,17) interfere with the formation of PGG_2. Several investigators (12,20,54) have demonstrated that treatment with aspirin or aspirin-like drugs results in a lower yield of metabolites from pathways 2 and 3, which implies inhibition at an early stage in the PG synthetase reaction. Results of experiments where PG synthetase has been partially resolved into the constituent enzymes (35) agree with this idea. Aspirin-like drugs also cause a greater yield of the metabolite from the lipoxygenase pathway (i.e., pathway 1; see ref. 20). This confirms that the acyl hydrolase reaction is rate-limiting in the metabolism of arachidonic acid. The foregoing data on the site of action of the blockers have been obtained in nonneural tissues, but conceivably they apply to the CNS as well.

BIOLOGICAL INACTIVATION OF THE PROSTAGLANDINS

The concept that PG inactivation is primarily enzymatic is firmly established (for review see ref. 49). Figure 2 illustrates the initial steps in the metabolism of PGE_2 and $PGF_{2\alpha}$ in organs other than the CNS. Both PGs undergo a rapid sequence of transformations, which are catalyzed by two specific enzymes: the 15-hydroxyprostaglandin dehydrogenase (15-PGDH) and the prostaglandin-Δ^{13}-reductase (13-PGR). The endproduct of the

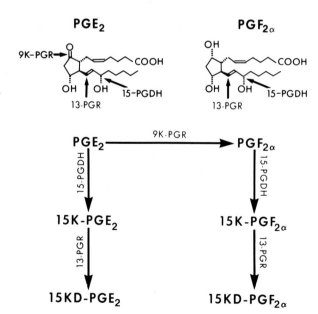

FIG. 2. Initial steps in the metabolism of PGE_2 and $PGF_{2\alpha}$. 15-PGDH, 15-hydroxyprostaglandin dehydrogenase. 13-PGR, prostaglandin-Δ^{13}-reductase. 9K-PGR, prostaglandin E-9-keto(α)-reductase. 15K-PG, 15-ketoprostaglandin. 15KD-PG, 15-keto-13,14-dihydroprostaglandin.

reaction is the inactive 15-keto-13,14-dihydro derivative. Further, PGE_2 is converted directly to $PGF_{2\alpha}$ by a third enzyme, the prostaglandin E-9-keto (α)-reductase (9K-PGR). This reaction is regarded as an inactivation at some sites (see below). PGD_2 is also reduced enzymatically to $PGF_{2\alpha}$ (25). Surprisingly, PGD_2 is a poor substrate for the 15-PGDH (F. F. Sun, *personal communication*).

The question of PG inactivation in the CNS is a moot point because of our incomplete knowledge of metabolic transformations of arachidonic acid (and the resulting uncertainty on the number and type of active products formed) as well as species and age differences in the activity of the 15-PGDH. All studies, whether performed in the intact (57) or homogenized (2,37,40) tissue, concur in showing that the mature mammalian brain has exceedingly low 15-PGDH activity. The 15-PGDH reaction is rate-limiting in the catabolic sequence (Fig. 2). By contrast, the foetal brain contains high levels of the enzyme, at least in some species (40,43; reviewed in ref. 8). A detailed analysis of the ontogenetic development of 15-PGDH was carried out in the lamb and proved that the activity of the enzyme is inversely related to the maturity of the tissue (40,43). Surprisingly, the CNS of the adult frog is a site of active PG catabolism (4). Perhaps 15-PGDH has been lost in the course of evolution from amphibians to mammals. Unlike 15-PGDH, 9K-PGR is present in the CNS of all species examined (4,32,33,57) regardless of their phylogenetic condition.

From the foregoing, one may conclude that the mature CNS in mammals lacks the prime path for PG inactivation. This condition, however, does not reconcile with the high biosynthetic activity of the tissue, which presupposes the occurrence of a widespread and efficient mechanism for the disposal of active PG products. This is especially true considering some of the functions attributed to the PGs (see below). The apparent inconsistency is possibly resolved by the presence in the CNS of alternative means for PG inactivation. The 9K-PGR reaction (Fig. 2) may function as an inactivation step because adenylate cyclase, a presumptive target for PG action in neural (reviewed in ref. 8) and nonneural (reviewed in ref. 27) tissues, is not affected by PGF compounds. However, this reaction is slow (4,32) and furthermore concerns PGE (and PGD) compounds only. Alternatively, PGs may be inactivated through their removal from the extracellular fluid. Several investigators have demonstrated that PGs are not taken up by neurons and glia (4,6,57), but there are reports of an active PG transport across the choroidal (5,6) and extrachoroidal (6) regions of the blood-brain barrier. Finally, a novel scheme of PG inactivation stems from work indicating that the PG endoperoxides (e.g., PGG_2 and PGH_2) and the thromboxanes (e.g., thromboxane A_2) are the active species of the PG system in certain organs. If the same happens in the CNS, these labile compounds could be inactivated through their conversion to inactive PG and/or non-PG derivatives. Such conversion may be enzymatic or nonenzymatic (Fig. 1, Table 2). Preliminary findings in our laboratory (I. Bishai, F. Coceani,

TABLE 2. *Nonenzymatic degradation of some biologically active derivatives of arachidonic acid*

Compound	Half-life in aqueous medium (37°C; pH 7.4)	Product formed
Thromboxane A_2[a]	30 sec	Thromboxane B_2
PGH_2[b]	5 min	PGE_2, PGD_2
PGE_2[c]	>6 hr	PGA_2, PGB_2
$PGF_{2\alpha}$[d]	Stable	—

[a] Data from Svensson et al. (54) and Hamberg et al. (21).
[b] Data from Hamberg et al. (19,22) and Nugteren and Hazelhof (39). PGE_2 and PGD_2 account for more than 90% of the product formed.
[c] See Monkhouse et al. (36).
[d] See Karim et al. (30).

and J. Tse, *unpublished*) suggesting that PGH_2 is a pyretic agent by itself are in accord with the idea that PG endoperoxides play a role in the CNS. The last hypothesis is particularly attractive not only because it is supported by experimental data but also because it affords an explanation for ontogenetic and phylogenetic differences in 15-PGDH activity. Since it is implicit in this hypothesis that the organization of the "PG synthetase" (and the active PG species) changes between organs and animal species, one may speculate that in the case of the CNS the PG system has grown in complexity from amphibians to mammals. In amphibians the PGs proper may be the active species of the system, and consequently high 15-PGDH activity is required for their disposal. Conversely, the PG endoperoxides and/or the thromboxanes may have a more central role in mammals. In the latter event the 15-PGDH would not be essential. Ontogenetic changes can be similarly explained. As pointed out earlier, 15-PGDH levels are inversely related to the maturity of the CNS, at least in one species. According to present reasoning, the loss of enzyme activity during neurogenesis would reflect the progressively greater importance of the PG endoperoxides and the thromboxanes over the PGs proper.

In sum, several different mechanisms may account for the termination of PG effects in the mature mammalian CNS, and they are not mutually exclusive. In fact, it is appealing to think that all these mechanisms work in concert to adjust the time course of PG action to diverse functional demands.

PROSTAGLANDIN SYSTEM: CELLULAR AND SUBCELLULAR LOCALIZATION

Although current methodologies are not suited to analysis of PG distribution in a polycellular tissue, sufficient indirect evidence has accumulated to prove that PGs are endogenous to several cell types within the CNS. Many investigators (reviewed in ref. 8) have shown that PG (PGEs and PGFs) release from the CNS is enhanced during stimulation of neural pathways, which implies a neuronal localization for the synthetic enzymes. Consistent with this view is the demonstration of PGE synthesis in cultured neuroblastoma cells (23). Glial tumors produce PGE_2 and $PGF_{2\alpha}$ in vitro (23,57), and this property is likely shared by normal glial cells in vivo. Vascular smooth muscle and leucocytes are a possible additional source of PGs. The occurrence of continuous PG biosynthesis in cerebral vessels is proved by the release of a PG-like material in vitro (45) and by the demonstration of effects of indomethacin on the vascular tone in vivo (44) and in vitro (45). Leucocytes produce E- and F-type PGs (tentatively identified with PGE_1, PGE_2, and $PGF_{2\alpha}$) during phagocytosis (26), and this event has been linked with the pathogenesis of pyrogen fever (see ref. 9 and Cooper et al., this volume).

Subcellular fractionation of different organs (including brain) has established that PG synthetase is located in the microsomes. By contrast, PG-metabolizing enzymes (15-PGDH, 13-PGR, and 9K-PGR) are recovered from a particle-free fraction. These findings form the basis for a scheme of the functional organization of the PG system in cells, which in its essential aspects was first proposed by Änggård (1) some years ago. According to this scheme, the PGs proper and other active derivatives of arachidonic acid are synthesized in the plasma membrane and exert an effect primarily in situ. As pointed out earlier there are several mechanisms for PG disposal in cells, and their relative importance varies with the type of cell and the particular spectrum of active compounds formed. For example, the PGs proper are inactivated most efficiently through their conversion to the 15-keto and the 15-keto-13,14-dihydro derivatives. These enzyme reactions are thought to take place in the cytosol. Whatever the mechanism, a variable fraction of the active compound(s) escapes inactivation and is released extracellularly. As inferred from Table 2, active compounds have a different life span in the extracellular fluid. PGE_2 and $PGF_{2\alpha}$, whether they are released from cells or originate from the nonenzymic breakdown of the endoperoxides, are stable and may gain access to distant structures. The opposite happens with thromboxane A_2.

The data presented in this and previous sections strongly suggest that the functional organization of the PG system differs between organs or even between cells of the same organ. Equal (if not greater) variability likely exists in the CNS, but at the present state of our knowledge any discussion of this subject is necessarily speculative. For example, neurons may be subcategorized in two classes depending on the ability to degrade PGs by the 15-PGDH pathway. According to the above scheme, the 15-PGDH determines the site and time course of action of PGs. Thus PGs would function as short-lived intracellular effectors in neurons containing the enzyme (e.g., in Purkinje cells; see below), whereas they may also function as intercellular effectors with the remaining neurons. More complex models of organization are envisaged should the PG endoperoxides and the thromboxanes play an active role in the CNS.

PROSTAGLANDINS AND NEURONAL FUNCTION

It is now generally believed that PGs are implicated in cell function either as "messengers" of extra- to intracellular (or intercellular) events, or as "modulators" of responses to external stimulation. PGs may play either or both roles in the CNS, and supporting evidence is best examined through the discussion of pertinent experimental models.

Modulatory Role of Prostaglandins

In a series of investigations Bloom and his associates (7,51) developed a theory of the operation of central noradrenergic synapses which implicates the PGs (specifically E-type PGs) in the role of modulators. In brief, they postulate that neurally released norepinephrine (NE) triggers a reaction sequence in the postsynaptic region involving, in order, the formation of cyclic adenosine 3',5'-monophosphate (cAMP), activation of a protein kinase, and phosphorylation of a specific membrane protein. The end result of the reaction is hyperpolarization of the cell membrane and consequently depression of neuronal activity. As a corollary to this scheme, they also postulate that the synaptic event elicits formation of an E-type PG in the receptor cell, which in turn exerts a control action on the above sequence by inhibiting the cAMP-generating mechanism. Although this model of PGE-mediated modulation is supported by findings in peripheral synapses (15), it has been challenged on several grounds (reviewed in ref. 8). In particular, different investigators have been unable to confirm that cAMP is as effective in depressing neurons as NE, and that PGEs consistently antagonize the action of NE. Technical factors may explain some of the inconsistencies (7). Further, it must be emphasized that while this model is based on work in the cerebellum (Purkinje cells) and the hippocampus (pyramidal cells) many of the negative findings have been obtained in other regions of the CNS. Thus it is possible that this model of NE-cAMP-PGE interaction applies only to some of the cell systems receiving a noradrenergic input. Relevant to this point is recent work of Stitt and Hardy (53), which demonstrates antagonism between PGE_1 and NE on Purkinje cells but not on anterior hypothalamic neurons (see also ref. 52). In this context it is also significant that Purkinje cells are seemingly unique among central neurons for their ability to degrade PGs by the 15-PGDH pathway (52). Thus they are optimally equipped to perform the function described here.

An alternative model of PG-mediated modulation was formulated by Hedqvist (24) on the basis of findings in the peripheral nervous system; possibly it may apply also to the CNS (3). There are several features in common between this and the former model, i.e., the neurohumoral mechanism being affected, the site of PG release, and the character of the active PG. Unlike Bloom's model, however, Hedqvist's model assumes that PGE action is exerted presynaptically on the release of NE.

Messenger Role of Prostaglandins

Current concepts on the pathogenesis of pyrogen fever afford the best-documented model of a messenger role of PGs in the CNS. As reported more extensively by others in this volume (Cooper et al. and Milton), this model states that pyrogen action on anterior hypothalamic neurons is mediated by an E-type PG. Since the PG in question may originate from neural (neurons, glia) and nonneural (leucocytes) elements, the messenger function postulated here may take place intra- and/or intercellularly.

PGs (specifically PGEs) may also play a messenger function for adenylate cyclase during neuronal growth and differentiation (reviewed in ref. 8). However, the experimental evidence supporting this concept is too tenuous to warrant discussion here.

CONCLUDING REMARKS

The data presented here indicate that PG synthetase is distributed diffusely throughout the CNS and that the enzyme(s) becomes functional at an early stage of neurogenesis. Several cellular types likely form PGs in the living animal, and their synthetic activity is conditioned by a variety of factors that may or may not be physiological. An important concept emerging from this review is that the PG biosynthetic process is potentially very flexible and may yield several active products of unequal potency and half-lives. Their action is likely exerted at both intra- and extracellular sites. Thus PG compounds can serve not only as "local effectors" within the cell of origin but also as "messengers" of complex interactions among neurons and between neural and nonneural elements. Clearly these compounds are optimally suited to play a central role in the control of neuronal function under normal and pathological conditions.

ACKNOWLEDGMENTS

This chapter and the experimental work of the author was supported by the Medical Research Council of Canada.

REFERENCES

1. Änggård, E. (1971): Studies on the analysis and metabolism of the prostaglandins. *Ann. NY Acad. Sci.,* 180:200–217.
2. Änggård, E., Larsson, C., and Samuelsson, B. (1971): The distribution of 15-hydroxy prostaglandin dehydrogenase and prostaglandin-Δ^{13}-reductase in tissues of the swine. *Acta Physiol. Scand.,* 81:396–404.
3. Bergström, S., Farnebo, L. O., and Fuxe, K. (1973): Effect of prostaglandin E_2 on central and peripheral catecholamine neurons. *Eur. J. Pharmacol.,* 21:362–368.
4. Bishai, I., and Coceani, F. (1976): Presence of 15-hydroxy prostaglandin dehydrogenase, prostaglandin-Δ^{13}-reductase and prostaglandin E-9-keto(α)-reductase in the frog spinal cord. *J. Neurochem.,* 26:1167–1176.
5. Bito, L. Z., and Davson, H. (1974): Carrier-mediated removal of prostaglandins from cerebrospinal fluid. *J. Physiol. (Lond.),* 234:39–40P.
6. Bito, L. Z., Davson, H., and Hollingsworth, R. (1976): Facilitated transport of prostaglandins across the blood-cerebrospinal fluid and blood-brain barriers. *J. Physiol. (Lond.),* 256:273–285.
7. Bloom, F. E., Siggins, G. R., Hoffer, B. J., Segal, M., and Oliver, A. P. (1975): Cyclic nucleotides in the central synaptic actions of catecholamines. *Adv. Cyclic Nucleotide Res.,* 5:603–618.
8. Coceani, F., and Pace-Asciak, C. R. (1976): Functional correlates of the prostaglandin system in central nervous tissue. In: *Prostaglandins Physiological, Pharmacological and Pathological Aspects,* edited by S. M. M. Karim. Medical and Technical Publishing Co., Oxford *(in press)*.
9. Cooper, K. E., Pittman, Q. J., and Veale, W. L. (1975): Observations on the development of the "fever" mechanism in the fetus and newborn. In: *Temperature Regulation and Drug Action,* edited by P. Lomax, E. Schönbaum, and J. Jacob, pp. 43–50. Karger, Basel.
10. Cooper, M. F., and Webster, G. R. (1970): The differentiation of phospholipase A_1 and A_2 in rat and human nervous tissue. *J. Neurocheri.,* 17:1543–1554.
11. Cooper, M. F., and Webster, G. R. (1972): On the phospholipase A_2 activity of human cerebral cortex. *J. Neurochem.,* 19:333–340.
12. Flower, R. J. (1974): Drugs which inhibit prostaglandin biosynthesis. *Pharmacol. Rev.,* 26:33–67.
13. Flower, R. J., and Vane, J. R. (1974): Some pharmacologic and biochemical aspects of prostaglandin biosynthesis and its inhibition. In: *Prostaglandin Synthetase Inhibitors,* edited by H. J. Robison and J. R. Vane, pp. 9–18. Raven Press, New York.
14. Gorman, R. R., Hamberg, M., and Samuelsson, B. (1975): Inhibition of basal and hormone-stimulated adenylate cyclase in adipocyte ghosts by the prostaglandin endoperoxide prostaglandin H_2. *J. Biol. Chem.,* 250:6460–6463.
15. Greengard, P. (1975): Cyclic nucleotides, protein phosphorylation, and neuronal function. *Adv. Cyclic Nucleotide Res.,* 5:585–601.
16. Gullis, R. J., and Rowe, C. E. (1975): The stimulation by transmitter substances and putative transmitter substances of the net activity of phospholipase A_2 of synaptic membranes of cortex of guinea-pig brain. *Biochem. J.,* 148:197–208.
17. Hamberg, M., and Samuelsson, B. (1974): Prostaglandin endoperoxides: Novel transformations of arachidonic acid in human platelets. *Proc. Natl. Acad. Sci. USA,* 71:3400–3404.
18. Hamberg, M., and Samuelsson, B. (1974): Prostaglandin endoperoxides. VII. Novel transformations of arachidonic acid in guinea pig lung. *Biochem. Biophys. Res. Commun.,* 61:942–949.
19. Hamberg, M., Hedqvist, P., Strandberg, K., Svensson, J., and Samuelsson, B. (1975): Prostaglandin endoperoxides. IV. Effects on smooth muscle. *Life Sci.,* 16:451–462.
20. Hamberg, M., Svensson, J., and Samuelsson, B. (1974): Prostaglandin endoperoxides: A new concept concerning the mode of action and release of prostaglandins. *Proc. Natl. Acad. Sci. USA,* 71:3824–3828.
21. Hamberg, M., Svensson, J., and Samuelsson, B. (1975): Thromboxanes: A new group of biologically active compounds derived from prostaglandin endoperoxides. *Proc. Natl. Acad. Sci. USA,* 72:2994–2998.
22. Hamberg, M., Svensson, J., Wakabayashi, T., and Samuelsson, B. (1974): Isolation and

structure of two prostaglandin endoperoxides that cause platelet aggregation. *Proc. Natl. Acad. Sci. USA*, 71:345–349.

23. Hamprecht, B., Jaffe, B. M., and Philpott, G. W. (1973): Prostaglandin production by neuroblastoma, glioma and fibroblast cell lines; stimulation by N^6,O^2-dibutyryl adenosine 3':5'-cyclic monophosphate. *FEBS Lett.*, 36:193–198.

24. Hedqvist, P. (1973): Autonomic neurotransmission. In: *The Prostaglandins*, Vol. 1, edited by P. W. Ramwell, pp. 101–131. Plenum Press, New York.

25. Hensby, C. N. (1974): The enzymatic conversion of prostaglandin D_2 to prostaglandin $F_{2\alpha}$. *Prostaglandins*, 8:369–372.

26. Higgs, G. A., McCall, E., and Youlten, L. J. F. (1975): A chemotactic role for prostaglandins released from polymorphonuclear leucocytes during phagocytosis. *Br. J. Pharmacol.*, 53:539–546.

27. Hittelman, K. J., and Butcher, R. W. (1973): Cyclic AMP and the mechanism of action of the prostaglandins. In: *The Prostaglandins, Pharmacological and Therapeutic Advances*, edited by M. F. Cuthbert, pp. 151–165. Heinemann, London.

28. Holmes, S. W. (1970): The spontaneous release of prostaglandins into the cerebral ventricles of the dog and the effect of external factors on this release. *Br. J. Pharmacol.*, 38:653–658.

29. Horton, E. W. (1972): Prostaglandins. *Monogr. Endocrinol.*, 7:11–12.

30. Karim, S. M. M., Devlin, J., and Hillier, K. (1968): The stability of dilute solutions of prostaglandins E_1, E_2, $F_{1\alpha}$ and $F_{2\alpha}$. *Eur. J. Pharmacol.*, 4:416–420.

31. Kunze, H., and Vogt, W. (1971): Significance of phospholipase A for prostaglandin formation. *Ann. NY Acad. Sci.*, 180:123–125.

32. Lee, S-C., and Levine, L. (1974): Prostaglandin metabolism. I. Cytoplasmic reduced nicotinamide adenine dinucleotide phosphate-dependent and microsomal reduced nicotinamide dinucleotide-dependent prostaglandin E 9-ketoreductase activities in monkey and pigeon tissues. *J. Biol. Chem.*, 249:1369–1375.

33. Leslie, C. A., and Levine, L. (1973): Evidence for the presence of a prostaglandin E_2-9-keto reductase in rat organs. *Biochem. Biophys. Res. Commun.*, 52:717–724.

34. Malmsten, C., Hamberg, M., Svensson, J., and Samuelsson, B. (1975): Physiological role of an endoperoxide in human platelets: Hemostatic defect due to platelet cyclo-oxygenase deficiency. *Proc. Natl. Acad. Sci. USA*, 72:1446–1450.

35. Miyamoto, T., Yamamoto, S., and Hayaishi, O. (1974): Prostaglandin synthetase system-resolution into oxygenase and isomerase component. *Proc. Natl. Acad. Sci. USA*, 71:3645–3648.

36. Monkhouse, D. C., Van Campen, L., and Aguiar, A. J. (1973): Kinetics of dehydration and isomerization of prostaglandins E_1 and E_2. *J. Pharm. Sci.*, 62:576–580.

37. Nakano, J., Prancan, A. V., and Moore, S. E. (1972): Metabolism of prostaglandin E_1 in the cerebral cortex and cerebellum of the dog and rat. *Brain Res.*, 39:545–548.

38. Nicosia, S., and Galli, G. (1975): A mass fragmentographic method for the quantitative evaluation of brain prostaglandin biosynthesis. *Prostaglandins*, 9:397–403.

39. Nugteren, D. H., and Hazelhof, E. (1973): Isolation and properties of intermediates in prostaglandin biosynthesis. *Biochim. Biophys. Acta*, 326:448–461.

40. Pace-Asciak, C. R. (1976): Biosynthesis and catabolism of prostaglandins during animal development. In: *Advances in Prostaglandin and Thromboxane Research*, Vol. 1, edited by B. Samuelsson and R. Paoletti, pp. 35–46. Raven Press, New York.

41. Pace-Asciak, C., and Nashat, M. (1975): Catabolism of an isolated, purified intermediate of prostaglandin biosynthesis by regions of the adult rat kidney. *Biochim. Biophys. Acta*, 388:243–253.

42. Pace-Asciak, C. R., and Nashat, M. (1976): Catabolism of 15-hydroxy-9,11-cyclic prostadienoate endoperoxide by homogenates of rat kidney, brain and stomach. In: *Advances in Prostaglandin and Thromboxane Research*, Vol. 2, edited by B. Samuelsson and R. Paoletti, p. 859. Raven Press, New York.

43. Pace-Asciak, C. R., Coceani, F., and Olley, P. M. (1974): Age-dependent decrease in the in vitro inactivation of prostaglandin $F_{2\alpha}$ by foetal lamb brain. *Trans. Am. Soc. Neurochem.*, 5:120.

44. Pickard, J. D., and Mackenzie, E. T. (1973): Inhibition of prostaglandin synthesis and the response of baboon cerebral circulation to carbon dioxide. *Nature [New Biol.]*, 245:187–188.

45. Pickard, J. D., Simeone, F., and Vinall, P. (1976): The effects of indomethacin on elements of the cerebral circulation in vitro and in vivo. In: *Advances in Prostaglandin and Thromboxane Research,* Vol. 2, edited by B. Samuelsson and R. Paoletti, pp. 918–919. Raven Press, New York.
46. Piper, P. J., and Vane, J. R. (1969): Release of additional factors in anaphylaxis and its antagonism by anti-inflammatory drugs. *Nature (Lond.),* 223:29–35.
47. Piper, P., and Vane, J. (1971): The release of prostaglandins from lung and other tissues. *Ann. NY Acad. Sci.,* 180:363–385.
48. Ramwell, P. W., Shaw, J. E., and Jessup, R. (1966): Spontaneous and evoked release of prostaglandins from frog spinal cord. *Am. J. Physiol.,* 211:998–1004.
49. Samuelsson, B., Granström, E., Green, K., Hamberg, M., and Hammarström, S. (1975): Prostaglandins. *Ann. Rev. Biochem.,* 44:669–695.
50. Shio, H., Shaw, J., and Ramwell, P. (1971): Relation of cyclic AMP to the release and actions of prostaglandins. *Ann. NY Acad. Sci.,* 185:327–335.
51. Siggins, G. R., and Henriksen, S. J. (1975): Analogues of cyclic adenosine monophosphate: Correlation of inhibition of Purkinje neurons with protein kinase activation. *Science,* 189:559–561.
52. Siggins, G., Hoffer, B., and Bloom, F. (1971): Prostaglandin-norepinephrine interactions in brain: Microelectrophoretic and histochemical correlates. *Ann. NY Acad. Sci.,* 180:302–323.
53. Stitt, J. T., and Hardy, J. D. (1975): Microelectrophoresis of PGE_1 onto single units in the rabbit hypothalamus. *Am. J. Physiol.,* 229:240–245.
54. Svensson, J., Hamberg, M., and Samuelsson, B. (1975): Prostaglandin endoperoxides. IX. Characterization of rabbit aorta contracting substance (RCS) from guinea pig lung and human platelets. *Acta Physiol. Scand.,* 94:222–228.
55. Turner, S. R., Tainer, J. A., and Lynn, W. S. (1975): Biogenesis of chemotactic molecules by the arachidonate lipoxygenase system of platelets. *Nature (Lond.),* 257:680–681.
56. Tuvemo, T., Strandberg, K., Hamberg, M., and Samuelsson, B. (1976): Maintenance of the tone of the human umbilical artery by prostaglandin and thromboxane formation. In: *Advances in Prostaglandin and Thromboxane Research,* Vol. 1, edited by B. Samuelsson and R. Paoletti, pp. 425–428. Raven Press, New York.
57. Wolfe, L. S., Pappius, H. M., and Marion, J. (1976): The biosynthesis of prostaglandins by brain tissue in vitro. In: *Advances in Prostaglandin and Thromboxane Research,* Vol. 1, edited by B. Samuelsson and R. Paoletti, pp. 345–355. Raven Press, New York.

Note added in proof: Thromboxane B_2, the stable derivative of thromboxane A_2, has been recently identified in guinea pig and rat brain [L. S. Wolfe, K. Rostworowski, and J. Marion (1976): Endogenous formation of the prostaglandin endoperoxide metabolite, thromboxane B_2, by brain tissue. *Biochem. Biophys. Res. Commun.,* 70:907–913]. This finding proves the presence in the tissue of a major pathway (pathway 2 in Fig. 1) for the metabolism of arachidonic acid.

Brain Dysfunction in Infantile Febrile Convulsions, edited by M. A. B. Brazier and F. Coceani. Raven Press, New York © 1976.

Temperature Regulation: An Overall View

Peter Lomax

Department of Pharmacology, School of Medicine and the Brain Research Institute, University of California, Los Angeles, California 90024

The mechanisms involved in the regulation of internal body temperature continue to be studied by many investigators. Present concepts are critically examined in the extensive review by Bligh (3), and the general principles of bioenergetics are most scholarly presented in a recent monograph by Swan (14). More specific aspects of thermoregulation have been considered in several symposia, and the topics covered at two meetings concerned with the pharmacological aspects of temperature regulation (11,13) are of particular relevance to the present discussion.

Our present purpose is to examine those features of thermoregulatory physiology and pathology which may be of etiological importance in the pathogenesis of so-called infantile febrile convulsions. The basic question being asked is whether the seizures and fever stem from a common cause (i.e., nonspecific infection) or if the seizures are the result of a response to the neurophysiological and neurochemical changes occurring during the pyrexial response. In either case there is presumably some underlying brain dysfunction, genetic or otherwise. It would seem that in the design of the present volume the *ad hoc* assumption of a cause-and-effect relationship between the fever and the convulsions has been adopted. Thus the thrust of the discussions to follow is centered around the brain mechanisms mediating pyrexia, the development of these mechanisms, and their modification by drug therapy.

The importance of understanding the pathogenesis of febrile convulsions lies in their management. There are those who subscribe to the view that brief seizures in a 2-year-old with a cold are invariably benign, while others believe such convulsions are within the spectrum of epilepsy and should be managed on the same principles. Treatment based on the former conviction might affirm the use of antipyretics and antibiotics, whereas those motivated by anxiety about epilepsy might recommend continuous anticonvulsant administration (4).

It is the purpose of this chapter to provide the general framework of current ideas of the thermoregulatory mechanisms for others to clothe with detail, especially in relation to fever.

EFFECTOR MECHANISMS

In order to stabilize the body temperature under varying environmental conditions, several systems regulating heat production and heat loss are utilized. At rest, in the so-called thermoneutral zone for the species, the heat produced as a concomitant of the basal energy expended to maintain vital functions can be dissipated or maximally conserved by regulating heat loss. This is achieved mainly by autonomic control of nonevaporative heat loss by radiation, convection, and conduction from the skin, especially in the extremities. It is only when the thermal load imposed is outside the thermoneutral range or heat production is markedly above the basal level (during exercise) that additional mechanisms (e.g., shivering, sweating, and panting) need to be brought into play. Over the longer term, hormonal changes and nonshivering thermogenesis may also contribute to the overall heat production.

The selection or creation of an environment in which body temperature can be maintained appears to be one of the most primitive thermoregulatory capabilities. Such behavioral responses show their greatest diversity in man; the inability to control the immediate environment, due to immaturity or incapacity, may cause serious, even fatal disturbances in thermoregulation. Comparative studies in several species, including man, indicate that behavioral thermoregulation is essentially physiological in that complex central nervous responses to a thermal stimulus—a change in skin temperature—are involved. These are not fundamentally different from the autonomic responses usually associated with temperature control.

CENTRAL THERMOSTATS

That coordination of the processes of heat loss and conservation are dependent on central nervous control is beyond dispute. The integrity of the hypothalamus is essential for normal control of body temperature, although other regions of the brain and spinal cord also play a role. There are temperature-sensitive neurons in these centers, and there is basic agreement that temperature itself is the variable that activates the thermostats. Although there is controversy as to which temperature the thermostats are "looking at," the balance of evidence favors the transduced hypothalamic temperature as the regulated temperature. Possibly the autonomic responses mediated by changes in hypothalamic temperature are sensed at other loci and fed back to the controlling neurons (1).

Apart from local temperature there are other inputs to the controlling centers from superficial and deep thermoreceptors, muscle proprioceptors, and other regions of the central nervous system. The integration of these several inputs and the resulting thermoregulatory effects in the face of varying external heat loads has been studied extensively. Models based on control system theory have been constructed to explain the observed data. Although the resulting arguments give rise to considerable complexity, two basic systems are proposed:

1. The thermal controller regulates the central temperature by comparing it with an intrinsic "set" temperature. The set temperature itself is variable, being modulated by the various inputs. Appropriate thermoregulatory mechanisms are activated depending on the direction and magnitude of the difference between the set and actual brain temperatures.

2. Inputs from two types of thermal receptors ("warm" and "cold") situated throughout the body are fed to the central controllers where they activate thermoregulatory effector pathways. The total thermoregulatory response is determined by comparing these feedbacks. When information from both sets of sensors exactly balance (zero load error) there is zero output from the comparator.

These two systems are demonstrated in Fig. 1. The arguments underlying these concepts are more fully discussed in several recent reviews (5,7,8). To some extent the differences between these various models may be more semantic than real when reduced to the fundamental level of membrane

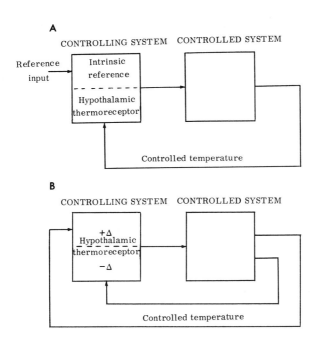

FIG. 1. Two models of central thermoregulation. **A:** A variable, intrinsically set level is compared to the transduced hypothalamic temperature, and appropriate responses to correct any deviation are activated. **B:** Peripheral and central "warm" and "cold" inputs are integrated, and the thermoregulatory effector responses depend on the load error between these inputs.

potentials of the thermoregulatory neurons. However, whichever model we adopt, similar mechanisms can explain the development of fever.

CENTRAL TRANSMITTERS

The demonstration of relatively high concentrations of the amines norepinephrine, 5-hydroxytryptamine, and acetylcholine in the hypothalamus, coupled with elucidation of the thermoregulatory function of this part of the brain, suggested that these amines might play an important role as neurotransmitters in thermoregulation. To this list should now be added histamine (10) and dopamine (6). Various neuronal models of temperature regulation have been developed to explain the role of these several amines (2), but it is not possible to construct any unified view or general hypothesis at the present time.

Several years ago prostaglandins were introduced into the field of thermoregulation when it was found that prostaglandin E_1 produced fever when injected in minute amounts into the ventricular system of unanesthetized cats (12). Thus prostaglandins may also be involved as neurotransmitters or neuromodulators in temperature regulation.

Since neuronal pathways are undoubtedly involved in thermoregulation, and since communication between neurons involves the release of excitatory or inhibitory neurotransmitters, it is to be expected that most or all of the various amines in the controlling centers and afferent and efferent pathways are involved in some stage or other of the thermoregulatory mechanisms. Indeed it is somewhat difficult to understand exactly why this subject has given rise to such debate and argument. Certainly the simple concept of the "balance" of one neurotransmitter versus another seems to be a most unlikely and naive explanation of the nature of the central thermoregulatory processes.

FEVER

For the purposes of the present discussion, attention must be directed to the mechanisms by which fever may occur and to consideration of temperature regulation during fever. Liebermeister in 1875 (9) appears to have been the first to suggest that body temperature continues to be regulated during pyrexia, but at a higher level than normal. On the basis of the two models expounded above, one would say that the set point had been raised or that there had been a change in gain of the feedback loops. Many studies, particularly during induced fever in man, have demonstrated that this concept is essentially correct.

The inflammatory process is the commonest cause of fever in man. The invading microorganisms liberate a heat-stable polysaccharide of high molecular weight (5×10^5 to 2×10^7) which can be extracted from practically all gram-negative bacteria (see Dinarello and Wolff, *this volume*). This compound, generally referred to as exogenous pyrogen, causes a rise in body temperature when as little as 1 ng is injected into man.

The onset of fever following administration of exogenous pyrogen is delayed and is characteristically biphasic. Repeated injections cause leucopenia, and tolerance to the pyrexial effect appears. It is now widely accepted that exogenous pyrogen does not act directly on the thermoregulatory centers (see Cooper et al., *this volume*). A variety of cells, including circulating leucocytes, Kupffer cells in the liver, and macrophages from the lung, spleen, and lymph nodes form, or release, a pyrogenic heat-labile protein in the presence of exogenous pyrogen. This substance, endogenous pyrogen, can be extracted from the blood of animals with bacterial or viral infections and gives rise to a monophasic fever of rapid onset and short duration. It is this endogenous pyrogen that causes the upward resetting of the thermoregulatory centers.

There is as yet no certainty as to the precise means by which the level of the thermoregulatory set point is elevated by endogenous pyrogen. A direct action on receptors in the controlling centers is possible since fever occurs after microinjection of endogenous pyrogen into the rostral hypothalamus. Alternative mechanisms include an effect of endogenous pyrogen on the release of endogenous amines in the hypothalamus or on the synthesis and release of pyrogenic prostaglandins (see Milton, *this volume*).

CONCLUSIONS

From this brief outline of thermoregulatory mechanisms, it is clear that fever is not due to inactivation or disorganization of the normal physiological controlling system but to a shift in the set level of the system. The central mechanisms involved in the development of fever are activated by a series of neurochemical changes in which several neuroamines, prostaglandins, and polypeptide pyrogens are involved. These various neurochemicals could well have effects on brain areas and functions other than those concerned with thermoregulation. Thus it might well be profitable, and certainly reasonable, to consider these compounds when studying the pathogenesis of the convulsions accompanying fever in newborns and infants.

In the chapters to follow these various factors are considered in greater detail. Perhaps as a final digression it might be noted that the survival value of fever in infective conditions is elusive. Although it seems unlikely that this universal response of homeotherms would have persisted if it had not conferred some advantages, the benefits of a raised temperature have yet to be demonstrated. The possibility that endogenous pyrogen exerts other, as yet unknown effects should not be neglected.

ACKNOWLEDGMENTS

Supported by NSF Grant GB-43531 and by Office of Naval Research Grant NR 201–066.

REFERENCES

1. Adair, E. R., and Rawson, R. O. (1975): Behavioral reduction of preoptic temperature — a closer look. *Physiologist,* 18:116 (abstract).
2. Bligh, J. (1972): Neuronal models of mammalian temperature regulation. In: *Essays on Temperature Regulation,* edited by J. Bligh, pp. 105–120. Elsevier, New York.
3. Bligh, J. (1973): *Temperature Regulation in Mammals and Other Vertebrates.* Elsevier, New York.
4. Editorial (1975): More about febrile convulsions. *Br. Med. J.,* 1:591–592.
5. Hensel, H. (1973): Neural processes in thermoregulation. *Physiol. Rev.,* 53:948–1016.
6. Horita, A., and Quock, R. M. (1975): Dopaminergic mechanisms in drug-induced temperature effects. In: *Temperature Regulation and Drug Action,* edited by P. Lomax, E. Schönbaum, and J. Jacob, pp. 75–84. Karger, Basel.
7. Horowitz, J. M. (1975): Neural models on temperature regulation for cold-stressed animals. In: *Temperature Regulation and Drug Action,* edited by P. Lomax, E. Schönbaum, and J. Jacob, pp. 1–10. Karger, Basel.
8. Houdas, Y., and Guieu, J-D. (1975): Physical models of human thermoregulation. In: *Temperature Regulation and Drug Action,* edited by P. Lomax, E. Schönbaum, and J. Jacob, pp. 11–21. Karger, Basel.
9. Liebermeister, C. (1875): *Handbuch der Pathologie und Therapie des Fiebers.* Vogel, Leipzig.
10. Lomax, P., and Green, M. D. (1975): Histamine and temperature regulation. In: *Temperature Regulation and Drug Action,* edited by P. Lomax, E. Schönbaum, and J. Jacob, pp. 85–94. Karger, Basel.
11. Lomax, P., Schönbaum, E., and Jacob, J., editors (1975): *Temperature Regulation and Drug Action.* Karger, Basel.
12. Milton, A. S., and Wendlandt, S. (1970): A possible role of prostaglandin E_1 as a modulator for temperature regulation in the central nervous system of the cat. *J. Physiol. (Lond.),* 207:76–77.
13. Schönbaum, E., and Lomax, P., editors (1973): *The Pharmacology of Thermoregulation.* Karger, Basel.
14. Swan, H. (1974): *Thermoregulation and Bioenergetics.* Elsevier, New York.

*Brain Dysfunction in Infantile Febrile
Convulsions*, edited by M. A. B. Brazier and
F. Coceani. Raven Press, New York © 1976.

Monoaminergic Mechanisms in Thermoregulation

E. Preston and E. Schönbaum

*Pharmacological Research and Development Laboratory,
Organon International B.V., Oss, The Netherlands*

The emphasis placed on fundamental biological problems in this volume concerned with infantile febrile convulsions — a very serious clinical problem — is witness of our minimal understanding of the pathology of thermoregulation. This approach also is an example of a well-coordinated effort to prevent the needless loss of young lives.

Liebermeister (57) argued in 1885 that the first, essential disturbance associated with fever should be sought in the central nervous system. He defined fever as a complex of symptoms involving a change in the regulation of body heat such that heat production and heat loss are balanced at an abnormally high body temperature. It is important therefore to consider central and peripheral neurohumoral mechanisms, and monoaminergic mechanisms in particular, involved in the regulation of heat production and heat loss. The monoamines of major physiological importance are dopamine, 5-hydroxytryptamine (serotonin, 5-HT), norepinephrine, and epinephrine. The first part of our discussion centers on the functions served by norepinephrine and epinephrine in the periphery. Neither dopamine nor 5-HT appears to play a major role in peripheral temperature regulation.

EARLY STUDIES OF NEUROTRANSMISSION IN THERMOREGULATION

The nineteenth century physiologist Pflueger (70) observed that animals become practically poikilothermic after treatment with curare. Claude Bernard (8) demonstrated in 1876 that an increase in heat production on exposure to cold may be derived not only from muscular activity but also from a nonmuscular chemical process which persists after spinal transection and curarization. Establishment of the importance of muscle contraction to thermoregulation, later shown by Loewi, Dale, and others to be acetylcholine-effected, and the suspicion that nonshivering heat production could take place preceded by many years recognition of the role played by the monoamines.

The discovery of epinephrine at the start of this century did not immediately contribute to the knowledge of thermoregulation. Only after the importance of epinephrine for energy production and metabolism had been realized, largely through Cannon's great contributions (16), did involvement of catecholamines in heat production become clear. Much research on the role of norepinephrine or epinephrine in thermoregulation in homeotherms centered on problems concerning the mechanism of adjustment to low ambient temperature, hypothermia, and hibernation. This was based on the reasoning that under such circumstances the necessity to raise metabolic rate would involve release of the catecholamines, and it was encouraged by the fact that adrenergically mediated heat production is a process of major importance in small rodents. Adrenergically mediated heat production also served as an important model for the study of adrenergic transmission. The results of such studies on peripheral neurotransmission has of course provided a basis for pharmacological investigations of central monoaminergic mechanisms under normal and pathological conditions.

MONOAMINES IN PERIPHERAL THERMOREGULATION

The most important physiological properties of epinephrine were established between 1895 and 1910 (53). Somewhat later Cannon included the adrenal medulla in his studies of the activities of endocrine glands; ever since the work of Cannon (16), exposure to cold has been known to be associated with activation of the adrenal medulla. Involvement of the sympathetic nervous system also was recognized (39) but could not be studied in detail until methodology for measurements of catecholamines and their metabolites had been suitably refined. As happens ever so often, turnover studies were preceded by straightforward quantitative analyses. Desmarais and Dugal (25) found higher levels of norepinephrine in rats acclimated to cold. In such animals heat production by shivering (a clearly cholinergically mediated process) was found to be complemented by nonshivering thermogenesis. Sellers (79) showed gradually decreasing electrical activity in skeletal muscle of rats during their acclimation to cold; i.e., heat production during acclimation to low environmental temperature increasingly occurs through processes other than shivering (48).

Carlson and his associates (17,47) showed that nonshivering heat production is accompanied by the release of norepinephrine from sympathetic nerve endings, epinephrine being released only in the adrenals. Increased production and excretion of norepinephrine during exposure to cold was demonstrated by several investigators (54,55,77). The metabolic response to norepinephrine infusion can be blocked with propranolol (9); in fact, nonshivering heat production in cold-acclimated animals can be blocked and shivering elicited through β-receptor blockade (78). Norepinephrine release from sympathetic nerves seems to be the primary mechanism of chemical thermogenesis. Release of epinephrine appears to be a second line of defence (55).

Acclimation to cold is characterized not only by the increased release of norepinephrine but also by the greater efficiency of noradrenergic transmission. The latter involves a change in either postsynaptic or presynaptic processes, or both. It has been shown that cold-adapted animals exhibit a heightened metabolic response to exogenous norepinephrine (24). There are at least two mechanisms that could account for this. It is certainly conceivable that more postsynaptic receptor sites develop. Alternatively, we are tempted to suggest that a reduced uptake of norepinephrine into the adrenergic nerve terminals might occur. Direct evidence of possible coupling of increased norepinephrine release with decreased norepinephrine uptake has been presented by Bruinvels (15) using rat brain synaptosomes. The experimental model developed by this author states that during depolarization of the nerve terminal there is relative deficiency of cations (Na^+, Ca^{2+}) in the extracellular medium, which in turn leads to acceleration of tyrosine (the norepinephrine precursor) uptake, acceleration of norepinephrine synthesis and release, and reduction of norepinephrine uptake. Opposite events would occur at rest. Thus the increase of sympathetic tone and the more frequent depolarization may be coupled, through cation influx, with reduced transmitter (re)uptake and therefore optimal stimulation of postsynaptic receptors.

It would be an oversimplification to assume that the process of acclimation to cold can be equated solely to an increase in the availability and efficacy of norepinephrine or epinephrine. Autonomic thermoregulatory responses involve more than merely postganglionic adrenergic activation; hypothalamic, endocrine, peripheral vasomotor, and many other adjustments occur that cannot be brought about by either sympathetic stimulation or catecholamine administration by whatever dosage schedule.

Brown adipose tissue has a profuse adrenergic innervation, and release of norepinephrine in this tissue has an important thermogenic role in certain newborn mammals in cold acclimation and hibernation. The thermoregulatory function of this tissue has been the subject of much research and also of several excellent reviews (11,47,58,71).

CENTRAL MONOAMINES AS MEDIATORS OF THERMOREGULATION

The first good evidence to suggest that norepinephrine, epinephrine, and 5-HT might serve as neurotransmitter chemicals in the hypothalamus was obtained during the 1950s. Vogt (81) showed that the catecholamines were present in extracts of hypothalamus; and Amin et al. (1) isolated 5-HT from the same tissue. Brodie and Shore (14) and Euler (28) suggested a possible role for these substances in thermoregulation, and Feldberg and Myers (32) developed a model of their function in the hypothalamus. According to this model, thermoregulation depends on a balance of opposing effects of catecholamines and 5-HT at hypothalamic sites. This hypothesis was made even more plausible by the finding that monoamines are mainly located within nerve fibers and endings in the hypothalamus (2,18,23), which is in agreement with a neurotransmitter function of these compounds.

The following criteria must be fulfilled to establish that a chemical serves as a neurotransmitter (60). (a) The chemical must be shown to be present within the nerve endings in question, and the enzymes for its synthesis and inactivation demonstrated. Monoamines occurring in the hypothalamus satisfy this condition (2,18,23, for review see ref. 30). (b) Effects of the exogenous application of the putative transmitter should mimic those of natural stimulation and release. (c) During such stimulation the chemical should be detectable in the extracellular fluid bathing the synaptic region. (d) Pharmacological manipulation should modify equally responses to the putative transmitter and to natural stimulation.

Our discussion of hypothalamic monoamines concerns mainly neuropharmacological work that reflects attempts to satisfy the latter three criteria. It should be anticipated that none of these criteria has been fully satisfied with any hypothalamic monoamine because little is known on the functional organization of brainstem monoaminergic pathways subserving thermoregulation. Experimental data on these substances have been gathered mainly through their injection into the ventricular spaces, microinjection or perfusion into discrete regions of the brain, and iontophoresis onto single neurons.

The following deals primarily with the role of norepinephrine, 5-HT, and dopamine in the hypothalamic control of body temperature. Although a possible role for epinephrine cannot be excluded, most research has focussed on norepinephrine, perhaps because the latter is more abundant in the hypothalamus (81). Most of the evidence reviewed here refers to the responses of the conscious animal in a thermoneutral environment.

Norepinephrine

Norepinephrine released in the anterior hypothalamus seems to be concerned with lowering body temperature. Feldberg and Myers (32) first showed that the injection of epinephrine or norepinephrine into the cerebral ventricles of the cat caused body temperature to fall. The catecholamines likely act in the anterior hypothalamic/preoptic area (AH/POA) since microinjection of these substances directly into this region also evoked a hypothermic response (34). Supportive results were obtained in the monkey (36,68), dog (36), rat (76), and chicken (41), as well as in the goat, sheep, and rabbit (12) exposed to a cold environment.

The above hypothesis is supported by results of the pharmacological manipulation of noradrenergic neurotransmission. 6-Hydroxydopamine, a stimulator of norepinephrine release from nerve terminals, causes a fall in body temperature after intraventricular injection in the cat (56,61) and rat (13,69,80). Milton and Harvey (61) showed that pretreatment of cats with 6-hydroxydopamine potentiates the febrile response to bacterial pyrogen, presumably due to depletion of the amine and destruction of noradrenergic terminals. Intraventricular injection of imipramine, a blocker of norepinephrine reuptake, also lowers the cat's body temperature (21).

Additional supporting evidence has come from the use of adrenergic receptor-blocking agents. Feldberg and Saxena (35) showed that intraventricular injections of α-receptor-blocking agents evoked a fever in the cat, presumably because of interference with the noradrenergic temperature-lowering mechanism. The hypothermic response to intracranial norepinephrine injections both in the cat (75) and the rat (76) is centrally antagonized by α-adrenergic-blocking agents.

Evidence for the release of endogenous norepinephrine in the AH/POA during activation of temperature-lowering pathways was provided by Myers and Chinn (65) in perfusion experiments with push-pull cannulas. They injected ^{14}C-norepinephrine intraventricularly in the cat to label the endogenous catecholamine stores. External warming of the cat increased the amount of radioactivity in the perfusate collected from the AH/POA but not from other brain areas.

If one accepts the concept that norepinephrine release in the AH/POA serves to lower body temperature, it still remains to be explained how the neurotransmitter functions in the thermoregulatory pathways. For example, does it excite synapses which activate heat-loss mechanisms; and if so, which mechanisms are affected (panting, sweating, or peripheral blood flow)? Alternatively, does the neurotransmitter act as an inhibitory substance, leading to disinhibition of heat loss or inhibition of heat production mechanisms? There is little firm evidence to answer these questions, but some tentative answers have been obtained. The neurotransmitter model based primarily on research in the cat and monkey (63,68) suggests that warm sensory input to the hypothalamus evokes release of norepinephrine in the AH/POA, which in turn causes inhibition of a serotonergic-cholinergic heat production pathway. In their neurotransmitter model based on experiments in the goat, sheep, and rabbit, Bligh et al. (12) envisioned a pathway from warm sensors to heat-loss effectors which exerts a cross-inhibitory influence on another pathway from cold sensors to heat production effectors. When activated, this crossed-inhibitory pathway releases norepinephrine, which suppresses activity of the temperature-raising mechanism.

A large number of investigations, which deserve consideration equal to those reviewed above, are not in agreement with the concept of a temperature-lowering role for hypothalamic norepinephrine. For example, in the ox the catecholamines had no effect on body temperature when injected into the cerebral ventricles (37). Although the rat exhibited a fall in body temperature after intraventricular or intrahypothalamic injection of high doses of norepinephrine (4,5,31,59), smaller doses evoked a rise in temperature when injected into the AH/POA (6,59) or intraventricularly (31,67). Satinoff and Cantor (76) concluded that the hypothermic response of the rat to intraventricular norepinephrine is due to the drug's action in a brain region other than the anterior hypothalamus since in the latter area the substance acts to evoke a rise in body temperature. Only when exposed to the cold does the rabbit exhibit a fall in body temperature after intraventricular injection of norepinephrine (12). In contrast, in a thermoneutral environment this species exhibits a fever after intraventricular injection of norepinephrine (19,46), desipramine, or 6-hydroxydopamine (56). The rise in body temperature appears to be mediated through central α-adrenergic receptors (27,35,72). It is a striking fact that all of these drug effects in the rabbit are completely opposite to those observed in cat. While there is convincing evidence from microinjection studies that the drug effects in the cat are exerted on noradrenergic synapses in the anterior hypothalamus, the site of drug action in the rabbit remains to be established. Norepinephrine has been microinjected into the anterior hypothalamus of the rabbit, but reports on its effect are conflicting (19,20,73). Other evidence arguing against a specific involvement of norepinephrine in thermoregulation was reviewed by Bligh (11).

Norepinephrine has been applied by microiontophoresis to neurons in the AH/POA of several species. In studies in the cat (7), rabbit (44), and rat (62), cold-sensitive neurons were excited and warm-sensitive neurons inhibited by norepinephrine. However, in one study in the cat no such correlation was found, and mixed responses were obtained with either group of neurons (49,50).

In summary, evidence obtained primarily from the cat and monkey supports the concept that the release of norepinephrine in the anterior hypothalamus serves to lower body temperature. Evidence obtained primarily from the rabbit and rat suggests that the neurotransmitter may serve to activate temperature-raising mechanisms. It may be that in any one species the neurotransmitter serves to influence both temperature-lowering and -raising mechanisms, depending on the environmental circumstances, as suggested by Bligh et al. (12). It remains unresolved whether the varied responses among species reflect physiological differences in the neurochemical coding of thermoregulatory pathways.

5-Hydroxytryptamine

As with norepinephrine, investigations of the role of 5-HT in central thermoregulatory pathways received impetus from the original experiments of Feldberg and Myers (32). These authors demonstrated that injection of

5-HT into the cerebral ventricles of the conscious cat produced a fever, an effect opposite to that of norepinephrine. A hyperthermic response was also obtained in the dog (36) and monkey (66). Microinjection experiments located the site of 5-HT action to the anterior hypothalamus (34,68). In their neurotransmitter model, Myers and Yaksh (68) and more recently Myers (63) proposed that 5-HT is released from nerve endings within the anterior hypothalamus in response to central and peripheral cold-sensory input. Serotonergic synapses in turn activate a cholinergically coded heat-production pathway. Several lines of evidence support this concept. Using push-pull cannulae, Myers and Beleslin (64) perfused the AH/POA of the conscious monkey and found that cooling the animal results in an increase of 5-HT in the perfusate. Conversely, warming the animal has no effect on 5-HT output. Milton and Harvey (61) observed that pretreatment of cats with parachlorophenylalanine, a depletor of 5-HT stores, attenuates the shivering and fever due to bacterial pyrogen or prostaglandin E_1 (PGE_1) injected intraventricularly. Methysergide, a 5-HT receptor blocker, exerted a similar effect.

That the role of 5-HT is to stimulate thermogenic pathways may be an oversimplified view of its action. The temperature response following intracranial injection in cats is often multiphasic. The response may begin as a rise in temperature, interrupted by a brief fall, and succeeded finally by a long-lasting hyperthermia (33,34); or it may consist of a fall in temperature followed by a long-lasting rise (61). Feldberg (30) attributed such falls in temperature to an overexcitation and blocking of serotonergic synapses by the high doses of 5-HT involved. However, the delayed fever produced in cats and monkeys by 5-HT is attenuated by treatment with antipyretic substances (61,82) and therefore may be a nonspecific fever involving the release of a prostaglandin (61).

The complexity of the problem is emphasized when one considers the experimental findings in other species. When injected intraventricularly, 5-HT lowers body temperature in the rabbit (19), sheep (10), goat (3), ox (38), and rat (31,67). In their neurotransmitter model of the role of central monoamines in thermoregulation, Bligh et al. (12) propose that 5-HT lowers body temperature by mediating the signals from warm sensors to heat-loss effectors, a role functionally opposite to that proposed from research in the cat and monkey (63,68). The weakness in this concept is that it has not been clearly established where the exogenous 5-HT acts when it is injected into the ventricular system. Cooper et al. (19) failed to see a fall in body temperature after microinjection of 5-HT into the AH/POA of the rabbit, except in a very few experiments when the animal was febrile. Also, Crawshaw (22) observed in the rat that microinjections of 5-HT into the anterior hypothalamus raised body temperature. On the basis of the effects of systemic drug injections, others have provided evidence in the rabbit for a temperature-raising role for 5-HT in the brain (26,29).

In iontophoresis studies Hori and Nakayama (44) observed in the rabbit that 5-HT excited warm-sensitive and inhibited cold-sensitive cells in the AH/POA, evidence consistent with the idea of a temperature-lowering role for the monoamine. On the other hand, in the cat Jell (49,50) reported no consistent relationship between the response of single units to 5-HT and the character of the response to local or peripheral temperature changes.

In conclusion, data obtained particularly from the cat and the monkey suggest that release of 5-HT in the AH/POA serves to raise body temperature. However, the effect of the drug in these species is complex and its interpretation difficult. Many data from other species suggest a temperature-lowering role for the transmitter, but the location of the serotonergic synapses remains to be established.

Dopamine

In recent years increasing attention has been focussed on the possibility that central dopaminergic mechanisms may be important in the control of body temperature. Systemic or intracranial injection of dopamine or dopamine-receptor agonists causes a fall in body temperature in a number of species including the mouse (40), rat (52), and cat (51). In the cat the hypothermic response to dopamine resulting from its intraventricular injection (51) or microinjection into the AH/POA (74) was blocked by treatment with the dopamine-receptor blocker haloperidol via the same routes. As with the other monoamines, responses are species-related. In the rabbit the pattern of responses to drugs which stimulate or block dopaminergic synapses is consistent with the concept that dopamine release mediates the elevation in body temperature (42,43,45).

CONCLUDING REMARKS

Two major problems arise from our current limited understanding of the role of central monoamines in thermoregulation: (a) What is the significance of species differences in the responsiveness to monoamines or to drugs which alter monoaminergic mechanisms? (b) What thermoregulatory mechanisms do each of the monoamines serve; i.e., do they mediate the thermosensory input, the putative set-point and comparator, or the effector functions of thermoregulation? These problems remain unanswered, in part because a major portion of the available data is based on the technique of intraventricular drug injection, which provides an indiscriminate pharmacological manipulation of brain structures. The logical follow-up approach of microinjection into the tissue to locate the site of drug action has often complemented the results of intraventricular injection but very often has provided contradictory results, leaving the researcher in a dilemma. The confusion that exists is not surprising when one considers that even the discrete microinjection of a drug into the brainstem may pharmacologically alter functionally opposing pathways at the same time. Such difficulties may be amplified in smaller species such as the rat because of their small brain size relative to injectate volumes. Whether the species differences represent true physiological differences in neurotransmitter organization of neural pathways or are solely artifacts inherent to the experimental conditions is a matter of contention and will probably continue to be so until more sophisticated pharmacological approaches are introduced to the field. A number of investigators have sought answers through the use of ionto-phoretic techniques for the analysis of monoamine action on thermoregulatory neurons. However, interpretation of such results is compromised by the facts that most of the studies have been carried out on anesthetized animals and that little is known of the role of the thermoresponsive units in the neuronal circuitry responsible for thermoregulation.

There has been much emphasis on body temperature as a measure of the central action of drugs. It is possible that a drug may alter one or more of the several physiological components that govern body temperature without evoking a change in the latter because compensatory mechanisms act to oppose the body temperature change. Thus it is important for researchers to monitor the activity of the major thermoregulatory effectors as well as body temperature to evaluate properly a drug's action on thermoregulation. Furthermore, drugs should be tested over a complete range of ambient temperatures because the level and pattern of neuronal activity, as well as responses to drugs, are influenced by the environmental conditions. It is an encouraging sign that experiments have been designed to measure changes in set-point. Likewise, it should be possible to design experiments that will reveal drug effects on the input (peripheral and central) and output components of the temperature control system. Such experiments should lead to a better understanding of the problem of species differences and the role of the monoamines in thermoregulation under normal and pathological conditions.

ACKNOWLEDGMENTS

The authors are indebted to Dr. W. Loskota for his critical reading of the manuscript and to Miss Monique van der Borg and Mrs. C. van Baaren for excellent secretarial assistance.

REFERENCES

1. Amin, A. N., Crawford, T. B. B., and Gaddum, J. H. (1954): The distribution of substance P and 5-hydroxytryptamine in the central nervous system of the dog. *J. Physiol. (Lond.)*, 126:596–618.
2. Andén, M. E., Dahlström, A., Fuxe, K., and Larsson, K. (1965): Mapping out of catecholamine and 5-hydroxytryptamine neurons innervating the telencephalon and diencephalon. *Life Sci.*, 4:1275–1279.
3. Andersson, B., Jobin, M., and Olsson, K. (1966): Serotonin and temperature control. *Acta Physiol. Scand.*, 67:50–56.

4. Avery, D. D. (1971): Intrahypothalamic adrenergic and cholinergic injection, effects on temperature and ingestive behavior in the rat. *Neuropharmacology*, 10:753–763.

5. Avery, D. D. (1972): Thermoregulatory effects of intrahypothalamic injections of adrenergic and cholinergic substances at different environmental temperatures. *J. Physiol. (Lond.)*, 220:257–266.

6. Beckman, A. L. (1970): Effects of intrahypothalamic norepinephrine on thermoregulatory responses in the rat. *Am. J. Physiol.*, 218:1596–1604.

7. Beckman, A. L., and Eisenman, J. S. (1970): Microelectrophoresis of biogenic amines on hypothalamic thermosensitive cells. *Science*, 170:334–336.

8. Bernard, C. (1876): *Leçons sur la Chaleur Animale.* Baillière, Paris.

9. Bertin, R., LeBlanc, J., Portet, R., and Chevillard, L. (1966): Effet d'inhibiteurs des récepteurs adrénergiques sur l'action calorigenique des catécholamines chez le rat adapté au froid. *J. Physiol. (Paris) (Suppl. 2)*, 60:349.

10. Bligh, J. (1966): The thermosensitivity of the hypothalamus and thermoregulation in mammals. *Biol. Rev.*, 41:317–367.

11. Bligh, J. (1973): *Temperature Regulation in Mammals and Other Vertebrates.* North Holland Publishing Co., Amsterdam.

12. Bligh, J., Cottle, W. H., and Maskrey, M. (1971): Influence of ambient temperature on the thermoregulatory response to 5-hydroxytryptamine, noradrenaline and acetylcholine injected into the lateral cerebral ventricles of sheep, goats and rabbits. *J. Physiol. (Lond.)*, 212:377–392.

13. Breese, G. R., Moore, R. A., and Howard, J. L. (1972): Central actions of 6-hydroxydopamine and other phenylethylamine derivatives on body temperature in the rat. *J. Pharmacol. Exp. Ther.*, 180:591–602.

14. Brodie, B. B., and Shore, P. A. (1957): A concept for a role of serotonin and norepinephrine as chemical mediators in the brain. *Ann. NY Acad. Sci.*, 66:631–642.

15. Bruinvels, J. (1975): Role of sodium in neuronal uptake of monoamines and amino acid precursors. *Nature (Lond.)*, 257:606–607.

16. Cannon, W. B., Querido, S., Britton, W., and Bright, E. M. (1927): Studies on conditions of activity in endocrine glands: The role of adrenal secretion in the chemical control of body temperature. *Am. J. Physiol.*, 79:466–507.

17. Carlson, L. D., and Hsieh, A. C. L. (1970): *Control of Energy Exchange.* Macmillan, New York.

18. Carlsson, A., Falck, B., and Hillarp, N. (1962): Cellular localization of brain monoamines. *Acta Physiol. Scand. [Suppl. 196]*, 56.

19. Cooper, K. E., Cranston, W. I., and Honour, A. J. (1965): Effects of intraventricular and intrahypothalamic injections of noradrenaline and 5-HT on body temperature in conscious rabbits. *J. Physiol. (Lond.)*, 181:852–864.

20. Cooper, K. E., Cranston, W. I., and Honour, A. J. (1967): Observations on the site and mode of action of pyrogens in the rabbit brain. *J. Physiol. (Lond.)*, 191:325–337.

21. Cranston, W. I., Hellon, R. F., Luff, R. H., and Rawlins, M. D. (1972): Hypothalamic endogenous noradrenaline and thermoregulation in the cat and rabbit. *J. Physiol. (Lond.)*, 223:59–68.

22. Crawshaw, L. I. (1972): Effects of intracerebral 5-hydroxytryptamine injection on thermoregulation in rat. *Physiol. Behav.*, 9:133–140.

23. Dahlström, A., and Fuxe, K. (1964): Evidence for the existence of monoamine-containing neurons in the central nervous system: Demonstration of monoamine in the cell bodies of brain stem neurons. *Acta Physiol. Scand. [Suppl. 232]*, 62.

24. Depocas, F. (1960): The calorigenic response of cold-acclimated white rats to infused noradrenaline. *Can. J. Biochem. Physiol.*, 38:107–114.

25. Desmarais, A., and Dugal, L. P. (1951): Circulation peripherique et teneur des surrénales en adrénaline et en artérénol (noradrénaline) chez le rat blanc exposé au froid. *Can. J. Med. Sci.*, 29:90–99.

26. DesPrez, R., Helman, R., and Oates, J. A. (1966): Inhibition of endotoxin fever by reserpine. *Proc. Soc. Exp. Biol. Med.*, 122:746–749.

27. Dhawan, B. N., and Dua, P. R. (1971): Evidence for the presence of alpha-adrenoceptors in the central thermoregulatory mechanism of rabbits. *Br. J. Pharmacol.*, 43:497–503.

28. Euler, C. von (1961): Physiology and pharmacology of temperature regulation. *Pharmacol. Rev.*, 13:361–398.
29. Fahim, I., Ismail, M., and Osman, O. H. (1972): The role of 5-hydroxytryptamine and noradrenaline in the hyperthermic reaction induced by pethidine in rabbits pretreated with pargyline. *Br. J. Pharmacol.*, 46:416–422.
30. Feldberg, W. (1968): The monoamines of the hypothalamus as mediators of temperature responses. In: *Recent Advances in Pharmacology*, edited by J. M. Robson and R. S. Stacey. pp. 349–397. Churchill, London.
31. Feldberg, W., and Lotti, V. J. (1967): Temperature responses to monoamines and an inhibitor of MAO injected into the cerebral ventricles of rats. *Br. J. Pharmacol.*, 31:152–161.
32. Feldberg, W., and Myers, R. D. (1963): A new concept of temperature regulation by amines in the hypothalamus. *Nature (Lond.)*, 200:1325.
33. Feldberg, W., and Myers, R. D. (1964): Effect on temperature of amines injected into the cerebral ventricles: A new concept of temperature regulation. *J. Physiol. (Lond.)*, 173:226–237.
34. Feldberg, W., and Myers, R. D. (1965): Changes in temperature produced by microinjection of amines into the anterior hypothalamus of cats. *J. Physiol. (Lond.)*, 177:239–245.
35. Feldberg, W., and Saxena, P. N. (1971): Effects of adrenoceptor blocking agents on body temperature. *Br. J. Pharmacol.*, 43:543–554.
36. Feldberg, W., Hellon, R. F., and Lotti, V. J. (1967): Temperature effects produced in dogs and monkeys by injections of monoamines and related substances into the third ventricle. *J. Physiol. (Lond.)*, 191:501–515.
37. Findlay, J. D., and Robertshaw, D. (1967): The mechanism of body temperature changes induced by intraventricular injections of adrenaline, noradrenaline and 5-hydroxytryptamine in the ox (Bos taurus). *J. Physiol. (Lond.)*, 189:329–336.
38. Findlay, J. D., and Thompson, G. E. (1968): The effects of intraventricular injections of noradrenaline, 5-hydroxytryptamine, acetylcholine and tranylcypromine on the ox at different environmental temperatures. *J. Physiol. (Lond.)*, 194:809–816.
39. Freund, H., and Janssen, S. (1923): Oxygen utilisation of skeletal muscle and its relation to heat regulation. *Pfluegers Arch. Gesamte Physiol.*, 200:96–118.
40. Fuxe, K., and Sjöqvist, F. (1972): Hypothermic effects of apomorphine in the mouse. *J. Pharm. Pharmacol.*, 24:702–705.
41. Grunden, L. R., and Marley, E. (1970): Effects of sympathomimetic amines injected into the third ventricle in adult chickens. *Neuropharmacology*, 9:119–128.
42. Hill, H. F., and Horita, A. (1971): Inhibition of d-amphetamine hyperthermia by blockade of dopamine receptors in rabbits. *J. Pharm. Pharmacol.*, 23:715–717.
43. Hill, H. F., and Horita, A. (1972): A pimozide-sensitive effect of apomorphine on body temperature of the rabbit. *J. Pharm. Pharmacol.*, 24:490–491.
44. Hori, T., and Nakayama, T. (1973): Effects of biogenic amines on central thermoresponsive neurones in the rabbit. *J. Physiol. (Lond.)*, 232:71–86.
45. Horita, A., and Quock, R. M. (1975): Dopaminergic mechanisms in drug-induced temperature effects. In: *Temperature Regulation and Drug Action*, edited by P. Lomax, E. Schönbaum, and J. Jacob, pp. 75–84. Karger, Basel.
46. Jacob, J., and Peindaries, R. (1973): Central effects of monoamines on the temperature of the conscious rabbit. In: *The Pharmacology of Thermoregulation*, edited by E. Schönbaum and P. Lomax, pp. 202–216. Karger, Basel.
47. Janský, L., editor (1971): *Nonshivering Thermogenesis*. Swets and Zeitlinger, Amsterdam.
48. Janský, L. (1973): Nonshivering thermogenesis and its thermoregulatory significance. *Biol. Rev.*, 48:85–132.
49. Jell, R. M. (1973): Responses of hypothalamic neurones to local temperature and to acetylcholine, noradrenaline and 5-hydroxytryptamine. *Brain Res.*, 55:123–134.
50. Jell, R. M. (1974): Responses of rostral hypothalamic neurones to peripheral temperature and to amines. *J. Physiol. (Lond.)*, 240:295–307.
51. Kennedy, M. S., and Burks, T. F. (1974): Dopamine receptors in the central thermoregulatory mechanism of the cat. *Neuropharmacology*, 13:119–128.
52. Kruk, Z. L. (1972): The effect of drugs acting on dopamine receptors on the body temperature of the rat. *Life Sci.*, 11:845–850.

53. Langley, J. N. (1921): *The Autonomic Nervous System.* Heffer and Sons, Cambridge.
54. LeBlanc, J. A., and Nadeau, G. C. (1961): Urinary excretion of adrenaline and noradrenaline in normal and cold-adapted animals. *Can. J. Biochem. Physiol.,* 39:215–218.
55. Leduc, J. (1961): Catecholamine production and release in exposure and acclimation to cold. *Acta Physiol. Scand. [Suppl. 183]*, 53.
56. Lewis, P. J., Rawlins, M. D., and Reid, J. L. (1975): Studies on central noradrenergic pathways in the control of body temperature. In: *Temperature Regulation and Drug Action,* edited by P. Lomax, E. Schönbaum, and J. Jacob, pp. 111–118. Karger, Basel.
57. Liebermeister, K. von (1875): *Handbuch der Pathologie und Therapie des Fiebers.* Vogel, Leipzig.
58. Lindberg, O., editor (1970): *Brown Adipose Tissue.* American Elsevier, New York.
59. Lomax, P., Foster, R., and Kirkpatrick, W. (1969): Cholinergic and adrenergic interactions in the thermoregulatory centers of the rat. *Brain Res.,* 15:431–438.
60. McLennan, H., editor (1963): *Synaptic Transmission.* Saunders, Philadelphia.
61. Milton, A. S., and Harvey, C. A. (1975): Prostaglandins and monoamines in fever. In: *Temperature Regulation and Drug Action,* edited by P. Lomax, E. Schönbaum, and J. Jacob, pp. 133–142. Karger, Basel.
62. Murakami, N. (1973): Effects of iontophoretic application of 5-hydroxytryptamine, noradrenaline and acetylcholine upon hypothalamic temperature-sensitive neurones in rats. *Jap. J. Physiol.,* 23:435–446.
63. Myers, R. D. (1975): An integrative model of monoamine and ionic mechanisms in the hypothalamic control of body temperature. In: *Temperature Regulation and Drug Action,* edited by P. Lomax, E. Schönbaum, and J. Jacob, pp. 32–42. Karger, Basel.
64. Myers, R. D., and Beleslin, D. B. (1971): Changes in serotonin release in hypothalamus during cooling or warming of the monkey. *Am. J. Physiol.,* 220:1746–1754.
65. Myers, R. D., and Chinn, C. (1973): Evoked release of hypothalamic norepinephrine during thermoregulation in the cat. *Am. J. Physiol.,* 224:230–236.
66. Myers, R. D., and Sharpe, L. G. (1968): Intracerebral injections and perfusions in the conscious monkey. In: *The Use of Non-human Primates in Drug Evaluation,* edited by Vagtborg. University of Texas Press, Austin.
67. Myers, R. D., and Yaksh, T. L. (1968): Feeding and temperature responses in the unrestrained rat after injections of cholinergic and aminergic substances into the cerebral ventricles. *Physiol. Behav.,* 3:917–928.
68. Myers, R. D., and Yaksh, T. L. (1969): Control of body temperature in the unanaesthetized monkey by cholinergic and aminergic systems in the hypothalamus. *J. Physiol. (Lond.),* 202:483–500.
69. Nakamura, K., and Thoenen, H. (1971): Hypothermia induced by intraventricular administration of 6-hydroxydopamine in rats. *Eur. J. Pharmacol.,* 16:46–54.
70. Pflueger (1878), cited by Sollmann, T. (1957): *A Manual of Pharmacology,* 8th ed., p. 689. Saunders, Philadelphia.
71. Precht, H., Christophersen, J., Hensel, H., and Larcher, W. (1973): *Temperature and Life,* Springer, New York.
72. Preston, E. (1973): Central effects of alpha-adrenergic blocking agents on thermoregulation against venous blood-stream cooling in unanaesthetized rabbits. *Can. J. Physiol. Pharmacol.,* 51:472–481.
73. Preston, E. (1975): Thermoregulation in the rabbit following intracranial injection of norepinephrine. *Am. J. Physiol.,* 229:676–682.
74. Quock, R. M., and Gale, C. C. (1974): Hypothermia-mediating dopamine receptors in the preoptic anterior hypothalamus of the cat. *Naunyn Schmiedebergs Arch. Pharmacol.,* 285:297–300.
75. Rudy, T. A., and Wolf, H. H. (1971): The effect of intrahypothalamically injected sympathomimetic amines on temperature regulation in the cat. *J. Pharmacol. Exp. Ther.,* 179:218–235.
76. Satinoff, E., and Cantor, A. (1975): Intraventricular norepinephrine and thermoregulation in rats. In: *Temperature Regulation and Drug Action,* edited by P. Lomax, E. Schönbaum, and J. Jacob, pp. 103–110. Karger, Basel.
77. Schönbaum, E., Johnson, G. E., and Sellers, E. A. (1966): Acclimation to cold and norepinephrine: Effects of immunosympathectomy. *Am. J. Physiol.,* 211:647–650.

78. Schönbaum, E., Johnson, G. E., Sellers, E. A., and Gill, M. J. (1966): Adrenergic β-receptors and non-shivering thermogenesis. *Nature (Lond.)*, 210:426.

79. Sellers, E. A., Scott, J. W., and Thomas, N. (1954): Electrical activity of skeletal muscle of normal and acclimatized rats on exposure to cold. *Am. J. Physiol.*, 177:372–376.

80. Simmonds, M. A., and Uretsky, N. J. (1970): Central effects of 6-hydroxydopamine on the body temperature of the rat. *Br. J. Pharmacol.*, 40:630–638.

81. Vogt, M. (1954): The concentration of sympathin in different parts of the central nervous system under normal conditions and after the administration of drugs. *J. Physiol. (Lond.)*, 123:451–481.

82. Waller, M. B., and Myers, R. D. (1974): Similar actions of intrahypothalamic 5,6-DHT and 5-HT in evoking hyperthermia in the monkey. *Res. Commun. Chem. Pathol. Pharmacol.*, 9:421–429.

Brain Dysfunction in Infantile Febrile
Convulsions, edited by M. A. B. Brazier and
F. Coceani. Raven Press, New York © 1976.

Central Cholinergic Mechanism of Pyrexia

*K. K. Tangri, Nisha Misra, and K. P. Bhargava

*Department of Pharmacology and Therapeutics, King George's Medical College,
Lucknow-226003, India*

Extensive experimental evidence implicates the hypothalamus in central thermoregulatory processes. Applying McLennan's (34) criteria, a number of chemical substances — viz., norepinephrine (NE), 5-hydroxytryptamine (5-HT), and acetylcholine (ACh) — are considered transmitters in the hypothalamus. Feldberg and Myers (17,18) suggested that central thermoregulation might result from a balance between the release of NE and 5-HT in the hypothalamus. Changes in body temperature have been observed after intracerebroventricular or intrahypothalamic injection of NE and 5-HT (3,4,8,12,14,20,21,40,45). A hypothalamic cholinergic mechanism for thermoregulation was also suggested because intracerebroventricular or intrahypothalamic injection of cholinomimetic agents resulted in thermal changes. With all substances, the sign of the response was species-dependent (2,3,6,22,28,32,40,41,46). Rabbits, however, failed to show consistent thermoregulatory responses to the cholinomimetics (6,25).

Central thermoregulation likely involves the integration of anterior and posterior hypothalamic functions and the interaction between monoaminergic and cholinergic mechanisms (5,12,39,41,43,54). However, the exact operation of the control system is not known.

Bacterial endotoxin (BE) has been shown to produce pyrexia in several species through an action on the preoptic area (POA) of the hypothalamus (1,13,42,44,53). Cabanac et al. (9), Eisenman (16), and Wit and Wang (54) observed stimulation of cold-sensitive neurons and depression of heat-sensitive neurons in the POA during BE fever. Blockade of BE pyrexia by cyproheptadine and reserpine in rabbits (10,33) suggested the involvement of hypothalamic 5-HT. Further, the inhibition of BE pyrexia in rabbits with α-methyl-p-tyrosine (50) and α-adrenergic blocking agents (29) pointed to a role of hypothalamic NE. The involvement of a hypothalamic cholinergic mechanism in the pathogenesis of fever was indicated by findings with atropine (52). Therefore the present study was undertaken to determine the effects of intracerebroventricular injection of cholinomimetic

* Present address: Dr. K. K. Tangri, Department of Clinical Pharmacology, Royal Postgraduate Medical School, Ducane Road, London W12, England.

agents on body temperature in rabbits and to elucidate the nature of the interaction between hypothalamic monoaminergic and cholinergic mechanisms in the thermoregulatory process. In the course of this study, the neurohumoral mechanism responsible for BE pyrexia was also investigated.

METHODS

Adult albino rabbits of either sex weighing 1.5–2 kg were used. The animals were kept at a constant ambient temperature using a B.O.D. incubator (Toshniwal) set at 72° ± 1°F. The incubator allowed free circulation of air. In some experiments animals were subjected to heat (95° ± 1°F) or cold (41° ± 1°F) stress. The core temperature was recorded every 30 min for 6 hr by means of a clinical thermometer or by a thermistor probe introduced 3 cm into the rectum. The output of the thermistor probe was recorded on an APLAB Telethermometer.

Drug Administration

Drugs were injected into the lateral cerebral ventricle according to the technique of Feldberg and Myers (17). A stainless steel template cannula with a rubber diaphragm was screwed into the skull taking care not to injure the meninges. Subsequently the wound was allowed to heal, and penicillin (200,000 IU/day) was injected intramuscularly for 5 days. The animals were used for the temperature studies 10 days after surgery. The intracerebroventricular injections were made with a 24-gauge hypodermic needle introduced through the rubber diaphragm of the template cannula. Drugs were dissolved in pyrogen-free distilled water, and the volume of injectate never exceeded 0.2 ml. Pyrogen-free glassware and syringes were used throughout the study. Glassware was heated at 160°C for 2 hr in an oven and then rinsed with pyrogen-free distilled water. Double-distilled water was irradiated with ultraviolet light for 15 min and then passed through a Seitz filter (0.5 μm pore size).

Analysis of Temperature Responses to Drugs

The time course of temperature responses to intracerebroventricular injection of drugs was plotted and the hypo- or hyperthermic indices measured according to the planimetric technique of Hall and Atkins (23). Means ± SE were calculated for each group of experiments, and values were subjected to Student's *t*-test.

The drugs used were: *l*-norepinephrine bitartrate, 5-hydroxytryptamine creatinine sulphate, acetylcholine hydrochloride, carbachol, pilocarpine hydrochloride, oxotremorine sesqueoxalate, physostigmine salicylate, phenoxybenzamine hydrochloride, hemicholinium-3, (±) propranolol hydrochloride, α-methyl-*m*-tyrosine (α-MMT), reserpine, atropine sulphate, ethybenztropine bromide, chlorisondamine chloride, cyproheptadine, and methysergide bimaleate. Doses of drugs refer to their salts.

The BE consisted of a suspension of attenuated *Salmonella typhi* "O" cells. All blockers except hemicholinium, α-MMT, and reserpine were given 1 hr prior to the injection of a putative transmitter or BE. Hemicholinium and α-MMT treatment preceded the test injection by 5 and 24 hr, respectively. All compounds were administered by the ventricular route with the exception of reserpine, which was given intramuscularly for 3 days prior to the experiment.

RESULTS

Effect of Intracerebroventricular Injection of Cholinergic Drugs on the Core Temperature of Rabbits

Intracerebroventricular injection of ACh (10 μg), carbachol (10 μg), and physostigmine (100 μg) produced hyperthermia in rabbits. Figure 1 shows the time course of the response to these agents. The maximum increase in the core temperature with these three agents was 2.1° ± 0.2°, 1.5° ± 0.4°, and 2.6° ± 0.4°F, respectively. Furthermore, the hyperthermia

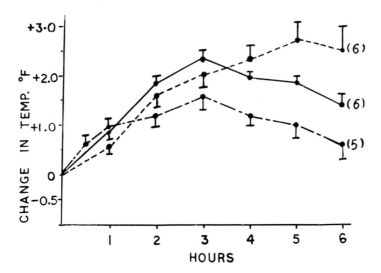

FIG. 1. Time course of hyperthermia induced by intracerebroventricular injection of ACh (●——●), carbachol (●---●), and physostigmine (●-----●) in rabbits. In this and subsequent figures, the number of animals is given in parentheses. Note the gradual development of hyperthermia. Maximal response was observed at 3 hr for ACh (10 μg) and carbachol (10 μg), and at 5 hr for physostigmine (100 μg). Partial recovery occurred in 6 hr. (From Tangri et al., ref. 48.)

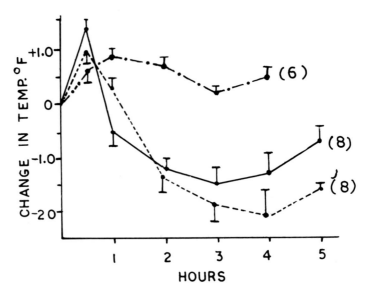

FIG. 2. Time course of thermal responses to intracerebroventricular injection of pilocarpine (6 mg) and oxotremorine (100 μg) in normal and atropine (500 μg) pretreated rabbits. Note the biphasic thermal response to pilocarpine (●-----●) and oxotremorine (●——●), consisting of an initial hyperthermia of short duration followed by a delayed hypothermia. Partial recovery of the core temperature occurred in 5 hr. Note also the disappearance of the hypothermic response to pilocarpine in atropinized animals (●—·—●). (From Tangri et al., ref. 48.)

induced by ACh injected into the lateral ventricle was dose-dependent. The hyperthermic indices for 5, 10, and 20 μg ACh were 23.6 ± 5.4, 43.1 ± 2.7, and 74.4 ± 4.2 cm^2, respectively.

On the other hand, intracerebroventricular injection of the muscarinic agents pilocarpine (6 mg) and oxotremorine (100 μg) elicited a biphasic thermal response consisting of an initial short-lived hyperthermia followed by prolonged hypothermia (Fig. 2). Mean increases in the core temperature were $0.9° \pm 0.2°$ and $1.4° \pm 0.2°$F with pilocarpine and oxotremorine, respectively. The hypothermia due to these agents began approximately 1 hr after the injection and reached a peak within 3–4 hr. The maximum falls in core temperature were $2.0° \pm 0.5°$ and $1.5° \pm 0.3°$F, respectively.

Effect of Pretreatment with Cholinergic Blocking Agents on Thermal Responses to Cholinergic Drugs

Figure 3 shows the effect of intracerebroventricular pretreatment with cholinergic blocking agents—viz., chlorisondamine (100 μg) and atropine (500 μg)—on the hyperthermia induced by ACh (10 μg) administered by the same route. Chlorisondamine blocked the ACh hyperthermia ($p < 0.01$).

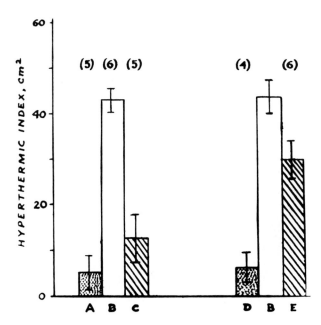

FIG. 3. Hyperthermic indices following intracerebroventricular injection of ACh in normal and chlorisondamine- and atropine-pretreated rabbits. A, chlorisondamine (100 µg). B, ACh (10 µg). C, ACh after chlorisondamine pretreatment. D, atropine (500 µg). E, ACh after atropine pretreatment. Note the disappearance of ACh-induced hyperthermia after chlorisondamine and the lack of effect of atropine.

The hyperthermic indices for intracerebroventricular ACh were 43.1 ± 5.2 and 12.9 ± 5.6 cm², respectively, in the control and chlorisondamine-pretreated animals. In contrast, ACh hyperthermia was essentially the same in atropine-treated animals and in controls ($p > 0.1$).

Atropine was also tested on the thermal response to intracerebroventricular pilocarpine. As shown in Fig. 2, the delayed hypothermia induced by pilocarpine (6 mg) was blocked by prior atropinization (500 µg) while the initial hyperthermia remained unaltered.

Effect of Intracerebroventricular Injection of NE on the Core Temperature of Rabbits: Interaction with Adrenergic and Cholinergic Blocking Agents

Intracerebroventricular injection of NE elicited a dose-dependent hyperthermia. The hyperthermic indices observed with 10, 20, and 40 µg NE were 19.0 ± 3.4, 25.8 ± 5.3, and 36.6 ± 4.3 cm², respectively. The effect of pretreatment with adrenergic and cholinergic blocking agents on NE-induced hyperthermia is shown in Fig. 4. Phenoxybenzamine (500 µg) abolished the hyperthermic response to NE (20 µg), whereas propranolol was ineffective. The hyperthermic indices due to NE were 25.8 ± 5.2 and 6.0 ± 4.5 cm², respectively, before and after treatment with phenoxybenzamine ($p < 0.05$).

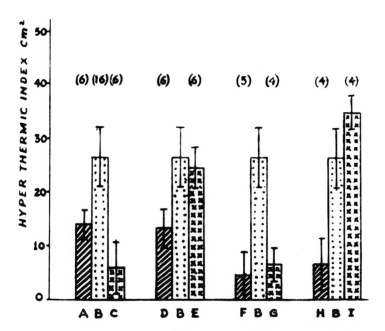

FIG. 4. Hyperthermic indices following intracerebroventricular injection of NE in normal rabbits and those pretreated with adrenergic and cholinergic blocking agents. A, Phenoxybenzamine (500 μg). B, NE (20 μg). C, NE after phenoxybenzamine pretreatment. D, propranolol (1 mg). E, NE after propranolol pretreatment. F, chlorisondamine (100 μg). G, NE after chlorisondamine. H, atropine (500 μg). I, NE after atropinization. Note that NE-induced hyperthermia is blocked by phenoxybenzamine and chlorisondamine but not by propranolol and atropine.

Further, chlorisondamine (100 μg) blocked ($p < 0.05$) the hyperthermia evoked by NE (hyperthermic indices were 5.7 ± 3.2 and 25.8 ± 5.3 cm^2 in chlorisondamine-pretreated and control animals, respectively). In contrast, atropinized animals (500 μg) behaved as controls in their response to NE ($p > 0.6$).

Effect of Intracerebroventricular Injection of 5-HT on the Core Temperature of Rabbits: Interaction With Cholinergic Blocking Drugs

Intracerebroventricular injection of 5-HT produced a dose-dependent hypothermia in rabbits. The hypothermic indices due to 5-HT were 12.2 ± 1.2 (100 μg), 21.2 ± 2.8 (200 μg), and 33.6 ± 2.2 (400 μg) cm^2. Figure 5A shows the time course of the hypothermic response to 5-HT (200 μg). Hypothermia had a fast onset, reached a peak ($1.3° \pm 0.5°$F) within 30 min, and subsided in 3 hr. Unlike controls, cyproheptadine-treated animals (100 μg) developed hyperthermia ($2.2° \pm 0.6°$F) following administration of 5-HT. Further, pretreatment with the muscarinic blocking agent ethybenztropine (100 μg) resulted in blockade of 5-HT hypothermia. Chlorisonda-

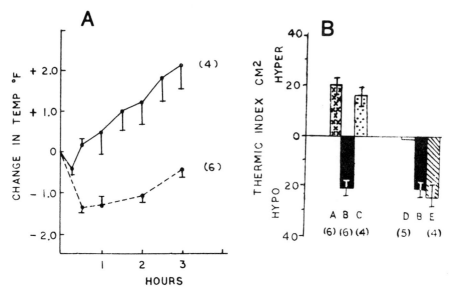

FIG. 5. A: Time course of thermal responses to intracerebroventricular injection of 5-HT (200 μg) in normal rabbits (●-----●) and those pretreated with 100 μg cyproheptadine (●——●). Note the immediate onset of 5-HT hypothermia and complete recovery within 5 hr. Note also the opposite effect of 5-HT in animals pretreated with cyproheptadine. **B:** Thermic indices due to intracerebroventricular injection of 5-HT in normal and ethybenztropine- and chlorisondamine-pretreated rabbits. A, ethybenztropine (100 μg). B, 5-HT (200 μg). C, 5-HT after ethybenztropine pretreatment. D, chlorisondamine (100 μg). E, 5-HT after chlorisondamine pretreatment. Note that only ethybenztropine blocks 5-HT hypothermia.

mine (100 μg), however, did not modify ($p > 0.6$) the central action of 5-HT. The hypothermic indices obtained with 5-HT were 24.5 ± 3.6 and 21.2 ± 2.8 cm², respectively, before and after treatment with chlorisondamine. Figure 5B illustrates the response to 5-HT in the presence of ethybenztropine and chlorisondamine.

Effect of Intracerebroventricular Injection of Cholinergic Blocking Agents on the Core Temperature of Rabbits at Different Ambient Temperatures

The thermal effects of intracerebroventricular cholinergic blocking agents were investigated at different ambient temperatures (T_A) in rabbits. Both atropine (200 μg) and chlorisondamine (100 μg) failed to produce any significant change in the core temperature at a neutral T_A (72°F). On the other hand, at a high T_A (95°F), when the warm sensor-heat loss mechanism is maximally active, atropine at the same dose induced a progressive hyperthermia. The maximal rise in the core temperature with atropine was $2.7° \pm 0.4°$F as compared to $0.8° \pm 0.2°$F in controls ($p < 0.01$). Again, chlorisondamine had no effect. The results of this study are shown in Fig. 6.

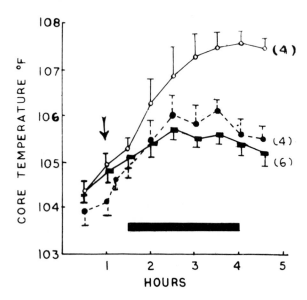

FIG. 6. Temperature changes in normal rabbits (■——■) and those pretreated with atropine (200 μg) (O——O) and chlorisondamine (100 μg) (●-----●) during exposure to a high T_A (95°F). The black horizontal bar and the arrow indicate, respectively, the period of heat stress and the time of drug injection. Note the progressive hyperthermia in the atropine-treated but not in chlorisondamine-treated animals.

The magnitude and time course of thermal changes induced by cholinergic blocking agents in rabbits exposed to cold (41°F) are shown in Fig. 7. At a low T_A, when the cold sensor-heat production mechanism is maximally active, chlorisondamine produced a rapidly developing hypothermia. The maximal fall in the core temperature was 3.8° ± 1.4°F in chlorisondamine-treated animals as compared to 1.1° ± 0.6°F in controls. In contrast, atropine had no effect.

Effect of Intracerebroventricular Injection of BE on the Core Temperature of Rabbits: Interaction With Physostigmine

In order to elucidate the central neurohumoral mechanism responsible for BE pyrexia, graded doses of BE (10^4–10^6 bacterial cells) were injected into the lateral cerebral ventricle of normal and physostigmine-treated rabbits. BE was found to elicit a dose-dependent pyrexia in normal animals. The maximum rise in the core temperature was 1.8° ± 0.3°F (hyperthermic index 27.2 ± 3.0 cm²), 2.1° ± 0.1°F (hyperthermic index 54.5 ± 3.4 cm²), and 3.2° ± 0.17°F (hyperthermic index 68.2 ± 3.2 cm²), respectively, with 10^4, 10^5, and 10^6 bacterial cells. The time course of BE (10^5 cells) and physostigmine (50 μg) pyrexia is shown in Fig. 8. BE pyrexia reached a maximum after 3 hr and abated within 24 hr. The response to physostigmine was

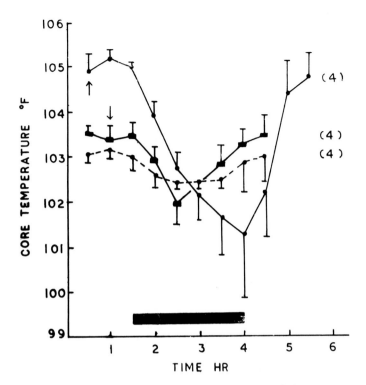

FIG. 7. Temperature changes in normal rabbits (●-----●) and those pretreated with intracerebroventricular chlorisondamine (●——●) and atropine (■——■) during exposure to a low T_A (41°F). The dark horizontal bar indicates the period of cold stress. Note the rapidly developing hypothermia in animals treated with chlorisondamine (100 μg) during exposure to cold and the quick reversal of the effect when the animal is returned to a T_A of 72°F.

slower and reached a peak (2.6° ± 0.4°F) after 5 hr. However, recovery from physostigmine action was complete by 24 hr. BE pyrexia was enhanced by pretreatment with physostigmine. As shown in Fig. 8, BE fever was maximal after 5 hr in physostigmine-treated animals (2.9° ± 0.5°F). Unlike controls, however, the core temperature of physostigmine-treated animals was still significantly ($p < 0.01$) elevated (2.9° ± 0.3°F) 24 hr after BE injection.

Effects of Pretreatment With Cholinergic Blocking Agents on BE Pyrexia in Rabbits

The effects of pretreatment with hemicholinium, chlorisondamine, and atropine on BE (10^5 cells) pyrexia are shown in Fig. 9. Hemicholinium (100 μg) induced a mild hyperthermia (hyperthermic index 14.0 ± 2.8 cm²) in normal rabbits while chlorisondamine (100 μg) and atropine (500 μg)

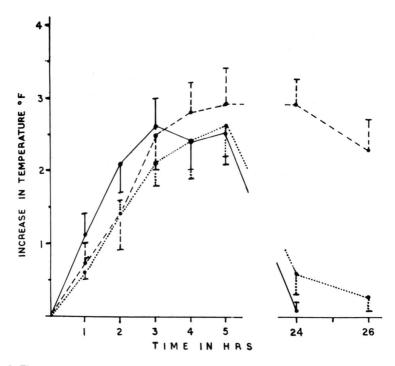

FIG. 8. Time course of hyperthermia induced by intracerebroventricular injection of BE (●——●), physostigmine (●·····●), and BE after treatment with physostigmine (●-----●). Note that the peak effect of BE (10^5 cells) and physostigmine (50 μg) occurred within 3 and 5 hr, respectively. With either compound, recovery was complete by 24 hr. Note also the enhancement of BE hyperthermia in physostigmine-pretreated animals. (From Tangri et al., ref. 49.)

were without effect. However, BE pyrexia was blocked by pretreatment with hemicholinium and chlorisondamine ($p < 0.01$). The hyperthermic indices due to BE in hemicholinium- and chlorisondamine-pretreated animals were, respectively, 22.7 ± 7.0 and 4.6 ± 3.7 cm^2, compared to 54.5 ± 3.4 cm^2 in the untreated group. Atropine did not alter significantly ($p > 0.1$) the BE pyrexia (hyperthermic index 38.5 ± 4.4 cm^2).

Effect of Monoamine Depletion on BE Pyrexia in Rabbits

BE action (10^5 cells) was investigated in reserpinized rabbits (15 mg/day i.m.) and in animals pretreated with α-MMT (10 mg). The results are shown in Fig. 10. Neither α-MMT nor reserpine modified the pyrexia induced by intracerebroventricular injection of BE. BE hyperthermic indices were 43.8 ± 5.8 and 49.5 ± 4.2 cm^2 in animals pretreated with α-MMT and reserpine, respectively, compared to 54.5 ± 3.4 cm^2 in controls ($p > 0.1$).

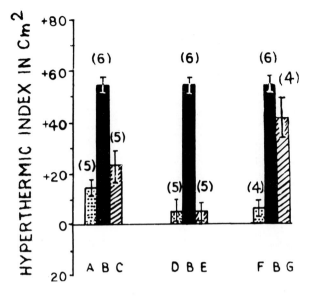

FIG. 9. Hyperthermic indices due to intracerebroventricular injection of BE in normal and hemicholinium-, chlorisondamine-, and atropine-pretreated rabbits. A, hemicholinium (100 μg). B, BE (10^5 cells). C, BE after hemicholinium pretreatment. D, chlorisondamine (100 μg). E, BE after chlorisondamine pretreatment. F, atropine (500 μg). G, BE after atropinization. Note the blockade of BE hyperthermia in hemicholinium- and chlorisondamine-treated animals but not in atropine-treated animals. (From Tangri et al., ref. 49.)

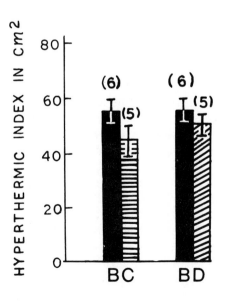

FIG. 10. Hyperthermic indices due to intracerebroventricular BE in normal and reserpine- or α-MMT-pretreated rabbits. B, BE (10^5 cells). C, BE after α-MMT (10 mg) pretreatment. D, BE after reserpinization (15 mg/day i.m.). Note that BE pyrexia is not affected by these drugs.

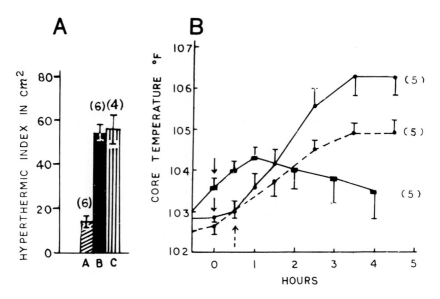

FIG. 11. A: Hyperthermic indices due to intracerebroventricular BE in normal and phe-noxybenzamine-pretreated rabbits. A, phenoxybenzamine (500 µg). B, BE (10^5 cells). C, BE after phenoxybenzamine pretreatment. Note that BE pyrexia is not blocked by phenoxy-benzamine. **B:** Time course of temperature changes in animals given BE (10^5 cells) (●-----●), methysergide (■——■), and BE plus methysergide (●——●). Methysergide (*solid arrow*) was given 1 hr prior to endotoxin (*broken arrow*). Note the greater potency of BE in methysergide-treated animals.

Effect of Pretreatment With Monoaminergic Blocking Agents on BE Pyrexia in Rabbits

The possible involvement of hypothalamic monoamines in the patho-genesis of BE fever was also examined by treating the animals with an α-adrenergic blocker (phenoxybenzamine) and a 5-HT antagonist (methy-sergide). The results of this study are shown in Fig. 11. Both phenoxy-benzamine (500 µg) and methysergide (1 mg) induced an insignificant hyperthermic response in rabbits (hyperthermic indices were, respectively, 13.5 ± 2.7 and 17.4 ± 7.1 cm²). Phenoxybenzamine did not modify the pyrexia induced by intracerebroventricular injection of BE. The fever indices due to BE (10^5 cells) pyrexia were 55.7 ± 6.8 cm² in phenoxy-benzamine-treated animals and 54.5 ± 3.4 cm² in controls ($p > 0.1$). In contrast, methysergide potentiated BE pyrexia. The maximum rise in the core temperature induced by BE (10^5 cells) was $1.8° \pm 0.3°F$ and $3.3° \pm 0.3°F$, respectively, before and after treatment with methysergide. The difference was significant ($p < 0.01$).

DISCUSSION

Pharmacological Characterization of Hypothalamic Receptors Concerned in Thermoregulation

The present study showed that intracerebroventricular injection of acetylcholine, carbachol, and physostigmine evokes a hyperthermic response in rabbits. A similar hyperthermia has been reported with intracerebroventricular or intrahypothalamic injection of cholinomimetic agents in cats (46), sheep, goats (6,28), monkeys (41), and rats (3,30,40). These observations, together with the demonstration of ACh in perfusates of the hypothalamus in monkeys subjected to cold stress (39) and the presence of synthetic and metabolic enzymes for ACh in the hypothalamus (19), suggested that a cholinergic mechanism contributes to central thermoregulation. The blockade of ACh hyperthermia with chlorisondamine, but not with atropine, indicated the involvement of a nicotinic receptor. That a hypothalamic nicotinic receptor is concerned with heat production in rabbits was further demonstrated in this study by the hypothermic action of chlorisondamine only in cold-stressed animals. The heat production mechanism is maximally active during exposure at a low ambient temperature. Both nicotinic and muscarinic receptors are known to be present in the hypothalamus. Hall and Myers (24) demonstrated nicotinic receptors in the caudal hypothalamus of monkeys. Muscarinic receptors (27) account for the hyperthermic response to intracerebroventricular carbachol and physostigmine in cats and sheep.

Muscarinic agents (pilocarpine and oxotremorine) induced a biphasic thermal response consisting of initial hyperthermia followed by hypothermia. Activation of a muscarinic receptor mediated the delayed hypothermia due to pilocarpine since it was blocked by treatment with atropine. Atropinization also evoked a hyperthermic response in heat-stressed rabbits but had no effect in animals exposed to a neutral or cold ambient temperature. These observations indicate that a hypothalamic muscarinic receptor is concerned in the activation of heat-loss processes.

Work in monkeys is consistent with the idea that a cholinergic mechanism is involved in both thermogenic and thermolytic processes. Microinjection of ACh into the hypothalamus elicited hyperthermia or hypothermia depending on the site (41). Similarly, ACh release from the hypothalamus is either increased or inhibited by peripheral cold stress (39). Bligh et al. (6) also suggested an excitatory role of ACh in the heat production mechanism of sheep and goats.

Interaction of Cholinergic and Monoaminergic Mechanisms in Thermoregulation

Several lines of evidence indicate a neurotransmitter role of the monoamines in the neuronal circuitry responsible for thermoregulation. Monoamines are present in the hypothalamus along with the enzymes for their synthesis and degradation (7,11,51). Monoamines, whether injected into the cerebral ventricles or applied directly to the hypothalamus, modify body temperature. The sign of their action is species-related (3,6,20,21, 40,41,45). Thermal stress stimulates the release of the appropriate mono-amines from the POA of cats and monkeys (37,38). Thermosensitive neurons in the POA respond to iontophoretically applied monoamines. 5-HT stimulated "cold"-sensitive neurons in the POA of monkeys (5) and "heat"-sensitive neurons in rabbits (26). NE has an opposite effect in the two species.

In the present investigation, intracerebroventricular injection of NE and 5-HT evoked hyperthermia and hypothermia, respectively. The hyper-thermic response to NE was due to the activation of α-adrenergic receptors because it was blocked by phenoxybenzamine and not by propranolol. Treatment with cyproheptadine changed the sign of 5-HT action, i.e., from hypothermia to hyperthermia. The 5-HT hyperthermia in cyproheptadine-treated animals could be mediated by an E-type prostaglandin. Intracere-broventricular injection of 5-HT has been shown to elicit the release of a PGE compound into the ventricular system, at least in the dog (25).

The present study also suggested that cholinergic and monoaminergic systems interact in the hypothalamus. NE hyperthermia was blocked by treatment with a nicotinic blocker, chlorisondamine, whereas atropine was ineffective. Further, 5-HT hypothermia was blocked by a muscarinic blocker, ethybenztropine, and not by chlorisondamine. Thermosensitive neurons responding to the monoamines are located in the POA (5,41,54), while cholinoceptive neurons involved in temperature responses occur predominantly in the caudal hypothalamus (40,41). Thermal stimulation of the POA results in the activation of neurons in the caudal hypothalamus (43), and injection of 5-HT in the POA releases ACh in the caudal hy-pothalamus (36). According to a hypothetical model of the neurohumoral control of body temperature which integrates these observations, the central "thermodetector" mechanism sensitive to monoamines and the central cholinergic integrating mechanism are located, respectively, in the POA and the caudal hypothalamus. "Cold" stress, whether central or peripheral, would activate the NE-sensitive neurons (α-adrenergic) in the POA through the release of NE. These "cold"-sensitive neurons, in turn, would activate cholinoceptive neurons (nicotinic) in the caudal hypothalamus, which would result in activation of heat-production mechanisms. Conversely, "heat"-sensitive neurons in the POA would be activated by the release of 5-HT, which would lead to stimulation of cholinoceptive neurons (muscarinic) and activation of heat-loss mechanisms. A similar interaction between monoaminergic and cholinergic neurons has been proposed in the monkey (35), but monkeys and rabbits respond to the amines in an opposite manner.

Neurohumoral Mechanism of BE Pyrexia

The neurohumoral mechanism subserving BE hyperthermia was also investigated in the light of this hypothetical model. Microinjection studies (13,53) have proved that endotoxin acts on neurons in the anterior hypothalamus. The sign of endotoxin action correlates with the character of the neuronal response to thermal stimuli (9,16,54). Our finding that BE action was potentiated by physostigmine indicated that hypothalamic cholinoceptor neurons are involved in the pathogenesis of fever. Evidence from experiments with the blockers suggested that the neurons in question are nicotinic. Further, it was shown that BE pyrexia is blocked by hemicholinium. Since hemicholinium inhibits ACh synthesis, it follows that the activation of nicotinic receptors in the caudal hypothalamus during BE fever involved the release of ACh.

In view of the postulated interaction between monoaminergic and cholinergic systems in the control of body temperature, the release of ACh in the caudal hypothalamus in response to BE might result from the activation of "norepinephrine"- or "cold"-sensitive neurons in the POA. Consistent with this idea is the finding (50) that BE pyrexia is abolished by depletion of the catecholamines with α-methyl-p-tyrosine. However, this seems unlikely because pyrexia was not blocked by treatment with phenoxybenzamine, whereas the same treatment inhibited NE pyrexia. Further, the catecholamine depletors α-MMT and reserpine did not modify BE pyrexia. Similar findings with the depletors have been reported by Des Prez et al. (15).

Kroneberg and Kurbjuweit (31), Takagi and Karuma (47), and Des Prez et al. (15) proposed that BE pyrexia is mediated by 5-HT because it is associated with a fall of 5-HT levels in brain and is blocked by reserpine and not by guanethidine or α-MMT. The finding, presented here, that methysergide potentiates BE pyrexia argues against this idea. The potentiation of BE pyrexia by methysergide could be due to the blockade of tryptaminergic receptors in POA concerned in the activation of heat loss. In this connection it should be added that the blockade of BE fever by cyproheptadine (10) could be due to a peripheral action of the drug. Thus it may be concluded that BE pyrexia results from the release of ACh in the caudal hypothalamus, which activates nicotinic receptors concerned in thermogenesis.

REFERENCES

1. Allen, I. V. (1965): The cerebral effects of endogenous serum and granulocytic pyrogen. *Br. J. Exp. Pathol.*, 46:25–34.
2. Avery, D. D. (1970): Hyperthermia induced by direct injection of carbachol in the anterior hypothalamus. *Neuropharmacology*, 9:175–178.
3. Avery, D. D. (1972): Thermoregulatory effects of intrahypothalamic injections of adrenergic and cholinergic drugs at different ambient temperature. *J. Physiol. (Lond.)*, 220:257–266.

4. Beckman, A. L. (1970): Effect of intrahypothalamic norepinephrine on thermoregulatory responses in the rat. *Am. J. Physiol.,* 218:1596–1604.
5. Beckman, A. L., and Eisenman, J. S. (1970): Microelectrophoresis of biogenic amines on hypothalamic thermosensitive cells. *Science,* 170:334–336.
6. Bligh, J., Cottle, W. H., and Maskrey, M. (1971): The influence of ambient temperature on the thermoregulatory responses to 5-hydroxytryptamine, noradrenaline and acetylcholine injected into the lateral cerebral ventricles of sheep, goats and rabbits. *J. Physiol. (Lond.),* 212:377–392.
7. Bogdanski, D. F., Weissbach, H., and Udenfriend, S. (1957): The distribution of serotonin, 5-hydroxytryptophan decarboxylase and monoamine oxidase in brain. *J. Neurochem.,* 1:272–278.
8. Brittain, R. T., and Handley, S. L. (1967): Temperature changes produced by injection of catecholamines and 5-hydroxytryptamine into cerebral ventricle of conscious mouse. *J. Physiol. (Lond.),* 192:805–814.
9. Cabanac, M., Stolwijk,J. A. J., and Hardy, J. D. (1968): Effect of temperature and pyrogens on single unit activity in the rabbit's brain stem. *J. Appl. Physiol.,* 24:645–652.
10. Canal, N., and Ornesi, A. (1961): La serotonina quale agente ipertermizzante. *Atti Accad. Med. Lomb.,* 16:64–69.
11. Carlsson, A., Falck, B., and Hillarp, N. A. (1962): Cellular localization of brain monoamines. *Acta Physiol. Scand. [Suppl. 196],* 56.
12. Cooper, K. E., Cranston, W. I., and Honour, A. J. (1965): Effect of intracerebral and intrahypothalamic injection of norepinephrine and 5-HT on body temperature in conscious rabbits. *J. Physiol. (Lond.),* 181:852–864.
13. Cooper, K. E., Cranston, W. I., and Honour, J. A. (1967): Observations on the site and mode of action of pyrogens in the rabbit brain. *J. Physiol. (Lond.),* 191:325–338.
14. Cranshow, L. I. (1972): Effects of intracerebral 5-hydroxytryptamine injection on thermoregulation in rat. *Physiol. Behav.,* 9:133–140.
15. Des Prez, R., Helman, R., and Oats, J. A. (1966): Inhibition of endotoxin fever with reserpine. *Proc. Soc. Exp. Biol. Med.,* 122:746–749.
16. Eisenman, J. S. (1969): Pyrogen-induced changes in the thermosensitivity of septal and preoptic neurons. *Am. J. Physiol.,* 216:330–334.
17. Feldberg, W., and Myers, R. D. (1964): Effect on temperature of amines injected into the cerebral ventricles: A new concept of temperature regulation. *J. Physiol. (Lond.),* 173:226–237.
18. Feldberg, W., and Myers, R. D. (1965): Changes in temperature produced by microinjection of amines in the anterior hypothalamus of cats. *J. Physiol. (Lond.),* 177:239–250.
19. Feldberg, W., and Vogt, M. (1948): Acetylcholine synthesis in different regions of the central nervous system. *J. Physiol. (Lond.),* 107:372–381.
20. Feldberg, W., Hellon, R. F., and Lotti, V. J. (1967): Temperature effects produced in dogs and monkeys by injections of monoamines and related substances into the third ventricle. *J. Physiol. (Lond.),* 191:501–515.
21. Feldberg, W., Hellon, R. F., and Myers, R. D. (1966): Effect on temperature of monoamines injected into the cerebral ventricle of anaesthetized dog. *J. Physiol. (Lond.),* 186:416–423.
22. Ford, D. M., Hellon, R. F., and Luff, M. N. (1973): Cholinergic pathways in the brain stem subserving thermoregulatory mechanisms in the cat. *J. Physiol. (Lond.),* 231:34–35.
23. Hall, G. H., Jr., and Atkins, L. (1959): Studies on tuberculin fever. I. The mechanism of fever in tuberculin hypersensitivity. *J. Exp. Med.,* 119:339–359.
24. Hall, G. H., and Myers, R. D. (1972): Temperature changes produced by nicotine injected into the hypothalamus of conscious monkey. *Brain Res.,* 37:241–251.
25. Holmes, S. W. (1970): The spontaneous release of prostaglandins into the cerebral ventricles of the dog and the effect of external factors on this release. *Br. J. Pharmacol.,* 38:653–658.
26. Hori, T., and Nakayama, T. (1973): Effects of biogenic amines on central thermoresponsive neurons in the rabbit. *J. Physiol. (Lond.),* 232:71–86.
27. Johnson, K. G. (1975): Thermoregulatory changes induced by cholinomimetic substances introduced into the cerebral ventricles of sheep. *Br. J. Pharmacol.,* 53:489–497.

28. Johnson, K. G., and Smith, C. A. (1974): The nature of the thermoregulatory sensitivity to cholinomimetic drugs in the cerebral ventricles of sheep. *J. Physiol. (Lond.)*, 236:31–32.
29. Kandasamy, B., Girault, J. M., and Jacob, J. (1974): Central effects of a purified bacterial pyrogen, prostaglandin E_1 and biogenic amines on the temperature in the awake rabbit. In: *Temperature Regulation and Drug Action*, edited by P. Lomax, E. Schönbaum, and J. Jacob, pp. 124–132. Karger, Basel.
30. Knox, G. V., Campbell, C., and Lomax, P. (1973): The effects of acetylcholine and nicotine on unit activity in the hypothalamic thermoregulatory centres of the rat. *Brain Res.*, 51:215–223.
31. Kroneberg, G., and Kurbjuweit, H. G. (1959): Die Beeinflussung von experimentellem Fieber durch Reserpin und sympatholytica auf Kaninchen. *Arzneim. Forsch.*, 2:536–538.
32. Lomax, P., Foster, R. S., and Kirkpatrick, W. E. (1969): Cholinergic and adrenergic interactions in the thermoregulatory centres. *Brain Res.*, 15:431–438.
33. Masek, K., Raskova, H., and Rotta, J. (1968): The mechanism of the pyrogenic effect of streptococcus cell wall mucopeptide. *J. Physiol. (Lond.)*, 198:345–353.
34. McLennan, H. (1963): *Synaptic Transmission*, p. 23. Saunders, Philadelphia.
35. Myers, R. D. (1971): Hypothalamic mechanism of pyrogen action in cat and monkeys. In: *Pyrogens and Fever*, edited by G. E. W. Wolstenholme and J. Birch, pp. 131–153. Churchill and Livingstone, London.
36. Myers, R. D. (1973): The role of hypothalamic serotonin in thermoregulation. In: *Serotonin and Behaviour*, edited by J. Barchas and E. Usdin, pp. 293–302. Academic Press, New York.
37. Myers, R. D., and Beleslin, D. B. (1971): Changes in serotonin release in hypothalamus during cooling and warming of monkeys. *Am. J. Physiol.*, 220:1846–1854.
38. Myers, R. D., and Chinn, C. (1973): Evoked release of hypothalamic norepinephrine during thermoregulation in the unanaesthetized cats. *Am. J. Physiol.*, 224:230–236.
39. Myers, R. D., and Waller, M. B. (1973): Differential release of acetylcholine from the hypothalamus and mesencephalon of monkeys during thermoregulation. *J. Physiol. (Lond.)*, 230:273–294.
40. Myers, R. D., and Yaksh, T. L. (1968): Feeding and temperature responses in the unrestrained rat after injections of cholinergic and aminergic substances into the cerebral ventricles. *Physiol. Behav.*, 3:917–928.
41. Myers, R. D., and Yaksh, T. L. (1969): Control of body temperature in the unanaesthetized monkeys by cholinergic and aminergic systems in the hypothalamus. *J. Physiol. (Lond.)*, 202:483–500.
42. Myers, R. D., Rudy, T. A., and Yaksh, T. L. (1971). Fever in the monkey produced by the direct action of pyrogen on the hypothalamus. *Experientia*, 27:160–161.
43. Nutik, S. L. (1971): Posterior hypothalamic neurons responsive to preoptic region thermal stimulation. *J. Neurophysiol.*, 36:238–249.
44. Rosendorff, C., and Mooney, J. J. (1971): Central nervouś system sites of action of a purified leucocyte pyrogen. *Am. J. Physiol.*, 220:597–603.
45. Rudy, T. A., and Wolf, H. H. (1971): The effects of intrahypothalamically injected sympathomimetic amines on temperature regulation in the cat. *J. Pharmacol. Exp. Ther.*, 179:218–235.
46. Rudy, T. A., and Wolf, H. H. (1972): Effects of intracerebral injections of carbamylcholine and acetylcholine in temperature regulation in the cat. *Brain Res.*, 38:117–130.
47. Takagi, K., and Karuma, J. (1966): Effect of bacterial lipopolysaccharide on the content of serotonin and norepinephrine in rabbit brain. *Jap. J. Pharmacol.*, 18:478–479.
48. Tangri, K. K., Bhargava, A. K., and Bhargava, K. P. (1974): Interrelation between monoaminergic and cholinergic mechanisms in the hypothalamic thermoregulatory centre of rabbits. *Neuropharmacology*, 13:333–346.
49. Tangri, K. K., Bhargava, A. K., and Bhargava, K. P. (1975): Significance of central cholinergic mechanism in pyrexia induced by bacterial pyrogen in rabbits. In: *Temperature Regulation and Drug Action*, edited by P. Lomax, E. Schönbaum, and J. Jacob, pp. 65–74. Karger, Basel.
50. Teddy, P. J. (1971): Discussion contribution. In: *Pyrogens and Fever*, edited by G. E. W. Wolstenholme and J. Birch, pp. 124–127. Churchill and Livingstone, Edinburgh.

51. Udenfriend, S., and Creveling, C. R. (1959): Location of dopamine beta-oxidase in brain. *J. Neurochem.,* 4:350–352.
52. Veale, W. L., and Cooper, K. E. (1974): Comparison of sites of action of prostaglandin E₁ and leucocyte pyrogen in brain. In: *Temperature Regulation and Drug Action,* edited by P. Lomax, E. Schönbaum, and J. Jacob, pp. 218–226. Karger, Basel.
53. Villablanca, J., and Myers, R. D. (1965): Fever produced by microinjection of typhoid vaccine into hypothalamus of cats. *Am. J. Physiol.,* 208:703–707.
54. Wit, A., and Wang, S. C. (1968): Temperature-sensitive neurons in preoptic anterior hypothalamic region: Actions of pyrogen and acetylsalicylate. *Am. J. Physiol.,* 215:1160–1169.

Brain Dysfunction in Infantile Febrile Convulsions, edited by M. A. B. Brazier and F. Coceani. Raven Press, New York © 1976.

Pathogenesis of Fever

K. E. Cooper, W. L. Veale, and Q. J. Pittman

Division of Medical Physiology, University of Calgary, Calgary, Canada

Some of the earliest observations on the nature of fever were made in 1797 by James Currie (9), who was a surgeon, physician, and epidemiologist. He was the first to make quantitative observations using thermometry, and he drew attention to the need to record patients' temperatures in order to monitor the progress of their febrile illnesses. He was also one of the earliest to draw attention to the need to "observe and delineate" rather than to "explain and to systematize" in the study of this branch of science. With the exception of the detailed study of the types of fever in different diseases presented by Wunderlich (24) and the measurements which demonstrated an apparent elevation of body temperature set point in fever by Liebermeister (15), both in the mid-1800s, the study of fever did not progress very far until the discovery by Beeson and Bennett (2,3) that a pyrogenic material could be extracted from the leucocytes of rabbits, even though those cells had not been in contact with any bacterial product. Later Grant and Whalen (13) showed that in the rabbit the time of onset of fever was significantly greater if bacterial pyrogen was injected intravenously than if an incubate of bacterial pyrogen and rabbit blood was injected. Further, the work of Gerbrandy et al. (12) in man demonstrated the production of a substance on incubating whole blood or leucocytes with bacterial products, which caused a fever with a very much shorter latency than was obtainable by injecting bacterial pyrogen intravenously into the human recipient. The evidence then developed along these lines that bacterial products, now known to be lipopolysaccharides with a molecular weight of approximately 10^6, interact with leucocytes, causing them to secrete a new substance called leucocyte pyrogen or endogenous pyrogen. This material was purified in the laboratory of the late Dr. Barry Wood by Murphy et al. (18) and was shown to be a polypeptide of molecular weight in the order of 10^4. There is other evidence that interaction between viruses and monocytes results in the release of an endogenous pyrogen also, as happens with the monocytes during some allergic responses (1). Further evidence from the laboratory of Atkins and from the work of Gander and Goodale (11) demonstrates the probability of the release of endogenous pyrogen from cells of the reticuloendothelial system. It thus appears that the initial reaction during fever is the release of one or a family of polypeptides having surprisingly high biological activity and capable of producing fever.

Cooper et al. (7) demonstrated that injection of endogenous pyrogen into patients with spinal cord transections above the outflow of the sympathetic nervous system did not cause fever. Interestingly, the skin blood vessels did not constrict, and therefore the drive for skin vasoconstriction normally seen in fever appears to be derived from a region above the cervical level of the spinal cord. Shivering was not seen below the level of the lesion, but it did occur in the few muscles innervated from above the level of the lesion; and, interestingly enough, the patients did not suffer the usual headache which follows a pyrogen injection.

Cooper et al. (5) further investigated the site of action of leucocyte pyrogens, prepared in a very crude form within the rabbit brain. They found that there was a site in the anterior hypothalamus/preoptic region (AH/POA) close to the wall of the third ventricle at which microinjection of pyrogen caused fever after a minimal latency. They could find no evidence of fever due to microinjecting leucocyte pyrogen at loci outside the AH/POA. This study provided results in agreement with those of Repin and Kratskin (19) on the rabbit and of Jackson (14) on the cat. However, further studies were made on a more purified leucocyte pyrogen by Rosendorff and Mooney (20), and they found an additional site from which leucocyte pyrogen microinjections appeared to produce a slow-onset type of fever, this site being in the midbrain. These observations should be repeated with the more highly purified endogenous pyrogen. We then have the picture built up of bacterial lipopolysaccharides interacting with leucocytes and other cells of the reticuloendothelial system, which produce an endogenous pyrogen that would get into and act in the AH/POA, principally to induce fever.

Evidence adduced by the studies (6) of vasomotor responses to body warming suggested that in man, at least, the central action of leucocyte pyrogen was such that the thermoregulatory mechanism appeared to work at a new high level but with its usual sensitivity, rather than by altering the sensitivity of the central warm receptors.

The thesis that naturally occurring fever is mediated in part through release of an endogenous type of pyrogen has been based on artificial experimental situations and on the ability to extract such pyrogen from leucocytes and other tissues. We attempted to demonstrate the presence of leucocyte pyrogen in the circulation during the naturally occurring disease in man. Assays using intravenous injections of patient's plasma into rabbits were too insensitive. We were, however, able, by microinjecting minute amounts of plasma into the AH/POA, to detect a circulating pyrogen in the plasma of a number of patients during the rapidly rising phase of fever. The blood containing this fever-producing substance did not appear to have any bacterial endotoxin in it, as judged by the limulus assay (16), which in our hands is sensitive enough to detect a few picograms of endotoxin. The fever-producing material in these patients was also heat-labile and so by these crude tests appears to be of the endogenous type. Further work is continuing in an attempt to find and characterize more definitively fever-producing substances in the blood of patients suffering natural febrile illnesses.

The next question that arose in our studies was whether the endogenous pyrogen reached the AH/POA via the bloodstream, or whether it was secreted into the cerebrospinal fluid (CSF) and found its way to the locus of action via the CSF. We performed a series of experiments in which the cerebral ventricular system was filled with a sterile, pyrogen-free mineral oil (4). This of itself did not produce any noticeable effect on body temperature or behaviour of the conscious recipient rabbits. Nevertheless, when rabbits were given a dose of pyrogen intravenously that had previously caused them to have a moderate fever lasting approximately 1 hr, they suffered significantly higher fevers, which in some instances lasted up to 48 hr. Furthermore, if the animals were given a priming dose of leucocyte pyrogen followed by a steady infusion of leucocyte pyrogen so as to maintain a steady high level of body temperature, injection of oil into the ventricular system during such a maintained fever led to another abrupt rise in body temperature which lasted a very long time. The evidence therefore was that the filling of the ventricular system with mineral oil, which prevented the normal circulation of CSF from the lateral ventricles to the fourth ventricle, did not prevent fever due to intravenous pyrogen, but rather prolonged it. This suggests that leucocyte pyrogen reaches the active site within the brain via the bloodstream, and that either leucocyte pyrogen or some other substance it causes to be released within the brain is excreted into the ventricular system. It also suggests that the substance excreted is not a normal product of thermoregulation since the oil injections were without effect on the animal's normal temperature.

At about this time the work of Feldberg, Milton, and Wendlandt (10,17) demonstrated that the injection of minute quantities of prostaglandins of the E series (PGEs) into the ventricular system or tissue of the AH/POA caused fever. Furthermore, Vane (21) demonstrated that the well-known antipyretic substances inhibit the formation of PGs. There is now growing evidence to suggest that the fever process, at least in part, may be mediated by the release of a PGE, possibly PGE_2, into the tissue of the brain, and that nerve cells in the region of the AH/POA are sensitive to this released material, which excites neurons involved in driving the processes of heat production and heat conservation. Additional evidence for this hypothesis derives from the studies of Feldberg and Milton (10) and their colleagues, who demonstrated the presence of a PGE in CSF withdrawn from the third ventricle. The PG concentration increased when the animal was made febrile and decreased again when the fever was reduced by administration of an antipyretic. These observations would be compatible with the suggestion made from our oil experiments: i.e., that some substance connected with fever would be released into the ventricular system. If PGs are released within the substance of the AH/POA, it should be possible to show that they can diffuse through the ependyma into the ventricular system. We have perfused the region of the AH/POA using the push-pull cannula technique (22) with tritiated PGE_1, and simultaneously perfused the ventricular system from a lateral ventricle to the cisterna magna in the rabbit (23). It was possible at the start of the fever to measure the injected radioactive label present in the perfusate from the ventricular system, and this label was shown by thin-layer chromatography to be attached to the PG that had been injected. Thus it was shown that if PG is placed into the AH/POA tissue a proportion of it can diffuse directly into the ventricular system. The evidence to date supports the view that the "prostaglandin" mechanism of fever represents a pathological response superimposed on, but distinct from, normal thermoregulation.

In a further series of experiments we found some evidence suggesting that there may be a component of fever mediated elsewhere in the brain than in the AH/POA, and that this part of the fever process may be independent of the release of a PG. Rabbits were anaesthetized and placed in stereotaxic holders. Heat coagulation electrodes were lowered into the AH/POA or the posterior hypothalamus, as desired, and lesions were made. The animals were subsequently allowed to recover; because of the relatively enormous size of the lesions, a number of animals did not survive the procedure. Those which did survive were subsequently tested for their ability to maintain their temperatures during exposure in a hot or a cold room. Animals were selected in which large AH/POA lesions had been made and which subsequently were unable to regulate their temperatures during hot or cold water exposure. An example of such a lesion is shown in Fig. 1; the extent of this lesion is shown in two sections histologically evaluated after the experiment. These animals had previously been shown to respond with fever to intravenous administration of pyrogen or to injection of PGs either into a lateral cerebral ventricle or the substance of the AH/POA. In this group of animals intravenous leucocyte pyrogen produced a fever following the large lesions made in the AH/POA, although the fever was slower in onset and took longer to reach a maximum than it did in the animals before the lesions were made. The mean maximal fever heights for a representative animal (rabbit No. 45) and for this group of animals before and after the lesions are shown in Figs. 2 and 3. It can be seen that there is only a small reduction in mean fever height in response to intravenous pyrogen following AH/POA lesions sufficiently large to prevent the animal from regulating its body temperature in an adverse climatic condition. However, neither administration of PGs into a lateral cerebral ventricle or into the centre of the lesion area produced any fever at all. Lesions made in the posterior hypothalamus completely abolished the fever due to both intravenous pyrogen (Figs. 4 and 5) and intraventricular PG or that administered

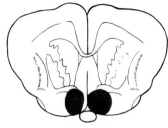

FRONTAL A

FIG. 1. Sections of the brain of rabbit No. 45 at the preoptic (frontal A) and anterior hypothalamic (frontal B) levels. Dark patches show the extent of the heat-coagulation lesion.

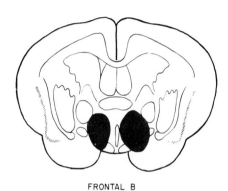

FRONTAL B

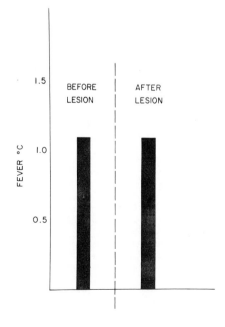

FIG. 2. Maximum fever height following intravenous injection of leucocyte pyrogen in rabbit No. 45, before and after AH/POA lesioning.

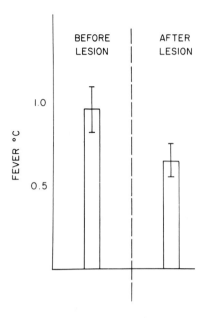

FEVER °C

1.0

0.5

BEFORE
LESION

AFTER
LESION

FIG. 3. Means of maximum fever heights in response to standard intravenous doses of leucocyte pyrogen in a group of rabbits, before and after AH/POA lesioning. Short vertical bars represent the SEM.

into the AH/POA. Thus it may be that there is another region of the brain sensitive to the action of leucocyte pyrogen where fever is induced without PG involvement.

Pyrogen acting on this region would produce a fever of slower onset and of a character different from that produced by the action of pyrogens in releasing PG in the AH/POA. Lesions of the posterior hypothalamus could destroy an efferent final common pathway for these fevers. Another series of experiments are underway to determine if the slow-onset fever due to intravenous leucocyte pyrogen following large AH/POA lesions is sensitive to the antipyretics known to be PG synthetase inhibitors.

It has been known since the work of Cooper et al. (5) in 1967 that rabbits given intraventricular reserpine in quantities sufficient to deplete the AH/POA of its monoamine content are still capable of developing fever

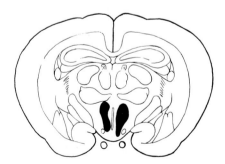

FIG. 4. Site of lesion (*black patch*) in the posterior hypothalamus in a representative experiment (rabbit No. 2).

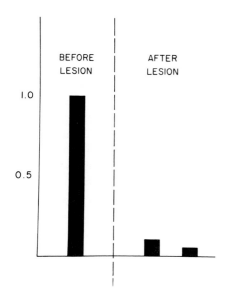

FIG. 5. Maximum fever heights due to standard doses of leucocyte pyrogen injected intravenously in rabbit No. 2, before and after posterior hypothalamic lesioning.

following intravenous leucocyte pyrogen. Again, the fever produced is of slow and gradually climbing onset, although this may be because the animals have maximally vasodilated skins and it is impossible for them to use modifications of vasomotor tone to prevent heat loss. It is known that administration of PGs into the ventricular system produces fever despite depletion of the hypothalamic monoamines by reserpine (8). We measured the febrile responses to both intravenous leucocyte pyrogen and intraventricular PGE_1 with concomitant or previous intraventricular administration of atropine. Atropine administered intraventricularly to rabbits in a cool environment caused a fall in body temperature, partly brought about by an increase of peripheral blood flow and partly by a reduction in heat production. The effect is fairly transient, lasting approximately 30 min before the body temperature is restored towards its normal level. Atropine given to the lateral cerebral ventricle 15 min before the administration of either leucocyte pyrogen or PGE_1 into the ventricular system causes a fall in body temperature on which the subsequent febrile response begins to be superimposed. The result is a net reduction in the fever response. If, however, atropine administration into the lateral cerebral ventricle is delayed until the febrile response has just begun, the temperature immediately returns to the baseline level and no fever subsequently develops. This suggests either that the fever is mediated through a cholinergic pathway which drives the elements of heat production and conservation, or that atropine inhibits the activity of a cholinergic pathway which acts separately from and similar to the fever-stimulated pathway but with more vigour. Atropine microinjected into the AH/POA did not affect the fever due to intravenous pyrogen or intraventricular PGE_1. This suggests that the muscarinic cholinergic synapses involved in suppression of fever by intraventricular atropine are outside the AH/POA.

The identification of PGs as mediators of the febrile process and the discovery of the mechanism of aspirin antipyresis have contributed much to our understanding of the pathogenesis of fever. Several questions remain unanswered. What is the specific brain tissue (neurons, glia, leucocytes) that elaborates the PG involved in fever? Does fever from other agents develop along the same lines as endotoxin fever? It would also be helpful to have more reliable and sensitive methods for detecting circulatory endogenous pyrogen and endotoxin. Finally, it will be necessary to identify by electrophysiological techniques the neural afferent and efferent connections involved in both fever and normal thermoregulation.

ACKNOWLEDGMENTS

This work was supported by the Medical Research Council of Canada. Prostaglandins were provided by Dr. J. Pike of the Upjohn Company, Kalamazoo, Michigan. The authors are indebted to T. Malkinson for his technical assistance.

REFERENCES

1. Atkins, E., Bodel, P., and Francis, L. (1967): Release of an endogenous pyrogen in vitro from rabbit mononuclear cells. *J. Exp. Med.,* 126:357–384.
2. Beeson, P. B. (1948): Temperature-elevating effect of a substance obtained from polymorphonuclear leukocytes. *J. Clin. Invest.,* 27:524.
3. Bennett, I. L., and Beeson, P. B. (1953): Studies on the pathogenesis of fever. I. The effect of injection of extracts and suspensions of uninfected rabbit tissues upon the body temperatures of normal rabbits. *J. Exp. Med.,* 98:477–492.
4. Cooper, K. E., and Veale, W. L. (1972): The effect of an inert oil in the cerebral ventricular system upon fever produced by intravenous pyrogen. *Can. J. Physiol. Pharmacol.,* 50: 1066–1071.
5. Cooper, K. E., Cranston, W. I., and Honour, A. J. (1967): Observations on the site and mode of action of pyrogens in the rabbit brain. *J. Physiol. (Lond.),* 191:325–337.
6. Cooper, K. E., Cranston, W. I., and Snell, E. S. (1964): Temperature regulation during fever in man. *Clin. Sci.,* 27:345–354.
7. Cooper, K. E., Johnson, R. H., and Spalding, J. M. K. (1964): Thermoregulatory reactions following intravenous pyrogen in a subject with couple transection of the cervical cord. *J. Physiol. (Lond.),* 171:55–56P.
8. Cooper, K. E., Preston, E., and Veale, W. L. (1976): Effects of atropine, injected into a lateral cerebral ventricle of the rabbit, on fevers due to intravenous leucocyte pyrogen and hypothalamic and intraventricular injections of prostaglandin E_1. *J. Physiol. (Lond.),* 254:729–741.
9. Currie, J. (1797): *The Effects of Water, Cold and Warm, as a Remedy in Fever.* Medical Reports, J. M'Creery, Liverpool.
10. Feldberg, W., and Milton, A. S. (1973): Prostaglandin fever. In: *The Pharmacology of Thermoregulation,* edited by P. Lomax and E. Schönbaum, pp. 302–310. Karger, Basel.
11. Gander, W., and Goodale, F. (1973): Studies on the endogenous pyrogen released in response to poly 1: poly C^1. In: *The Pharmacology of Thermoregulation,* edited by P. Lomax and E. Schönbaum, pp. 255–263. Karger, Basel.

12. Gerbrandy, J., Cranston, W. I., and Snell, E. S. (1954): The initial process in the action of bacterial pyrogens in man. *Clin. Sci.,* 13:453–459.
13. Grant, R., and Whalen, W. J. (1953): Latency of pyrogen fever: Appearance of a fast-acting pyrogen in the blood of febrile animals and in plasma incubated with bacterial pyrogen. *Am. J. Physiol.,* 173:47–54.
14. Jackson, D. L. (1967): A hypothalamic region responsive to localized injection of pyrogens. *J. Neurophysiol.,* 30:586–602.
15. Liebermeister, C. (1875): *Handbuch der Pathologie und Therapie des Fiebers.* Vogelwelt, Leipzig.
16. Mears, G. J., Cooper, K. E., and Veale, W. L. (1976): The *in vitro* limulus assay for detection and measurement of bacterial pyrogens. In: *Biogenic Amines, Drugs and Thermoregulation,* edited by P. Lomax, E. Schönbaum, and K. Cooper. Karger, Basel (*in press*).
17. Milton, A. S., and Wendlandt, S. (1971): Effects on body temperature of prostaglandins of the A, E and F series on injection into the third ventricle of unanaesthetized cats and rabbits. *J. Physiol. (Lond.),* 218:325–336.
18. Murphy, P. A., Chesney, J. P., and Wood, W. B., Jr. (1974): Further purification of rabbit leucocyte pyrogen. *J. Lab. Clin. Med.,* 85:310–322.
19. Repin, I. S., and Kratskin, I. L. (1967): An analysis of hypothalamic mechanisms of fever. *Fiziol. Zh., SSSR,* 53:1206–1211.
20. Rosendorff, C., and Mooney, J. J. (1971): Central nervous system sites of action of a purified leucocyte pyrogen. *Am. J. Physiol.,* 220:597–603.
21. Vane, J. R. (1971): Inhibition of prostaglandin synthesis as a mechanism of action for aspirin-like drugs. *Nature [New Biol.],* 231:232–235.
22. Veale, W. L. (1972): A stereotaxic method for the push-pull perfusion of discrete regions of brain tissues of the unanesthetized rabbit. *Brain Res.,* 42:479–481.
23. Veale, W. L., and Cooper, K. E. (1974): Prostaglandin in cerebrospinal fluid following perfusion of hypothalamic tissue. *J. Appl. Physiol.,* 37:942–945.
24. Wunderlich (1871): *On the Temperature in Diseases. A Manual of Medical Thermometry.* New Sydenham Society, London.

Brain Dysfunction in Infantile Febrile Convulsions, edited by M. A. B. Brazier and F. Coceani. Raven Press, New York © 1976.

Exogenous and Endogenous Pyrogens

C. A. Dinarello and S. M. Wolff

Laboratory of Clinical Investigation, National Institute of Allergy and Infectious Diseases, National Institutes of Health, Bethesda, Maryland 20014

Pyrogens are substances of diverse chemical structure having in common the ability to produce fever. Most of the pyrogens which have been available for study are exogenous; i.e., they occur outside the subject in which they induce fever. Conversely, endogenous pyrogens are produced by the host. Most investigators now accept the concept that exogenous pyrogens, regardless of their source or chemical nature, stimulate appropriate cells within the host to synthesize and release endogenous pyrogen. Endogenous pyrogen then acts on the temperature-regulating centers in the hypothalamus to produce fever. Thus endogenous pyrogen is regarded as the mediator substance of all fevers, regardless of source.

EXOGENOUS AND ENDOGENOUS PYROGENS

The sequence by which exogenous pyrogens are thought to elicit the release of endogenous pyrogen and produce fever is illustrated in Fig. 1. Following activation of phagocytic leukocytes, there is a period of m-RNA and protein synthesis before the endogenous pyrogen is released. Endogenous pyrogen enters the circulation and exerts an effect on the hypothalamus, which results in fever. Neurotransmitters (e.g., monoamines), cyclic nucleotides, and particularly the prostaglandins (Cooper et al., *this volume*) are possibly involved in the central action of pyrogen. Several investigators have localized the responsive sites to the anterior hypothalamus-preoptic region (AH/POA) by using microinjections of purified endogenous pyrogens (27,50). This region also contains clusters of temperature-sensitive neurons (31,35).

Until recently human endogenous pyrogen was thought to be a single protein with a molecular weight of 12,000–15,000 (21); lipid or carbohydrate moieties are not required for pyrogenicity. A second human endogenous pyrogen was recently described. This material, also a protein, has a molecular weight of 38,000 and is produced by human blood monocytes (29).

Exogenous Pyrogens: Endotoxin and Etiocholanolone

Exogenous pyrogens differ markedly with regard to biologic and chemical properties, and consequently they could act on the hypothalamus only

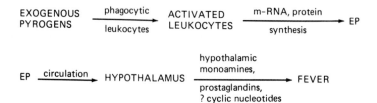

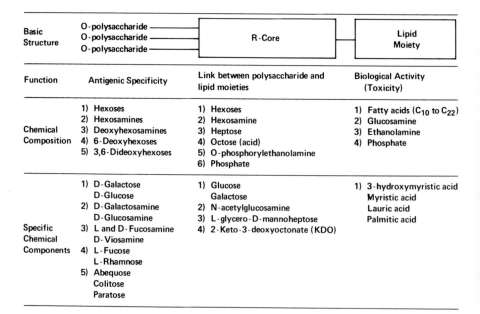

FIG. 1. Hypothesis for the pathogenesis of fever. EP, endogenous pyrogen.

through distinct receptor sites. This is an unlikely occurrence. In fact, because of their size most exogenous pyrogens do not gain access to the hypothalamus from the systemic circulation (26).

If we consider the most potent exogenous pyrogen, endotoxin, which is a lipopolysaccharide derived from gram-negative bacteria, we can appreciate the great complexity of the molecule with a molecular weight in excess of 1 million (Fig. 2). The lipid moiety is essential for many toxic properties and is composed of fatty acids bound to glucosamine units for structural integrity. This lipid is either covalently or ionically bound to a peptidoglycan in the bacterial cell wall.

Most investigators believe that the pyrogenic property of endotoxin depends on the lipid moiety (47). The second part of the endotoxin molecule

Basic Structure	O-polysaccharide ——— O-polysaccharide ——— O-polysaccharide ———	R-Core		Lipid Moiety
Function	Antigenic Specificity	Link between polysaccharide and lipid moieties		Biological Activity (Toxicity)
Chemical Composition	1) Hexoses 2) Hexosamines 3) Deoxyhexosamines 4) 6-Deoxyhexoses 5) 3,6-Dideoxyhexoses	1) Hexoses 2) Hexosamine 3) Heptose 4) Octose (acid) 5) O-phosphorylethanolamine 6) Phosphate		1) Fatty acids (C_{10} to C_{22}) 2) Glucosamine 3) Ethanolamine 4) Phosphate

Specific Chemical Components	1) D-Galactose
	   D-Glucose
	2) D-Galactosamine
	   D-Glucosamine
	3) L and D-Fucosamine
	   D-Viosamine
	4) L-Fucose
	   L-Rhamnose
	5) Abequose
	   Colitose
	   Paratose
		1) Glucose
		   Galactose
		2) N-acetylglucosamine
		3) L-glycero-D-mannoheptose
		4) 2-Keto-3-deoxyoctonate (KDO)
				1) 3-hydroxymyristic acid
				   Myristic acid
				   Lauric acid
				   Palmitic acid

FIG. 2. Schematic representation of lipopolysaccharide (endotoxin). (From Elin and Wolff, ref. 32.)

TABLE 1. *Febrile responses to endotoxin in different species*

Endotoxin	Dose (μg/kg)	Seven-hour fever index (cm²)	Maximum rise in temperature (°C)
S. abortus equi			
Rabbit (4)[a]	0.005	22.5	1.3
Man (7)	0.002	49.8	1.9
S. typhosa			
Rabbit (4)	0.05	27.8	1.3
Man (6)	0.005	32.7	1.3
E. coli			
Rabbit (6)	0.005	20.3	1.4
Monkey (5)	1.250	15.4	0.8

Data are from Wolff (52).
[a] Numbers of animals tested are given in parentheses.

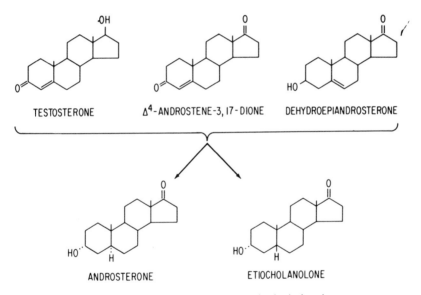

FIG. 3. Breakdown of androgens into androsterone and etiocholanolone.

is called the R-core and is composed of amino sugars, hexoses, and the oc-
tose KDO (2-keto-3-deoxyoctonate). The antigenic property of endotoxin lies in the third part of the molecule, the O-polysaccharide, which is
attached to the R-core and provides O-specificity for all gram-negative
bacteria (32).

When injected into the rabbit or man, endotoxin produces fever in micro-
gram quantities (52,54). For example, man is more sensitive than the rabbit
(Table 1) to the pyrogenic properties of endotoxin, whereas the monkey
develops little fever even when exposed to enormous doses of endotoxin
(51).

TABLE 2. *Exogenous pyrogens*

Exogenous pyrogen	Chemical nature	Probable mechanism of endogenous pyrogen induction	Reference
Viruses Myxoviruses, Coxsackie, New Castle disease	Coat protein; nucleic acids	Particulate nature; cell infection	5,36,40
Bacteria (killed) Gram-positive (staph., pneumo.)	Mucopeptide	Phagocytosis; heat- stable antigens	3,6,11
Gram-negative (typhoid vaccine)	Peptidoglycan; lipopolysaccharide	Phagocytosis + toxicity	7
Bacterial products Gram-positive (staph. products)	Large proteins	Cell-mediated immunity (I)	2,4,15,16
Gram-negative (endotoxin)	Lipopolysaccharide (? lipid A only)	Toxicity (? antigenicity)	8,13,49
Fungi Yeast cells (killed and live) cell products	Complex carbohydrates	Phagocytosis	24
	Proteins; polysaccharide	Cell-mediated I	33
Antigens Human serum albumin	Protein	Humoral-mediated I	48
Bovine serum globulin	Protein	Cell-mediated I (? lymphokines)	9
Penicillin	β-Lactam ring	Humoral-mediated I	25
Soluble Ag-Ab complexes	Protein	Immune clearance (complement consumption)	42,48
Tuberculin (OT, PPD)	Protein	Cell-mediated I (? cytophilic antibody)	1,4,34

Steroids			
Etiocholanolone	C_{19} steroid	Unknown	19, 53
5β-Androstane-3α-01-17-one	C_{19} steroid	Unknown	22
Pharmacologic agents			
Poly I:Poly C	Polynucleotides	Unknown	45
Bleomycin	Polypeptide	? DNA transferase inhibition	30
Colchicine, vinblastine	Plant alkaloids	Prevention of microtubule assembly	(P. Bodel, *personal communication*)

Another extensively studied exogenous pyrogen is etiocholanolone, which is a normal product of the metabolism of androgenic hormones. There are other pyrogenic steroids, e.g., pregnanediol, a metabolite of progesterone. Pyrogenic steroids have in common the 5-β hydrogen configuration; steroids of the 5-α hydrogen type are nonpyrogenic (38,53). In addition, pyrogenic steroids require a 3-α hydroxyl group, but this can be oxidized to a ketone with little loss in activity. Figure 3 demonstrates the structural requirements for pyrogen action. Testosterone, androstenedione, and dehydroepiandrosterone are metabolized to androsterone, a 5-α hydrogen compound which is nonpyrogenic, and an optical isomer of etiocholanolone, which is a 5-β hydrogen compound and a pyrogen. Etiocholanolone injected intramuscularly into normal human volunteers produces fever after a latent period of 6–8 hr, whereas it is inactive in rabbits and some other animals (22,37,39).

Table 2 provides a list of exogenous pyrogens that have been studied in man or animals. Although the mode of action of these agents is still largely unknown, their ability to induce the release of endogenous pyrogen has been repeatedly demonstrated both *in vivo* and *in vitro*. In what is now a classic experiment, Atkins and Wood (7) injected rabbits with endotoxin and bled the animals at different times during the ensuing fever. The plasma from febrile rabbits was then infused into normal or endotoxin-resistant animals and produced a monophasic fever after a 12- to 15-min delay. This finding clearly demonstrated a circulating endogenous pyrogen, and the experimental paradigm is currently used to establish the presence of circulating endogenous pyrogen following injection of viruses, bacteria, yeasts, bacterial products, antigen-antibody complexes, tuberculin, etc. (Table 2).

Production of Endogenous Pyrogen In Vitro

Endogenous pyrogen can also be formed *in vitro* when an exogenous pyrogen is incubated with host leukocytes. The endogenous pyrogen appears in the supernatant fluid after an incubation period of 6–8 hr and can be assayed in the rabbit (17,49). There is little host specificity for the endogenous pyrogens of cats, dogs, and rabbits (23); and human endogenous pyrogen causes fever in rabbits (17), mice (20), and the rhesus monkey (46). Although the formation of endogenous pyrogen was first demonstrated in the neutrophils of a rabbit peritoneal exudate (10), other cell types are known to produce pyrogen under the appropriate challenge. They are the monocyte (18), splenic macrophage (8), lung alveolar macrophage (8), eosinophil (41), and Kupffer cell of the liver (28). In contrast, the lymphocyte, either from peripheral blood or lymph nodes, does not release endogenous pyrogen in response to all known stimulating exogenous agents (14,49).

One of the most interesting aspects of the interaction between exogenous pyrogens and host cells is that endogenous pyrogen does not originate from preformed stores. Human and rabbit endogenous pyrogen production was shown to be dependent on m-RNA and protein synthesis since inhibition of m-RNA translation by actinomycin D or inhibition of protein synthesis by puromycin or cycloheximide prevents the production and release of endogenous pyrogen (12,44). Thus release of endogenous pyrogen requires *ex novo* synthesis of protein. This has obvious implications, since the delay between injection of exogenous pyrogens and the onset of fever is often great and exceeds the time required by the injected material to reach the hypothalamus via the circulation. This then supports the concept that exogenous pyrogens injected intravenously do not act directly on the hypothalamus.

Chemical Nature of Human Endogenous Pyrogen

As mentioned earlier, both neutrophils and monocytes from man release endogenous pyrogen *in vitro*. Recently, however, it was observed that monocytes produce more endogenous pyrogen than an equal number of neutrophils (13,29). Figure 4 illustrates the fever response to human endogenous pyrogen released from either neutrophils or monocytes incubated with heat-killed staphylococci. The monocyte releases 20 times more pyrogen on a cell-to-cell basis than does the neutrophil.

To characterize the human leukocytic pyrogen, whole blood from normal donors was centrifuged and the buffy coat incubated overnight with heat-killed staphylococci. Buffy coats were comprised of approximately 70% neutrophils and 5% monocytes. When the supernatant fluid containing human endogenous pyrogen was chromatographed over Sephadex G-50, a single peak of pyrogenic activity was found, corresponding to a molecular weight of 15,000. This confirmed previous studies using both human and rabbit leukocytes (21,43). However, when the mononuclear layer from Ficoll-Hypaque gradients was used, which increased the numbers of monocytes from 5% to 25%, the endogenous pyrogen showed two peaks of biologic activity (Fig. 5). These peaks corresponded to molecular weights of 38,000 and 15,000. Neither pyrogen is associated with a protein peak. We named the large- and the small-molecular-weight pyrogens, respectively, monocyte and neutrophil pyrogens.

We subjected these two molecules to isoelectric focusing on thin-layer Sephadex G-75 superfine and found that the smaller-molecular-weight pyrogen has a pI of 6.8–6.9 (Fig. 6). In contrast, the larger-molecular-weight pyrogen has a pI of 5.1.

Other chemical differences between the two pyrogenic molecules were found (29). At this time, however, it is difficult to say whether the larger-molecular-weight pyrogen, produced by monocytes, has an active site different from that of the smaller-molecular-weight pyrogen. These chemical differences may be restricted to the nonpyrogenic moiety.

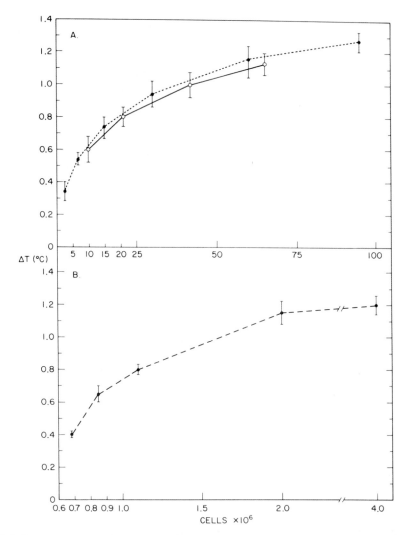

FIG. 4. Dose-response relationship for the action of human leukocytic pyrogen in rabbits. **A:** Neutrophil (O——O) or mixed buffy coat (●----●) preparations. **B:** Monocyte preparation separated on a Ficoll-Hypaque gradient. (From Dinarello et al., ref. 29.)

We recently tested the effect of a semipurified human neutrophil pyrogen on body temperature in the rhesus monkey (46). An interesting finding was that the monkey is as sensitive to human endogenous pyrogen as the rabbit, despite the fact that the two species differ markedly in their responsiveness to endotoxin (Table 1). From this we conclude that the relative insensitivity of the monkey to bacterial endotoxin is not due to unresponsiveness of the hypothalamus to endogenous pyrogen.

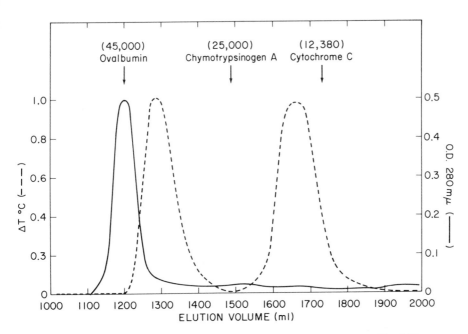

FIG. 5. Chromatography of human endogenous pyrogen prepared from Ficoll-Hypaque gradients on Sephadex G-50. (From Dinarello et al., ref. 29.)

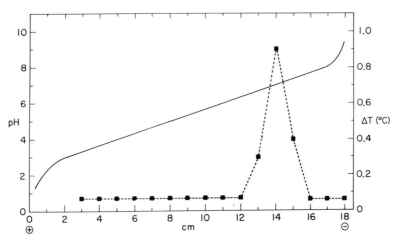

FIG. 6. Thin-layer isoelectric focusing on Sephadex G-75 superfine of human pyrogen (M.W. 15,000; ampholines 2%; 400 volts × 24 hr). Solid line, pH gradient. Dashed line, fever response. (From Dinarello et al., ref. 29.)

CONCLUSIONS

Exogenous pyrogens are substances of diverse biologic and chemical properties which have in common the ability to cause fever when injected into host animals. Endogenous pyrogens are proteins synthesized by the host's phagocytic cells in response to the injected exogenous pyrogen and serve as the final common mediator of fever. Endogenous pyrogens act on specific neurons in the AH/POA. Although there are at least two molecular species of human endogenous pyrogen, their mechanism of action in the hypothalamus is likely the same.

REFERENCES

1. Allen, I. V. (1965): The pathogenesis of fever in delayed hypersensitivity. *Irish J. Med. Sci.,* 6:247–254.
2. Atkins, E. (1963): Studies in staphylococcal fever. II. Responses to culture filtrate. *Yale J. Biol. Med.,* 35:472–488.
3. Atkins, E., and Freedman, L. E. (1963): Studies in staphylococcal fever. I. Responses to bacterial cells. *Yale J. Biol. Med.,* 35:451–471.
4. Atkins, E., and Heijn, C. (1965): Studies on tuberculin fever. III. Mechanism involved in the release of endogenous pyrogen in vitro. *J. Exp. Med.,* 122:207–235.
5. Atkins, E., and Huang, W. C. (1958): Studies on the pathogenesis of fever with influenza viruses. I. The appearance of an endogenous pyrogen in the blood following intravenous injection of virus. *J. Exp. Med.,* 107:383–435.
6. Atkins, E., and Morse, S. I. (1967): Studies in staphylococcal fever. VI. Responses induced by cell walls and various fractions of staphylococci and their products. *Yale J. Biol. Med.,* 39:297–311.
7. Atkins, E., and Wood, W. B., Jr. (1955): Studies on the pathogenesis of fever. I. The presence of transferable pyrogen in the blood stream following the injection of typhoid vaccine. *J. Exp. Med.,* 101:519–528.
8. Atkins, E., Bodel, P., and Francis, L. (1967): Release of an endogenous pyrogen in vitro from rabbit mononuclear cells. *J. Exp. Med.,* 126:357–386.
9. Atkins, E., Feldman, J. D., Francis, L., and Hursh, E. (1972): Studies on the mechanism of fever accompanying delayed hypersensitivity: The role of the sensitized lymphocyte. *J. Exp. Med.,* 135:1113–1132.
10. Bennett, I. L., Jr., and Beeson, P. B. (1953): Studies on the pathogenesis of fever. II. Characteristics of fever-producing substance from polymorphonuclear leukocytes and from the sterile exudates. *J. Exp. Med.,* 98:493–508.
11. Berlin, R. D., and Wood, W. B., Jr. (1964): Studies on the pathogenesis of fever. XIII. The effect of phagocytosis on the release of endogenous pyrogen by polymorphonuclear leukocytes. *J. Exp. Med.,* 119:715–726.
12. Bodel, P. (1970): Studies on the mechanism of endogenous pyrogen production. I. Investigation of new protein synthesis in stimulated human blood leukocytes. *Yale J. Biol. Med.,* 43:145–163.
13. Bodel, P. (1974): Studies on the mechanism of endogenous pyrogen production. III. Human blood monocytes. *J. Exp. Med.,* 140:943–965.
14. Bodel, P. (1974): Pyrogen release in vitro by lymphoid tissue from patients with Hodgkin's disease. *Yale J. Biol. Med.,* 47:101–112.
15. Bodel, P., and Atkins, E. (1964): Studies in staphylococcal fever. IV. Hypersensitivity to culture filtrates. *Yale J. Biol. Med.,* 37:130–144.
16. Bodel, P., and Atkins, E. (1965): Studies in staphylococcal fever. V. Staphylococcal filtrate pyrogen. *Yale J. Biol. Med.,* 38:282–298.
17. Bodel, P., and Atkins, E. (1966): Human leukocyte pyrogen producing fever in rabbits. *Proc. Soc. Exp. Biol. Med.,* 121:943–946.

18. Bodel, P., and Atkins, E. (1967): Release of endogenous pyrogen by human monocytes. *N. Engl. J. Med.,* 276:1002–1008.
19. Bodel, P., and Dillard, M. (1968): Studies on steroid fever. I. Production of leukocyte pyrogen in vitro by etiocholanolone. *J. Clin. Invest.,* 47:107–117.
20. Bodel, P., and Miller, H. (1976): Human endogenous pyrogen producing fever in mice. *Proc. Soc. Exp. Biol. Med.* (*in press*).
21. Bodel, P., Wechsler, A., and Atkins, E. (1969): Comparison of endogenous pyrogens from human and rabbit leukocytes utilizing Sephadex filtration. *Yale J. Biol. Med.,* 41:376–387.
22. Bondy, P. K., and Bodel, P. (1971): Mechanism of action of pyrogenic and antipyrogenic steroids in vitro. In: *Pyrogens and Fever,* edited by G. E. Wolstenholme and J. Birch, pp. 101–113. Churchill Livingston, Edinburgh.
23. Bornstein, D. L., and Woods, J. W. (1969): Species specificity of leukocytic pyrogens. *J. Exp. Med.,* 130:707–721.
24. Briggs, R. S., and Atkins, E. (1966): Studies in cryptococcal fever. I. Responses to intact organisms and to a soluble agent derived from cryptococci. *Yale J. Biol. Med.,* 38:431–448.
25. Chusid, M. J., and Atkins, E. (1972): Studies on the mechanism of penicillin-induced fever. *J. Exp. Med.,* 136:227–240.
26. Cooper, K. E., and Cranston, W. I. (1963): Clearance of radioactive bacterial pyrogen from the circulation. *J. Physiol.* (*Lond.*), 166:41–42P.
27. Cooper, K. E., Cranston, W. I., and Honour, A. J. (1967): Observations on the site and mode of action of pyrogens in the rabbit brain. *J. Physiol.* (*Lond.*), 191:325–337.
28. Dinarello, C. A., Bodel, P., and Atkins, E. (1968): The role of the liver in the production of fever and in pyrogenic tolerance. *Trans. Assoc. Am. Physicians,* 81:334–344.
29. Dinarello, C. A., Goldin, N. P., and Wolff, S. M. (1974): Demonstration and characterization of two distinct human leukocytic pyrogens. *J. Exp. Med.,* 139:1369–1381.
30. Dinarello, C. A., Ward, S. B., and Wolff, S. M. (1973): Pyrogenic properties of bleomycin. *Cancer Chemother. Rep.,* 57:393–398.
31. Eisenman, J. S., and Jackson, D. C. (1967): Thermal response patterns of septal and preoptic neurons in cats. *Exp. Neurol.,* 19:33–45.
32. Elin, R. J., and Wolff, S. M. (1973): Bacterial endotoxins. In: *CRC Handbook on Microbiology,* edited by A. I. Laskin and H. A. Lechevalier, pp. 215–239. CRC Press, Cleveland.
33. Haley, L. D., Meyer, R., and Atkins, E. (1966): Studies in cryptococcal fever. II. Responses of sensitized and unsensitized rabbits to various substances derived from cryptococcal cells. *Yale J. Biol. Med.,* 39:165–185.
34. Hall, W. J., Francis, L., and Atkins, E. (1970): Studies in tuberculin fever. IV. The passive transfer of reactivity with various tissues of sensitized donor rabbits. *J. Exp. Med.,* 131:483–498.
35. Hardy, J. D., Hellon, R. F., and Sutherland, K. (1964): Temperature-sensitive neurons in the dog's hypothalamus. *J. Physiol.* (*Lond.*), 175:242–253.
36. Kanoh, S., and Kawasaki, H. (1966): Studies on myxovirus pyrogen. I. Interaction of myxovirus and rabbit polymorphonuclear leukocytes. *Biken J.,* 9:177–184.
37. Kappas, A., and Ratkovits, B. (1960): Species specificity of steroid-induced fever. *J. Clin. Endocrinol. Metab.,* 29:898–900.
38. Kappas, A., Soybel, W., Glickman, P., and Fukushima, D. K. (1960): Fever-producing steroids of endogenous origin in man. *Arch. Intern. Med.,* 105:701–708.
39. Kimball, H. R., Vogel, J. M., Perry, S., and Wolff, S. M. (1967): Quantitative aspects of pyrogenic and hemologic responses to etiocholanolone in man. *J. Lab. Clin. Med.,* 69: 415–427.
40. King, M. K. (1964): Pathogenesis of fever in rabbits following intravenous injection of Coxsackie virus. *J. Lab. Clin. Med.,* 63:23–29.
41. Mickenberg, I. D., Root, R. K., and Wolff, S. M. (1972): Bactericidal and metabolic properties of human eosinophils. *Blood,* 39:67–80.
42. Mickenberg, I. D., Synderman, R., Root, R. K., Mergenhagen, S. E., and Wolff, S. M. (1971): The relationship of complement consumption to immune fever. *J. Immunol.,* 107:1466–1476.
43. Murphy, P. A., Chesney, J., and Wood, W. B., Jr. (1974): Further purification of rabbit leukocyte pyrogen. *J. Lab. Clin. Med.,* 83:310–322.
44. Nordlund, J. J., Root, R. K., and Wolff, S. M. (1970): Studies on the origin of human leukocytic pyrogen. *J. Exp. Med.,* 131:727–743.

45. Nordlund, J. J., Wolff, S. M., and Levy, H. B. (1970): Inhibition of biologic activity of Poly I:Poly C by human plasma. *Proc. Soc. Exp. Biol. Med.,* 133:439–444.
46. Perlow, M., Dinarello, C. A., and Wolff, S. M. (1975): A primate model for the study of human fever. *J. Infect. Dis.,* 132:157–164.
47. Rietschel, E. T., and Luederitz, O. (1975): Chemical structure of lipopolysaccharides and endotoxin immunity. *Z. Immunitaetsforsch.,* 149:201–213.
48. Root, R. K., and Wolff, S. M. (1968): Pathogenetic mechanisms in experimental immune fever. *J. Exp. Med.,* 128:309–323.
49. Root, R. K., Nordlund, J. J., and Wolff, S. M. (1970): Factors affecting the quantitative production and assay of human leukocytic pyrogen. *J. Lab. Clin. Med.,* 75:679–693.
50. Rosendorff, C., and Mooney, J. J. (1971): Central nervous system sites of action of a purified leukocyte pyrogen. *Am. J. Physiol.,* 220:597–603.
51. Sheagren, J. N., Wolff, S. M., and Shulman, N. R. (1967): Febrile and hematologic responses of rhesus monkeys to bacterial endotoxins. *Am. J. Physiol.,* 212:884–890.
52. Wolff, S. M. (1973): Biological effects of bacterial endotoxins in man. In: *Bacterial Lipopolysaccharides,* edited by E. H. Kass and S. M. Wolff, pp. 251–256. University of Chicago Press, Chicago.
53. Wolff, S. M., Kimball, H. R., Perry, S., Root, R., and Kappas, A. (1967): The biological properties of etiocholanolone. *Ann. Intern. Med.,* 67:1268–1295.
54. Wolff, S. M., Mulholland, J. H., and Ward, S. B. (1965): Quantitative aspects of the pyrogenic response of rabbits to endotoxin. *J. Lab. Clin. Med.,* 65:268–276.

Brain Dysfunction in Infantile Febrile Convulsions, edited by M. A. B. Brazier and F. Coceani. Raven Press, New York © 1976.

Prostaglandins in Fever

A. S. Milton

Department of Pharmacology, University Medical Buildings, Foresterhill, Aberdeen AB9 2ZD, Scotland

The first evidence that prostaglandins were hyperthermic and possibly involved in fever was provided by Milton and Wendlandt (17) in 1970 when they reported that prostaglandin E_1 (PGE_1) when injected directly into the third cerebral ventricle of the conscious cat produced vigorous shivering, ear skin vasoconstriction, and a rapid rise in deep body temperature. The threshold dose needed to produce a rise in deep body temperature was extremely small, in the order of 3×10^{-11} mole, and the duration of the response was short, particularly when compared with the long-lasting fever produced by the intraventricular injection of bacterial pyrogens. In all other respects the hyperthermia produced by PGE_1 resembled that produced by bacterial pyrogens, both behaviourally and autonomically. Milton and Wendlandt found that prostaglandins A_1, $F_{1\alpha}$, and $F_{2\alpha}$ were inactive at the same dose levels as PGE_1 with respect to thermoregulatory effects. In a more detailed investigation published in 1971 Milton and Wendlandt (19) showed that prostaglandin E_2 (PGE_2) had almost identical actions to PGE_1, and that PGE_1 was hyperthermic in the rabbit. In another publication in 1971 Milton and Wendlandt (18) reported on the hyperthermic effects of PGE_1 in the rat.

In their original publication in 1970, Milton and Wendlandt (17) reported that although the fever produced by the intraventricular injection of pyrogen was abolished by the antipyretic drug 4-acetamidophenol [first reported in 1968 (16)] the hyperthermia produced by PGE_1 was not affected, and they put forward the theory that PGE_1 might be a modulator of body temperature and, more important, that bacterial pyrogens might produce fever by causing the release of prostaglandin and that antipyretic drugs might act by preventing that release.

By 1971 Feldberg and Saxena (9,10) had confirmed the original observations of Milton and Wendlandt on the hyperthermic effects of PGE_1 in the cat and had also shown that this substance was hyperthermic in the rabbit and rat. In addition they had made two most important discoveries. The first was that when PGE_1 was infused into the cerebral ventricular system of the cat the hyperthermia produced was sustained for only as long as the infusion lasted, and thereafter deep body temperature soon returned to the preinfusion level. Secondly, they located the site of action of PGE_1 to the preoptic area of the anterior hypothalamus.

These observations, then, of Milton and Wendlandt and of Feldberg and Saxena indicated that a prostaglandin of the E series would be an ideal substance for modulating increases in body temperature including fever, since it was active in very small amounts, its duration of action was short, it acted in the area of the brain considered to be the centre for thermoregulation, and it was hyperthermic in all the species in which it had been administered up to that time.

In 1971 Vane (24) showed that the synthesis of PGE_2 and $PGF_{2\alpha}$ from arachidonic acid by guinea pig lung homogenate was inhibited by aspirin-like drugs. Vane suggested that not only the analgesic and anti-inflammatory action of these drugs but also their antipyretic action could be explained by an inhibition of prostaglandin synthesis, a view that is now widely accepted. In 1971 Piper and Vane (21) indicated that since there is little preformed prostaglandin in body tissues PG synthesis could be equated with PG release; consequently Vane's observations on the inhibition of PG synthesis by aspirin-like drugs provided the explanation to the theory previously put forward by Milton and Wendlandt (1970) (17) that antipyretic drugs acted by preventing prostaglandin release in the central nervous system.

THERMOREGULATORY RESPONSES TO PROSTAGLANDINS OF THE E SERIES

In order to obtain information on the physiological responses to prostaglandins involved in the increase in deep body temperature Bligh and Milton (1973) (1) studied the effects of infusing PGE_1 into a lateral cerebral ventricle of the Welsh Mountain Sheep. The sheep was chosen as the experimental animal for these investigations since it can maintain a constant deep body temperature over a very wide range of ambient air temperatures by regulating its heat loss and heat gain mechanisms, and these can be readily monitored. Bligh and Milton recorded deep body temperature, ear skin temperature, respiratory rate, and shivering while the animals were subjected to different ambient temperatures.

At an ambient air temperature of 10°C the respiratory rate was low (approximately 35 min^{-1}); the ear skin temperature was the same as the air temperature, indicating vasoconstriction; and occasional bursts of activity were observed on the electromyograph recording from a thigh muscle, indicating shivering. These measurements showed that the animals were maintaining deep body temperature by minimizing heat loss and by occasionally increasing heat production. When PGE_1 was infused into a lateral ventricle, the respiratory rate dropped slightly, to approximately 30 min^{-1}; there was no change in ear skin temperature, but violent shivering was recorded and deep body temperature rose. As soon as the infusion was stopped, shivering ceased and the animal started to pant (respiratory rate approximately 100 min^{-1}) and continued to do so until the deep body temperature had returned to the preinfusion level.

When the ambient air temperature was raised to 45°C (that is, above the deep body temperature), the animals panted vigorously (respiratory rate approximately 200 min^{-1}), the ear vessels were dilated, and no shivering was recorded, indicating that the animals were actively preventing body temperature from rising primarily by evaporative heat loss. Under these conditions when the PGE$_1$ infusion was started there were no effects on ear skin temperature and no shivering was observed; however, the respiratory rate dropped dramatically, to about 30 min^{-1}. Consequently evaporative heat loss by panting was suppressed, and deep body temperature rose rapidly. On cessation of the PGE$_1$ infusion, panting was resumed and the respiratory rate rose well above the preinfusion level, to over 300 min^{-1}; this elevated panting continued until the body temperature had returned to normal.

When the animals were at room temperature (18°C), the respiratory rate was about 150 min^{-1}, with the ear skin temperature being between ambient air temperature and deep body temperature. No shivering was observed. Under these conditions the animals were maintaining deep body temperature by changes in vasomotor tone with some evaporative heat loss. At an ambient air temperature of 18°C, the PGE$_1$ infusion produced a fall in respiratory rate, to approximately 30 min^{-1}; the ear skin temperature dropped, indicating vasoconstriction; and occasional bursts of shivering were recorded. After the infusion of PGE$_1$ was stopped, shivering ceased; ear skin temperature increased, indicating vasodilatation; the respiratory rate rose to above 250 min^{-1}, indicating panting and evaporative heat loss; and deep body temperature quickly fell to normal. (The results of one such experiment are given in Table 1.)

These experiments on the Welsh Mountain Sheep showed that PGE$_1$ increased deep body temperature by inhibiting heat loss mechanisms, including evaporative heat loss and surface heat loss, and by stimulating heat gain

TABLE 1. *Effect of PGE$_1$ infusion into the lateral ventricle*

Parameter	Five minutes before infusion	At end of 45-min infusion[a]	One hour after cessation of infusion
Rectal temperature (°C)	39.5	41.2	40.5
Ear skin temperature (°C)	28.0	23.5	28.2
Respiration rate (min^{-1})	150	30	270
Shivering[b]	0	++	0

From Bligh and Milton (*unpublished data*).
[a] PGE$_1$ was infused at 2.5 μg min^{-1} into a lateral ventricle of a Welsh Mountain Sheep.
[b] 0, no shivering. ++, moderate shivering.

mechanisms such as shivering (metabolic heat production). The predominant effect depended upon the ambient air temperature, and therefore upon the thermoregulatory pathways being driven at any particular time. Of particular interest were the observations that as soon as the PGE_1 infusions were stopped the animals actively lost the heat they had gained during the infusion and deep body temperature was quickly restored to normal. This is very reminiscent of the effects of antipyretic drugs in reducing fever produced by bacterial pyrogens. Stitt in 1973 (22) carried out similar experiments in the rabbit and compared the effects of PGE_1 with bacterial pyrogens.

In the cat at an ambient temperature of 18–20°C, PGE_1 and PGE_2 both increase deep body temperature by producing shivering and ear skin vasoconstriction, and the animals take up a curled-up position to reduce heat loss. Body temperature returns to normal after the PGE_1 hyperthermia by active heat loss, including ear vasodilatation, occasional sweating from the paw pads, and occasional panting, and the animals resume their normal body positions [Milton and Wendlandt, 1971 (19); Feldberg and Saxena, 1971 (9,10)].

ROLE OF PROSTAGLANDINS OF THE E SERIES IN NORMAL THERMOREGULATION

As a result of the reported actions of prostaglandins of the E series in raising body temperature, the question arises as to whether they are involved in the maintenance of deep body temperature in normal as opposed to pathological conditions. Cammock, Dascombe, and Milton (1975) (2) subjected cats to different ambient temperatures, collected cerebrospinal fluid (CSF) from the cisterna magna, and assayed the CSF for PGE using radioimmunoassay.

During exposure to cold (0°C) the animals exhibited autonomic and behavioural thermoregulatory responses, including shivering and ear skin vasoconstriction, and the deep body temperature rose slightly. During exposure to heat (45°C) the animals were unable to control their deep body temperature; and though panting, sweating from the paw pads, and ear skin vasodilatation were observed, deep body temperature rose. However, Cammock, Dascombe, and Milton were unable to show any changes in the PGE content of the CSF collected from animals exposed to either cold or heat when compared with animals maintained at 25°C. It is of course possible that any changes in PGE release would occur in the region of the thermoregulatory area of the anterior hypothalamus, and such changes might be too small to produce significant changes in PGE levels in cisternal CSF.

In 1970 Feldberg and Saxena (8) showed that body temperature could be altered by perfusing the cerebral ventricles with artificial CSF containing different ratios of calcium and sodium ions. In the presence of sodium ions and in the absence of calcium ions, body temperature rose rapidly; whereas in the presence of sodium ions, increasing the calcium ion concentration to above normal values produced a fall in body temperature. Similar experiments were carried out by Myers and Veale (1971) (20), and the concept was put forward that body temperature was maintained by a balance between these two ions, and that fever resulted from an imbalance between the levels of these two cations. In 1974 Dey, Feldberg, Gupta, Milton, and Wendlandt (4) investigated the hyperthermia produced by lack of calcium ions to determine whether there was any evidence of PGE release which would account for the rise in deep body temperature. They found no evidence of PGE release when the ventricles of the conscious cat were perfused from the third ventricle to cisterna magna with artificial CSF containing no calcium ions. The PGE content was the same as when the ventricles were perfused with CSF containing normal calcium. During perfusion with calcium-free CSF there was violent shivering and initial vasoconstriction, and the deep body temperature rose rapidly; however, subsequently panting and vasodilatation were observed as the animal apparently attempted to dissipate the heat gained. The shivering continued throughout the perfusion but ceased when the perfusion was terminated. The prostaglandin synthetase inhibitors 4-acetamidophenol and indomethacin did not inhibit the hyperthermia produced by the calcium-free CSF perfusions. It was concluded from these results that the prostaglandins of the E series were not involved in this hyperthermic response.

Recently Milton (1975) (14) has investigated the hyperthermia produced by the intravenous and the intraventricular injection of morphine into the conscious cat. The hyperthermia produced was unaffected by prostaglandin synthetase inhibitors, though it was completely blocked by the specific morphine antagonist naloxone; it was concluded that the prostaglandins were not involved in morphine hyperthermia.

PROSTAGLANDIN E RELEASE DURING FEVER AND THE ACTION OF ANTIPYRETIC DRUGS

In 1970 Milton and Wendlandt (17) reported that a prostaglandin-like substance had been found in cat CSF during pyrogen fever, and in 1973 Feldberg and Gupta (6) obtained CSF from the third ventricle of the conscious cat and assayed it for contractile activity using the rat fundus strip preparation of Vane (1957) (23). They found that in afebrile animals the activity was very low or absent; in contrast, during fever produced by injecting pyrogen directly into the third ventricle, the activity was considerably greater. Following administration of the antipyretic drug 4-acetamidophenol, the fever abated and the contractile activity of the CSF was again low. From their results Feldberg and Gupta concluded that the contractile substance present in the CSF was a prostaglandin.

In 1973 Feldberg, Gupta, Milton, and Wendlandt (7) collected CSF from the cisterna magna of the conscious cat and assayed it for PGE-like activity. They found that the O-somatic antigen of *Shigella dysenteriae* produced a fever when administered into both the third ventricle and the cisterna magna and also when given intravenously. In all cases during the febrile response, the PGE-like activity of the CSF increased and the three anti-pyretic drugs acetylsalicylic acid (aspirin), 4-acetamidophenol (paracetamol, acetaminophen), and indomethacin all abolished fever, and at the same time the CSF content of PGE fell (Fig. 1). Thin-layer chromatography of the CSF samples followed by bioassay and radioimmunoassay indicated that the prostaglandin present in the CSF of the cat during fever was PGE_2.

Similar results were obtained by Harvey, Milton, and Straughan in 1975 (12) in the rabbit, in which they produced fever both with the O-somatic antigen of *S. dysenteriae* and with a purified pyrogen prepared from *Proteus vulgaris* ('E' Pyrogen, Organon) (Table 2). In addition, they found that if rabbits were made tolerant to the fever-producing effect of the 'E' Pyrogen by injecting it intravenously every day for 10 days, then on the tenth day when the animals were refractory to the pyrogenic action no increase in the PGE content of the CSF was found.

In 1974 Dey, Feldberg, and Wendlandt (5) injected purified lipid A pre-pared from a mutant strain of *Salmonella* into the conscious cat and showed that this substance also produced fever accompanied by an increase in the

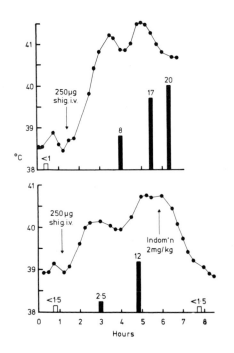

FIG. 1. Records of rectal temperatures from two unanaesthetised cats. The height of the columns and the values above them refer to PGE_1-like activity in $ng.ml^{-1}$ of cisternal CSF. The position of the columns refers to the time but not to the duration of the CSF collection. The first arrow in both records indicates an i.v. injection of 250 μg pyrogen and the second arrow in the bottom record an i.p. injection of indomethacin 2 $mg.kg^{-1}$ (Indom'n). (From Feldberg, Gupta, Milton, and Wendlandt, 1973, ref. 7.)

TABLE 2. *Prostaglandin E$_2$ content of rabbit CSF*

Control	Ninety minutes after saline i.v.	Ninety minutes after S. dys.[a] 15 μg kg^{-1} i.v.	Five hours after S. dys. 15 μg kg^{-1} i.v.
<1.0	<1.0	4.5	1.0
<1.0	<1.0	11.0	1.0
<1.0	<0.5	18.0	2.0
<0.5	<0.5	60.0	
<0.5	<0.5		

From Harvey, Milton, and Straughan (*unpublished data*).
PGE$_2$ content (ng ml^{-1}) was measured in rabbit CSF collected from the cisterna magna.
[a]*S. dys.*, O-somatic antigen of *Shigella dysenteriae.*

PGE content of cisternal CSF. In addition, they showed that antipyretic drugs inhibited both the fever and the release of PGE.

It is now generally considered that bacterial pyrogens activate neutrophils and possibly certain monocytes to synthesize and release a low-molecular-weight protein known as endogenous pyrogen (or leucocytic pyrogen). Harvey and Milton (1975) (11) prepared endogenous pyrogen from cat peritoneal exudate and found that when this material was infused intravenously into a conscious cat it produced fever which was associated with an increase in PGE of the cisternal CSF (Fig. 2); again this fever and the increase in PGE were inhibited by antipyretic agents. In contrast to these results, Cranston, Hellon, and Mitchell (1975) (3), carrying out similar experiments in the rabbit, showed that though endogenous pyrogen produced fever and a rise in the PGE content of the CSF, when they infused aspirin at the same time as the endogenous pyrogen no increase in the PGE levels of the CSF were observed though the dose of aspirin which they used had no antipyretic action and the fever still occurred. These authors maintained that since it was possible to dissociate the effect of aspirin on PGE release from its effect on fever the direct relationship between PGE and fever was in question. However, their experiments did not show whether,

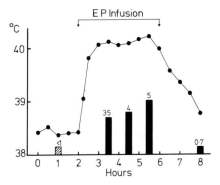

FIG. 2. Record of rectal temperature of an unanaesthetised cat. The height of the columns and the values above them refer to the PGE$_2$-like activity in ng.ml^{-1} of cisternal CSF. The position of the columns refers to the time but not to the duration of the CSF collection. Between the arrows endogenous pyrogen (EP; 2 × 10^6 cell equivalents min^{-1} for 5 min, then 2 × 10^5 cell equivalents min^{-1}) was infused into a saphenous vein. (From Harvey and Milton, *unpublished data*.)

though the PGE content of the CSF collected from the cisterna magna was reduced, sufficient PGE was still being synthesized and released in the temperature-regulating region of the anterior hypothalamus. The fact that the dose of aspirin they infused was not antipyretic could be used as an argument to support the view that sufficient PGE was still being synthesized to produce fever.

In 1975 Veale and Cooper (25) reported that when they made extensive lesions in the preoptic area of the anterior hypothalamus (PO/AH) of the rabbit and then applied PGE_1 locally it no longer produced a rise in deep body temperature. This observation provided further evidence that the site of action of the PGE_1 is the PO/AH; they also observed that in lesioned animals locally applied leucocytic pyrogen (LP) was ineffective in producing a fever. In contrast to these observations, when they injected PGE_1 and LP into a lateral cerebral ventricle, the hyperthermic effect of the PGE_1 was abolished by the lesion but the fever produced by the LP was not, although the onset of fever was more gradual. Similarly, LP given intravenously also produced fever in a lesioned animal.

The authors conclude from their results that LP also acts at a site other than the PO/AH to produce fever, and that this action is independent of the release of PGE, though in their investigations they were unable to find such a site. Unfortunately the authors did not investigate whether the fever produced by LP following lesioning of the PO/AH was inhibited by antipyretic agents. If this secondary site does exist, it is possible that LP, whether administered intravenously or intraventricularly, could reach the site and release a prostaglandin whereas PGE_1, when injected into the cerebral ventricles, would be unable to reach the site.

These experiments of Veale and Cooper and of Cranston, Hellon, and Mitchell obviously need further investigation, for if it were shown that the action of pyrogens and of prostaglandins in producing hyperthermia were unrelated then the present theory concerning pyrogens, prostaglandins, and the mode of action of antipyretic drugs becomes untenable.

Harvey and Milton (1975) (11) found that if plasma obtained from a donor cat, in which fever had been produced by intravenously administered *S. dysenteriae,* was injected into a recipient cat which had been made refractory to the pyrogen, then this recipient cat developed a fever accompanied by an increase in cisternal CSF PGE levels (Fig. 3). These experiments showed that during bacterial pyrogen fever there was a circulating pyrogenic material in the plasma which differed from the bacterial pyrogen and which was itself capable of producing PGE release. It is concluded that this circulating pyrogen is endogenous pyrogen. In contrast, when they injected bacterial pyrogen directly into the cerebral ventricular system to produce fever, no circulating pyrogenic material could be detected in the plasma. These results show, therefore, that centrally administered bacterial pyrogen does not activate the synthesis and release of endogenous pyrogen

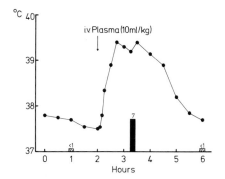

FIG. 3. Record of rectal temperature of an unanaesthetised cat tolerant to *S. dysenteriae*. At the arrow, plasma (10 ml/kg) obtained from a donor cat in which fever had been induced by the O-somatic antigen of *S. dysenteriae* was infused into a jugular vein. The height of the columns and the values above them refer to PGE_2-like activity in $ng.ml^{-1}$. The position of the columns refers to the time but not to the duration of the CSF collection. (From Harvey and Milton, *unpublished data*.)

peripherally and must produce fever by acting on cells within the central nervous system.

PROSTAGLANDIN RELEASE IN BRAIN INJURY AND "NONSPECIFIC" FEVERS

It was first noticed by Milton and Wendlandt (1968) (16) that the long-lasting hyperthermic response following the injection of 5-hydroxytryptamine into the cerebral ventricles was inhibited by the antipyretic drug 4-acetamidophenol. They also noticed to their surprise that following the injection of 4-acetamidophenol itself into the cerebral ventricular system there was, after a period of time, a hyperthermic response which was itself inhibited by an intraperitoneal injection of the antipyretic drug. In the light of our present knowledge and with subsequent experiments [Dey, Feldberg, Gupta, Milton, and Wendlandt, 1974 (4); Milton and Harvey, 1975 (15)], it would appear that these hyperthermic responses are not due to a direct action of the drugs themselves but are a "nonspecific" fever produced by interference with the central nervous system, and that in the absence of bacterial infection the slightest "injury" stimulus to the brain may result in fever consequent to the release of PGE.

HYPOTHERMIC EFFECTS OF ANTIPYRETIC DRUGS IN AFEBRILE STATES

Antipyretic drugs such as 4-acetamidophenol and indomethacin, but generally not salicylates, may produce a fall in deep body temperature when administered to both man and animals in the absence of fever, particularly when given in large doses. In addition, when given as antipyretics to reduce fever, the temperature may fall from the fever level to below that found in the afebrile state.

In 1973 Milton (13) investigated this phenomenon to determine whether the fall in body temperature in the absence of fever could be attributed to an inhibition of prostaglandin synthesis and release. Indomethacin (2–25 mg/kg^{-1}) and 4-acetamidophenol (50–100 mg/kg^{-1}) both produced a fall in deep body temperature when administered intraperitoneally to the conscious cat. This hypothermia was accompanied by ear skin vasodilatation and, when high doses were administered, by panting. When PGE$_1$ was infused into a lateral ventricle, shivering and ear vasoconstriction occurred and deep body temperature rose; when the temperature had reached a plateau and whilst the infusion of PGE$_1$ was continued, 4-acetamidophenol (50 and 100 mg/kg^{-1}) and indomethacin (2 mg/kg^{-1}) were administered. Both drugs produced vasodilatation and panting but had no effect on the shivering; deep body temperature fell slightly before reaching a new plateau level, which was sustained until the infusion was stopped. From these results it was considered that the effects of the two drugs to produce ear skin vasodilatation and panting were not mediated through inhibition of prostaglandin synthesis but were due to an action of the two drugs on the heat loss mechanisms concerned. Acetylsalicylic acid 25 mg/kg^{-1} did not affect deep body temperature in either the afebrile state or during PGE$_1$ infusion. These results are also regarded as further evidence that the prostaglandins are not involved in normal thermoregulation.

DISCUSSION

Since the possibility was first suggested by Milton and Wendlandt (17) just 5 years ago, the evidence that a prostaglandin of the E series, probably PGE$_2$, is a mediator of pyrogen fever is fairly convincing. When injected directly into the thermoregulatory area of the anterior hypothalamus, both PGE$_1$ and PGE$_2$ activate heat gain and inhibit heat loss mechanisms in a manner very similar to that produced by bacterial and endogenous pyrogens. PGE$_1$ and PGE$_2$ are among the most potent substances known which increase deep body temperature when injected directly into the central nervous system; the threshold dose for PGE$_1$ to produce a significant rise in deep body temperature is in the order of 3×10^{-11} mole (1 ng). They produce a rise in deep body temperature in all the placental mammals in which they have so far been studied. In this respect they differ from the monoamines, which appear to have different effects on deep body temperature in different species and under different ambient conditions.

Bacterial pyrogens, lipid A, and endogenous pyrogen—all of which produce fever—all increase the level of PGE found in the CSF. The concentration of PGE in the CSF found during fever would be sufficient to produce a rise in deep body temperature if it were applied to the region of the anterior hypothalamus.

During bacterial pyrogen fever a circulating pyrogenic material which is not the bacterial pyrogen administered and is of endogenous origin is found in the plasma, which when transferred to a recipient animal produces both fever and a rise in the PGE levels of the CSF. Not only does fever not develop in animals which have been made refractory to the pyrogenic action of bacterial pyrogen by chronic administration, but no increase in CSF PGE levels is seen.

The antipyretic drugs such as acetylsalicylic acid, 4-acetamidophenol, and indomethacin, which have been shown to inhibit the enzyme systems concerned with prostaglandin synthesis, all inhibit the rise in PGE levels of the CSF when administered during pyrogen fever at the same time as they produce antipyresis. This is true whether this fever is produced by bacterial pyrogens, lipid A, or endogenous pyrogens. It is therefore reasonable to assume that the antipyretic drugs produce their action by inhibiting prostaglandin synthesis and release. In contrast to their postulated role in fever, there is no evidence as yet that prostaglandins are involved in normal thermoregulation.

In their paper in 1973 Feldberg, Gupta, Milton, and Wendlandt (7) posed the intriguing question as to whether the general malaise seen in fever was due not to the increase in body temperature as has been suggested but to the action of prostaglandins released by the bacterial pyrogens acting on other areas of the brain. Also at the present time we do not know how bacterial or endogenous pyrogens activate the synthetic mechanisms responsible for prostaglandin synthesis; in addition, we have almost no information on the role of prostaglandins in fever in man. These are areas for future research.

REFERENCES

1. Bligh, J., and Milton, A. S. (1973): The thermoregulatory effects of prostaglandin E_1 when infused into a lateral cerebral ventricle of the Welsh Mountain Sheep at different ambient temperatures. *J. Physiol. (Lond.)*, 229:30–31P.
2. Cammock, S., Dascombe, M. J., and Milton, A. S. (1976): Prostaglandins in thermoregulation. In: *Advances in Prostaglandin and Thromboxane Research*, Vol. 1, edited by B. Samuelsson and R. Paoletti, pp. 375–380. Raven Press, New York.
3. Cranston, W. I., Hellon, R. F., and Mitchell, D. (1975): Fever and brain prostaglandin release. *J. Physiol. (Lond.)*, 248:27–28P.
4. Dey, P. K., Feldberg, W., Gupta, K. P., Milton, A. S., and Wendlandt, S. (1974): Further studies on the role of prostaglandins in fever. *J. Physiol. (Lond.)*, 241:629–646.
5. Dey, P. K., Feldberg, W., and Wendlandt, S. (1974): Lipid A and prostaglandin. *J. Physiol. (Lond.)*, 239:102P.
6. Feldberg, W., and Gupta, K. P. (1973): Pyrogen fever and prostaglandin-like activity in cerebrospinal fluid. *J. Physiol. (Lond.)*, 228:41–53.
7. Feldberg, W., Gupta, K. P., Milton, A. S., and Wendlandt, S. (1973): Effect of pyrogen and antipyretics on prostaglandin activity in cisternal CSF of unanaesthetised cats. *J. Physiol. (Lond.)*, 234:279–303.
8. Feldberg, W., and Saxena, P. N. (1970): Mechanism of action of pyrogen. *J. Physiol. (Lond.)*, 211:245–261.
9. Feldberg, W., and Saxena, P. N. (1974): Fever produced by prostaglandin E_1. *J. Physiol. (Lond.)*, 217:547–556.
10. Feldberg, W., and Saxena, P. N. (1971): Further studies on prostaglandin E_1 fever in cats. *J. Physiol. (Lond.)*, 219:739–745.
11. Harvey, C. A., and Milton, A. S. (1975): Endogenous pyrogen fever, prostaglandin release and prostaglandin synthetase inhibitors. *J. Physiol. (Lond.)*, 250:18–20P.

12. Harvey, C. A., Milton, A. S., and Straughan, D. W. (1975): Prostaglandin E levels in cerebrospinal fluid of rabbits and the effects of bacterial pyrogen and antipyretic drugs. *J. Physiol. (Lond.)*, 248:26–27P.
13. Milton, A. S. (1973): Prostaglandin E_1 and endotoxin fever and the effects of aspirin, indomethacin and 4-acetamidophenol. In: *Advances in Biosciences*, Vol. 9, pp. 495–500. Pergamon Press, Oxford.
14. Milton, A. S. (1975): Morphine hyperthermia, prostaglandin synthetase inhibitors and naloxone. *J. Physiol. (Lond.)*, 251:27–28P.
15. Milton, A. S., and Harvey, C. A. (1975): Prostaglandins and monoamines in fever. In: *Temperature Regulation and Drug Action*, edited by P. Lomax, E. Schönbaum, and J. Jacob, pp. 133–142. Karger, Basel.
16. Milton, A. S., and Wendlandt, S. (1968): The effect of 4-acetamidophenol in reducing fever produced by the intracerebral injection of 5-hydroxytryptamine and pyrogen in the conscious cat. *Br. J. Pharmacol.*, 34:215–216P.
17. Milton, A. S., and Wendlandt, S. (1970): A possible role for prostaglandin E_1 as a modulator for temperature regulation in the central nervous system of the cat. *J. Physiol. (Lond.)*, 207:76–77P.
18. Milton, A. S., and Wendlandt, S. (1971): The effects of 4-acetamidophenol (paracetamol) on the temperature response of the conscious rat to the intracerebral injection of prostaglandin E_1, adrenaline and pyrogen. *J. Physiol. (Lond.)*, 217:33–34P.
19. Milton, A. S., and Wendlandt, S. (1971): Effects on body temperature of prostaglandins of the A, E and F series on injection into the third ventricle of unanaesthetised cats and rabbits. *J. Physiol. (Lond.)*, 218:325–336.
20. Myers, R. D., and Veale, W. L. (1971): The role of sodium and calcium ions in the hypothalamus in the control of body temperature of the unanaesthetised cat. *J. Physiol. (Lond.)*, 212:411–430.
21. Piper, P., and Vane, J. (1971): The release of prostaglandins from lung and other tissues. *Ann. NY Acad. Sci.*, 180:363–385.
22. Stitt, J. T. (1973): Prostaglandin E_1 fever induced in rabbits. *J. Physiol. (Lond.)*, 232:163–179.
23. Vane, J. R. (1957): A sensitive method for the assay of 5-hydroxytryptamine. *Br. J. Pharmacol.*, 12:344–349.
24. Vane, J. R. (1971): Inhibition of prostaglandin synthesis as a mechanism of action for aspirin-like drugs. *Nature [New Biol.]*, 231:232–235.
25. Veale, W. L., and Cooper, K. E. (1975): Comparison of sites of action of prostaglandin E and leucocyte pyrogen in brain. In: *Temperature Regulation and Drug Action*, edited by P. Lomax, E. Schönbaum, and J. Jacob, pp. 218–226. Karger, Basel.

*Brain Dysfunction in Infantile Febrile
Convulsions,* edited by M. A. B. Brazier and
F. Coceani. Raven Press, New York © 1976.

Mechanisms of Action of Antipyretic Drugs

R. Ziel and P. Krupp

*Research Department, Pharmaceuticals Division, Ciba-Geigy Limited,
CH-4002 Basel, Switzerland*

Although antipyretics have been used in clinical medicine for over 200 years primarily on the basis of empirical knowledge, it is only during the last two decades that some progress has been made towards elucidating their mode of action. A distinctive feature of the therapeutic action of these compounds is that they relieve all febrile states, infectious and noninfectious, without necessarily affecting the cause of the disease. The antipyretic effect is primarily the result of augmented heat loss through the skin (50,61). By contrast, antipyretics in therapeutic doses do not lower the body temperature in afebrile persons, nor do they influence the normal temperature control mechanism (3,4,50).

Several substances of diverse chemical structure (Fig. 1) have in common the antipyretic property. The most commonly used preparations in clinical practice are derivatives of salicylic acid, pyrazolone, *p*-aminophenol, indole, and phenylacetic acid. It must be emphasized that all these drugs may exert additional effects; i.e., they are analgesics, antiphlogistics, and inhibitors of platelet aggregation.

Compounds differ with regard to the spectrum of their pharmacological actions; a simplified synopsis of their properties is given in Table 1. In addition to their antipyretic action, all the compounds listed have an analgesic effect. Among those displaying only antipyretic and analgesic properties are amidopyrine and paracetamol. Drugs that exert not only these two actions but also an anti-inflammatory effect are those described as nonsteroidal anti-inflammatory agents, examples of which are acetylsalicylic acid, phenylbutazone, indomethacin, and diclofenac sodium (10,36,37,58,63). *In vitro* at least, all the last-mentioned compounds have a clear-cut inhibitory action on platelet aggregation (43–45,49,53). Despite differences in the activity spectra, all antipyretic agents are thought to act as the salicylates, which are the most widely used drugs to counter fever and the most thoroughly investigated in man and animals (1,8,9,11,14,20,26,32,48). Certain other drugs also exert an antifebrile effect, but they are not included among the antipyretics. The glucocorticoids belong to the latter group. As is discussed later, these steroids differ in their mechanism of action from the antipyretics proper (2,28).

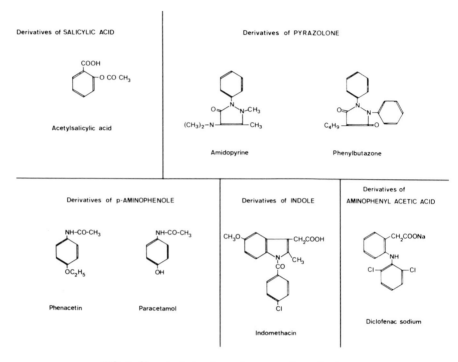

FIG. 1. Chemical structure of some antipyretic drugs.

TABLE 1. *Activity profile of some antipyretic agents*

Preparation	Antipyretic effect	Analgesic effect	Anti-inflammatory effect	Inhibition of platelet aggregation
Acetylsalicylic acid	++	++	+	+
Aminopyrine	++	++	+	−
Diclofenac sodium	+++	+++	+++	++
Indomethacin	+++	+++	+++	++
Paracetamol	++	++	+	−
Phenacetin	++	+	−	−
Phenylbutazone	++	+	++	++

+++, strong effect. ++, moderate effect. +, slight effect. −, no effect.

MODE OF ACTION

Current views on the mechanism of action of the antipyretics are based chiefly on animal experiments performed in various laboratories over the past few years. The observations made in animals, however, are largely consistent with the results obtained in pharmacological studies in man.

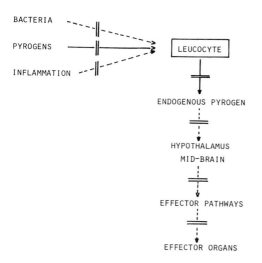

FIG. 2. Mechanism of the febrile reaction and possible target sites for antipyretics.

Theoretically there are a number of ways by which drugs could bring about an antipyretic effect. According to the prevalent view, as illustrated in Fig. 2, a febrile reaction is induced when in the course of an inflammatory process the leucocytes are stimulated, as by a bacterial pyrogen. This causes the formation and release of endogenous pyrogen (EP). This polypeptide is carried in the blood to the central nervous system, where it affects the thermoregulatory centres at the level of the hypothalamus and the mid-brain. The end-organs ultimately responsible for the development of fever are then activated via the effector pathways. The cross bars in Fig. 2 indicate theoretical target sites for the antipyretics. There are a number of different possibilities: (a) Interference with the formation of bacterial pyrogen or suppression of the inflammatory process. In this way causative factors in the development of fever could be eliminated. (b) Inhibition of the formation or release of EP from leucocytes and other phagocytic cells. (c) Inactivation or accelerated elimination of circulating EP or inhibition of its passage from the blood into the brain. (d) Interference with the effector pathways or organs. (e) Interference with the effect of EP on the thermoregulatory centres. The question to be considered here is which of these possibilities is the most likely to occur.

Interference With the Pyrogenic Stimulus

There is no indication that antipyretics administered in therapeutic dosage have any bacteriostatic or bactericidal effect that enables them to interfere with the formation of bacterial pyrogen. This is, however, the mechanism through which infectious fever is dispelled by antibiotics. The anti-inflammatory action of an antipyretic may also contribute to the normalization of body temperature, especially in a noninfectious inflammatory process. Although it is not easy to obtain quantitative data concerning the importance of anti-inflammatory activity to a given antipyretic effect, it must again be emphasized that certain antipyretics lack anti-inflammatory properties. Hence antipyretic activity is certainly independent of the anti-inflammatory activity to some degree.

Inhibition of the Formation or Release of Endogenous Pyrogen

The next possible explanation for the activity of antipyretics is that they may interfere with the formation or release of endogenous pyrogen from leucocytes and other phagocytic cells. In the peripheral blood, activation of leucocytes takes place in response to various stimuli (e.g., endotoxin or viral invasion) or in the process of phagocytosis. One of the ensuing reactions is the formation and release of endogenous pyrogen into the circulation (5,6,17,35). From the observations of Gander et al. (29) it appeared that antipyretics interfere with this process. These authors reported, for instance, that pretreatment with salicylate in the rabbit lessened the febrile reaction to an intravenous injection of a bacterial pyrogen; by contrast, salicylates failed to exert any antipyretic effect if the febrile reaction was induced by the systemic administration of homologous EP. Since other experiments *in vitro* had also demonstrated that sodium salicylate inhibited the release of leucocytic pyrogen from peritoneal cells, it seemed reasonable to conclude that salicylate antipyresis at least was brought about by the inhibition of EP release from leucocytes. According to more recent findings, however, this mechanism is not likely to be of major importance, for in both animals and man salicylates exert a rapid and dose-related suppressant effect on the febrile reaction induced by the infusion of EP (1,20). There are also reports indicating that neither sodium salicylate nor p-aminophenone or indomethacin inhibit the release of EP from leucocytes, either *in vitro* or *in vivo* (10,11,27,30,33,58).

Despite these partially contradictory findings, it now appears that the action of antipyretics is not solely attributable to inhibition of the release of EP from phagocytic cells. On the other hand, there is some evidence indicating, directly or indirectly, that the antipyretic effect of the glucocorticoids results from suppression of leucocyte activation, inhibition of EP release, or both. To what extent stabilization of the lysosomal membrane, which is apparently labilized by endotoxin, is also relevant to the antipyretic effect of these steroids still remains to be seen (59,60).

Interference With Circulating Endogenous Pyrogen

There is no conclusive evidence to support the view that antipyretic agents could inactivate or accelerate the elimination of EP from the blood or interfere with its passage from the blood into the brain. Although the possibility that circulating EP may be reversibly inactivated cannot be dismissed, the fact that the biological activity of EP *in vitro* is not affected by incubation with salicylates tends to argue against a mode of action of this sort (32,58). Besides, salicylates are consistently effective in inhibiting the febrile reaction to EP, whether it is injected into the blood or directly into the brain (10,12).

Interference With the Effector Pathways or Organs

It seems unlikely that antipyretics could interfere with the effector pathways or the end-organs ultimately responsible for the febrile reaction. They have no influence whatever on the physiological thermoregulatory functions, or affect them only under extreme thermal conditions. There is also no evidence that these drugs have any influence on the effector pathways that convey the signals initiating the dissipation or production of heat. It has been demonstrated that salicylates have no effect on the rise in temperature provoked in the rabbit by localized hypothermia of the hypothalamus, and it can be assumed that the increase in body temperature following hypothermia of the hypothalamic thermoregulatory centres is mediated by the same effector mechanisms as the febrile reaction occurring in response to the central injection of EP (18). It is thus more than improbable that the antipyretics act by modifying the activity of the effector pathways or the end-organs responsible for causing fever. It must be stressed, however, that various drugs (e.g., the neuroleptics) that are capable of inhibiting febrile reactions but also affect normal body temperature, do modify the activity of these systems. The drugs exerting such effects are predominantly those that interfere with various neurotransmitter substances, for the effector pathways initiating the production or the loss of heat are composed of cell systems containing 5-hydroxytryptamine, dopamine, norepinephrine, or acetylcholine (31,42). There is accordingly ample evidence that the antipyretics do not act by interfering with the activity of the effector pathways and end-organs concerned with thermoregulation.

Interference With the Effect of Endogenous Pyrogen on Thermoregulatory Centres

The last remaining plausible explanation for the action of antipyretics is therefore that they interfere with the effect of EP on the thermoregulatory centres of the hypothalamus and midbrain. There are several experimental observations that lend support to this assumption, even though the question of how EP ultimately affects the activity of the thermoregulatory centres is still partly obscure.

Of decisive importance in determining *where* the site of action of the antipyretics is located was the observation that the bilateral microinjection of salicylates into the preoptic area lowers body temperature in the febrile animal, whereas it does not affect thermoregulation in the afebrile animal. Microinjection experiments in which EP and salicylates were applied concurrently to the hypothalamus strongly suggest that antipyretics interfere, directly or indirectly, with the effect of EP on hypothalamic thermoregulatory centres (13,15,16,34,51,61).

With regard to *how* the antipyretics exert their action, two discoveries made during the last few years proved crucial. One was the observation that certain prostaglandins (PGs) play a determinant part in the initiation of a febrile reaction (7,39,40,47,54,55). The other was Vane's (24,57) demonstration that drugs belonging to the class of antipyretics inhibit the biosynthesis of PGs. All antipyretic agents, even though they are structurally different, exert a dose-related inhibitory effect *in vitro* on the PG synthetase system, which is responsible for the biosynthesis of PGs (Fig. 3). The enzyme system used to demonstrate this effect was the microsomal fraction of bovine cerebral cortex, and the substrate was ^{14}C-labelled arachidonic acid. The differences between the various drugs are merely quantitative. Inhibition of the PG synthetase system by antipyretics is of a competitive nature (25,38,63). Depending on the drug investigated, reversible and irreversible enzyme inactivation has been described (37). The effects of various antipyretics on the PG synthetase isolated from the seminal vesicle and from the cerebral cortex are shown in Table 2. Both enzyme preparations are inhibited by various antipyretics, although at different concen-

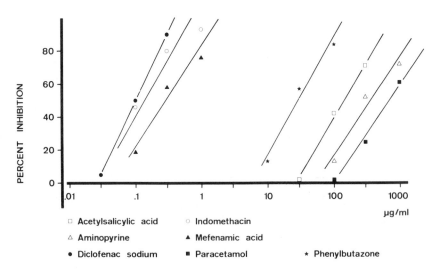

FIG. 3. Inhibition of the PG synthetase system *in vitro*. The enzyme was isolated from the bovine cerebral cortex. Abscissa: drug concentration. Ordinate: percent inhibition of PGE$_2$ formation.

TABLE 2. *Inhibition of the PG synthetase system in vitro*

Preparation	Seminal vesicle[a] (ID$_{50}$, μM)	Cerebral cortex[a] (ID$_{50}$, μM)
Phenacetin	>5,000	>5,000
Aminopyrine	4,300	1,300
Paracetamol	n.t.[b]	4,600
Acetylsalicylic acid	3,300	780
Phenylbutazone	490	100
Mefenamic acid	8.3	1.1
Indomethacin	5.6	0.4
Diclofenac sodium	1.6	0.3

The enzymatic assays were carried out according to a modification of the technique described by Takeguchi et al. (56). The incubation medium contained 3 mg of the lyophilized microsomal fraction of bovine seminal vesicle or cerebral cortex, 0.33 μM ^{14}C-labelled arachidonic acid with a specific activity of 58 mCi/mM and 9.85 μM unlabelled arachidonic acid as substrate, and 2.95 mM *l*-epinephrine and 2.93 mM reduced *l*-glutathione as cofactors in 5 ml Tris buffer at pH 8.3. Each of the compounds tested was added to the reaction mixture in three concentrations. After a 30-min incubation the reaction was stopped by adding one drop of concentrated hydrochloric acid, and the lipid fraction was extracted twice with ethyl acetate. Prostaglandins were separated by column chromatography according to Orczyk and Behrman (46), and the radioactivity in each fraction was counted with a liquid scintillation spectrometer. In preliminary experiments it has been shown that prostaglandin activity was attributable to PGE$_2$.
[a] Source of enzyme.
[b] n.t., not tested.

trations. A single exception is phenacetin, which, however, is rapidly converted to paracetamol *in vivo*. Under the given experimental conditions the synthetase system isolated from brain is inhibited at lower concentrations than that derived from the seminal vesicle (Table 2). In addition, it seems significant that antipyretics with anti-inflammatory properties (e.g., phenylbutazone, indomethacin, and diclofenac sodium) differ from the others in that they inhibit both enzyme preparations at low concentrations, indicating that these drugs suppress the biosynthesis of PGs in the brain and the peripheral organs alike. This may explain the spectrum of activity of this group of drugs (i.e., the nonsteroidal anti-inflammatory agents), which besides their antipyretic, analgesic, and anti-inflammatory effects also inhibit platelet aggregation. By contrast, antipyretics without anti-inflammatory properties inhibit the PG synthetase from the seminal vesicle only when used in high concentrations. The cerebral PG synthetase, on the other hand, is more susceptible to drugs of the latter type, which is a further indication that antipyretics act in the central nervous system.

In this connection it is important to note that there is a close correlation between the activity of the various antipyretics on the brain PG synthetase systems *in vitro* and their antipyretic activity. The yeast test in the rat (52) was employed as a means of assessing the antipyretic activity of the drugs. In this experimental model, body temperature rises to approximately 40°C after injection of yeast and remains almost unchanged at this level for 5 hr. When the animal is given an antipyretic, there is a dose-related decrease in body temperature. If the antipyretic potency demonstrated in this test system is plotted against the antisynthetase activity observed *in vitro*, a significant correlation emerges (Fig. 4). A high degree of structural specificity appears to be important to both antisynthetase activity *in vitro* and the antipyretic action. However, certain physicochemical properties (e.g., affinity for lipids) do not appear to have any bearing on either action of the compounds. No significant correlation exists between the partition coefficients in an octanol-water system (representing their lipid affinity) and their antisynthetase and antipyretic activity (Fig. 5). By contrast, lipid affinity conditions the analgesic potency of nonnarcotic analgesics, which can likewise be classed as antipyretics (64). This is an indication that however close the relation between analgesic and antipyretic activity may be these two effects are apparently not necessarily mediated by the same mechanism of action.

Numerous observations made by Feldberg and co-workers further confirm the decisive importance of inhibition of PG biosynthesis in relation to the antipyretic activity of the drugs in question (21–23,41). For example,

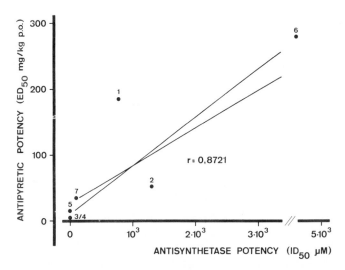

FIG. 4. Correlation between inhibition of PG synthetase *in vitro* and the antipyretic activity of various drugs. Abscissa: inhibition of the PG synthetase system (microsomal fraction of the bovine cerebral cortex). Ordinate: antipyretic activity against yeast-induced fever in the rat. 1, acetylsalicylic acid. 2, aminopyrine. 3, diclofenac sodium. 4, indomethacin. 5, mefenamic acid. 6, paracetamol. 7, phenylbutazone.

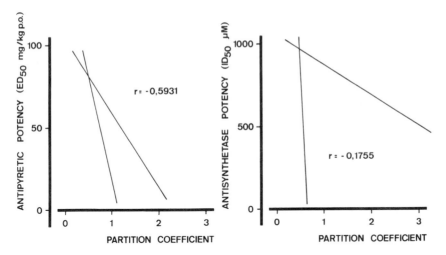

FIG. 5. Correlation between inhibition of PG synthetase *in vitro* or the antipyretic activity and partition coefficient of various drugs. Abscissa: logarithm of the partition coefficient as measured in an octanol-water system for the drugs listed in Fig. 4. Ordinate: (left) antipyretic activity against the yeast-induced fever and (right) inhibition of PG synthetase *in vitro* (microsomal fraction of the bovine cerebral cortex).

the concentration of PG-like material in the cerebrospinal fluid (CSF) of the cat is low at normal body temperature; it increases, however, if a febrile reaction is induced by the administration of bacterial pyrogen. Moreover, the defervescence subsequent to antipyretic treatment is accompanied by a decrease in the amount of PG-like material in the CSF. The concurrence of these changes indicates that there is probably a causal relationship between them. In addition it has been shown in the rabbit that arachidonic acid, a precursor of the PGs, is transformed to a PG (possibly PGE_2) when it is perfused through the ventricular system. The rate of its conversion varies with body temperature. It is low at normal rectal temperature but increases significantly during a febrile reaction. Antipyretics, while suppressing fever, inhibit the conversion of arachidonic acid to PGE_2 (62). An explanation of these phenomena is afforded by the preliminary observation that EP stimulates the cerebral PG synthetase *in vitro* (R. Ziel, *unpublished observations*). It can therefore be postulated that EP brings about a febrile reaction by stimulating this enzyme system, and that EP and antipyretic agents exert an antagonistic action on this enzyme.

CONCLUDING REMARKS

The various data discussed here provide solid grounds for the hypothesis that antipyretics act through inhibition of PG biosynthesis and consequently interfere with the action of EP on the thermoregulatory centres. Naturally this assumption presupposes that the action of EP in the hypothalamic thermoregulatory centres is mediated by an increase in the rate of PG synthesis, i.e., that augmented synthesis of PGs in the brain is an indispensable event in the initiation of a febrile reaction. Although numerous findings lend support to this hypothesis, recent observations cast some doubt on its validity (19). The mode of action of antipyretic drugs will consequently not be known for certain until the entire sequence of events occurring in the course of a febrile reaction is fully elucidated. However, even taking into account the findings that appear to contradict the PG theory, interference with PG biosynthesis in the brain seems, at present, to be the most plausible explanation for the antifebrile effect of antipyretic drugs.

REFERENCES

1. Adler, R. D., Rawlins, M., Rosendorff, C., and Cranston, W. I. (1969): The effect of salicylate on pyrogen-induced fever in man. *Clin. Sci.,* 37:91–97.
2. Atkins, E., Allison, M., Smith, M. R., and Wood, W. B. (1955): Studies on the antipyretic action of cortisone in pyrogen induced fever. *J. Exp. Med.,* 101:355–366.
3. Barbour, H. G. (1919): Antipyresis III, acetylsalicylic acid and heat regulation in fever cases. *Arch. Int. Med. Exp.,* 24:624–632.
4. Barbour, H. G., and Devenis, M. W. (1919): Acetylsalicylic acid and heat regulation in normal individuals. *Arch. Int. Med. Exp.,* 24:617–623.
5. Beeson, J. P. (1948): Temperature elevating effect of a substance obtained from polymorphonuclear leucocytes. *J. Clin. Invest.,* 27:524.
6. Berlin, R. D., and Wood, W. B. (1964): Studies on the pathogenesis of fever. XIII. The effect of phagocytosis on the release of endogenous pyrogen by polymorphonuclear leucocytes. *J. Exp. Med.,* 119:715–726.
7. Bligh, J., and Milton, A. S. (1973): The thermoregulatory effects of prostaglandin E_1 when infused into a lateral ventricle of the Welsh Mountain Sheep at different ambient temperatures. *J. Physiol. (Lond.),* 229:30–31P.
8. Chai, C. Y., Lin, M. T., Chen, H. J., and Wang, S. C. (1971): Site of action of leucocytic pyrogen and antipyresis of sodium acetylsalicylate in monkeys. *Neuropharmacology,* 10:715–723.
9. Clark, W. G., and Alderdice, M. T. (1972): Inhibition of leucocytic pyrogen induced fever by intracerebroventricular administration of salicylate and acetaminophen. *Proc. Soc. Exp. Biol. Med.,* 140:399–403.
10. Clark, W. G., and Cumby, H. R. (1975): The antipyretic effect of indomethacin. *J. Physiol. (Lond.),* 248:625–638.
11. Clark, W. G., and Moyer, S. G. (1972): The effect of acetaminophen and sodium salicylate on the release and activity of leucocytic pyrogen in the cat. *J. Pharmacol. Exp. Ther.,* 181:183–191.
12. Clark, W. G., Cumby, H. R., and Davis, H. E. (1974): The hyperthermic effect of intracerebroventricular cholera endotoxin in the unanaesthetized cat. *J. Physiol. (Lond.),* 240:493–504.
13. Cooper, K. E., Cranston, W. J., and Honour, A. J. (1967): Observations on the site and mode of action of pyrogen in the rabbit brain. *J. Physiol. (Lond.),* 191:325–337.
14. Cooper, K. E., Grundmann, M. J., and Honour, A. J. (1968): Observations on sodium salicylate as an antipyretic. *J. Physiol. (Lond.),* 196:56–57.
15. Cranston, W. I., and Rawlins, M. D. (1971): The site of salicylate-induced antipyresis in the central nervous system of the rabbit. *J. Physiol. (Lond.),* 215:27P.
16. Cranston, W. I., and Rawlins, M. D. (1972): Effects of intracerebral micro-injections of sodium salicylate on temperature regulations in the rabbit. *J. Physiol. (Lond.),* 222:257–266.

17. Cranston, W. I., Goodale, F., Snell, E. S., and Wendt, F. (1956): The role of leucocytes in the initial action of bacterial pyrogens in man. *Clin. Sci.,* 15:219–226.
18. Cranston, W. I., Hellon, R. F., Luff, R. H., Rawlins, M. D., and Rosendorff, C. (1970): Observations on the mechanism of salicylate-induced antipyresis. *J. Physiol. (Lond.),* 210:593–600.
19. Cranston, W. I., Hellon, R. F., and Mitchell, D. (1975): Fever and brain prostaglandin release. *J. Physiol. (Lond.),* 248:28–29P.
20. Cranston, W. I., Luff, R. H., Rawlins, R. H., and Rosendorff, C. (1970): The effects of salicylate on temperature regulation in the rabbit. *J. Physiol. (Lond.),* 208:251–259.
21. Feldberg, W., and Gupta, P. K. (1973): Pyrogen fever and prostaglandin-like activity in cerebrospinal fluid. *J. Physiol. (Lond.),* 228:41–53.
22. Feldberg, W., and Saxena, P. N. (1971): Further studies on prostaglandin E_1 fever in cats. *J. Physiol. (Lond.),* 219:739–745.
23. Feldberg, W., Gupta, P. K., Milton, A. S., and Wendlandt, S. (1972): Effect of bacterial pyrogen and antipyretics on prostaglandin activity in cerebrospinal fluid of unanesthetized cats. *Br. J. Pharmacol.,* 46:550–551.
24. Flower, R. J., and Vane, J. R. (1972): Inhibition of prostaglandin synthetase in brain explains the antipyretic activity of paracetamol (4-acetamidophenol). *Nature (Lond.),* 240: 410–411.
25. Flower, R. J., Cheung, H. S., and Cushman, D. W. (1973): Quantitative determination of prostaglandin and malondialdehyde formed by the arachidonate oxygenase system of bovine seminal vesicles. *Prostaglandins,* 4:325–341.
26. Fürbringer, P. (1875): Salicylsäure gegen Katarrhe der harnleitenden Organe mit ammoniakalischer Gärung des Harns. *Berl. Klin. Wochenschr.,* 12:249–250.
27. Gander, G. W., and Goodale, F. (1969): The mechanism of the antipyretic effect of several drugs. *Fed. Proc.,* 28:357.
28. Gander, G. W., Brown, R. E., and Goodale, F. (1968): Mechanism of action of glucocorticoids. *Endocrinology,* 82:195–198.
29. Gander, G. W., Chaffe, J., and Goodale, F. (1967): Studies upon the antipyretic action of salicylate. *Proc. Soc. Exp. Biol. Med.,* 126:205–209.
30. Gander, G. W., Milton, A. S., and Goodale, F. (1972): The antipyretic effect of N-acetyl-p-aminophenol. In: *Fifth International Congress of Pharmacology, San Francisco,* p. 76 (abstract).
31. Goodman, L. S., and Gilman, A., editors (1970): *The Pharmacological Basis of Therapeutics,* 4th ed., pp. 165 and 504. Macmillan, New York.
32. Grundmann, M. J. (1969): Studies on the action of antipyretic substances. Phil. thesis, Oxford.
33. Hoo, S. L., Lin, M. T., Wei, R. T., Chai, C. Y., and Wang, S. C. (1972): Effects of sodium acetylsalicylate on the release of pyrogen from leucocytes. *Proc. Soc. Exp. Biol. Med.,* 139:1155–1158.
34. Jackson, D. L. (1967): A hypothalamic region responsive to localized injection of pyrogens. *J. Neurophysiol.,* 30:586–602.
35. King, M. K., and Wood, W. B. (1958): Studies on the pathogenesis of fever. IV. The site of action of leucocyte and circulating endogenous pyrogen. *J. Exp. Med.,* 107:291–303.
36. Krupp, P. J., Menasse-Gdynia, R., Sallmann, A., Wilhelmi, G., and Ziel, R. (1973): Sodium [o-[2,6-dichlorophenyl-amino]-phenyl]-acetate (GP 45 850), a new non-steroidal antiinflammatory agent. *Experientia,* 29:450–452.
37. Ku, E. C., Wasvary, J. M., and Cash, W. D. (1975): Diclofenac sodium (GP 45 840, Voltaren) a potent inhibitor of prostaglandin synthetase. *Biochem. Pharmacol.,* 24:641–643.
38. Lands, W. E. M., LeTellier, P. R., Rome, L. H., and Vanderhoek, J. Y. (1973): Inhibition of prostaglandin biosynthesis. In: *Advances in the Biosciences,* Vol. 9, edited by S. Bergstrom, pp. 15–28. Pergamon Press Vieweg, Braunschweig.
39. Milton, A. S., and Wendlandt, S. (1970): A possible role for prostaglandin E_1 as a modulator for temperature regulation in the central nervous system of the cat. *J. Physiol. (Lond.),* 207:76–77P.
40. Milton, A. S., and Wendlandt, S. (1971): Effects on body temperature of prostaglandins of the A, E and F series on injection into the third ventricle of unanaesthetized cats and rabbits. *J. Physiol. (Lond.),* 218:325–336.

41. Milton, A. S., and Wendlandt, S. (1971): The effects of 4-acetamidophenol (paracetamol) on the temperature response of the conscious rat to the intracerebral injection of prostaglandin E_1, adrenaline and pyrogen. *J. Physiol. (Lond.)*, 217:33–34P.
42. Møller, K. O. (1966): *Pharmakologie*, p. 340. Schwabe and Co. Verlag, Basel/Stuttgart.
43. Mustard, J. F., Jenkins, C. S. P., and Packham, M. A. (1972): Modification of platelet function. *Ann. NY Acad. Sci.*, 201:343–359.
44. O'Brien, J. R. (1968): Effects of salicylates on human platelets. *Lancet*, 1:779–783.
45. O'Brien, J. R. (1968): Effect of anti-inflammatory agents on platelets. *Lancet*, 1:894–895.
46. Orczyk, G. P., and Behrman, H. R. (1972): Ovulation blockade by aspirin or indomethacin — in vivo evidence for a role of prostaglandin in gonadotrophin secretion. *Prostaglandins*, 1:3–20.
47. Potts, W. J., and East, P. F. (1972): Effects of prostaglandin E_2 on the body temperature of conscious rats and cats. *Arch. Int. Pharmacodyn. Ther.*, 197:31–36.
48. Rawlins, M. D. (1973): Mechanism of salicylate induced antipyresis. In: *The Pharmacology of Thermoregulation*, edited by E. Schönbaum and P. Lomax, pp. 311–324. Karger, Basel.
49. Renaud, S., and Lecompte, F. (1970): Thrombosis prevention by coagulation and platelet inhibition in hyperlipidemic rats. *Thromb. Diath. Haemorrh.*, 24:577–586.
50. Rosendorff, C., and Cranston, W. T. (1968): Effects of salicylate on human temperature regulation. *Clin. Sci.*, 35:81–91.
51. Rosendorff, C., and Mooney, J. J. (1971): Central nervous system sites of action of a purified leucocyte pyrogen. *Am. J. Physiol.*, 220:597–603.
52. Smith, P. K., and Hambourger, W. E. (1935): The ratio of the toxicity of acetanilid to its antipyretic activity in rats. *J. Pharmacol. Exp. Ther.*, 54:346–356.
53. Smith, J. B., and Willis, A. L. (1971): Aspirin selectively inhibits prostaglandin production in human platelets. *Nature [New Biol.]*, 231:235–237.
54. Splawinski, J. A., Reichenberg, K., Vetulani, J., Marchaj, J., and Kalaza, J. (1974): Hyperthermic effect of intraventricular injections of arachidonic acid and prostaglandin E_2 in the cat. *Pol. J. Pharmacol. Pharm.*, 26:101–107.
55. Stitt, J. T. (1973): Prostaglandin fever induced in rabbits. *J. Physiol. (Lond.)*, 233:163–179.
56. Takeguchi, C., Kokno, E., and Sih, C. J. (1971): Mechanism of prostaglandin biosynthesis. I. Characterization and assay of bovine prostaglandin synthetase. *Biochemistry*, 10:2372–2376.
57. Vane, J. R. (1971): Inhibition of prostaglandin synthesis as a mechanism of action for aspirin-like drugs. *Nature [New Biol.]*, 231:232–235.
58. van Miert, A. S. J. P. A. M., van Essen, J. A., and Tromp, G. A. (1972): The antipyretic effect of pyrazolone derivatives and salicylates on fever induced with leucocytic or bacterial pyrogen. *Arch. Int. Pharmacodyn. Ther.*, 197:388–391.
59. Weissman, G. (1965): Studies of lysosomes. VI. The effect of neutral steroids and bile acids on lysosomes in vitro. *Biochem. Pharmacol.*, 14:525–535.
60. Weissman, G., and Thomas, L. (1962): Studies on lysosomes. I. The effects of endotoxin tolerance and cortisone on the release of acid hydrolases from a granular fraction of rabbit liver. *J. Exp. Med.*, 116:433–450.
61. Woodbury, D. M. (1970): Analgesia-antipyresis, anti-inflammatory agents and inhibition of urine acid synthesis. In: *The Pharmacological Basis of Therapeutics*, 4th ed., edited by L. S. Goodman and A. Gilman. Macmillan, New York.
62. Ziel, R., and Krupp, P. (1975): Effect on prostaglandin synthesis and antipyretic activity of non-steroidal anti-inflammatory agents. In: *Temperature Regulation and Drug Action*, edited by P. Lomax, E. Schönbaum, and J. Jacob, pp. 233–240. Karger, Basel.
63. Ziel, R., and Krupp, P. (1975): The significance of inhibition of prostaglandin synthesis in the selection of non-steroidal anti-inflammatory agents. *Int. J. Clin. Pharmacol.*, 12:186–191.
64. Ziel, R., and Krupp, P. (1976): The significance of the membrane-stabilizing effect of non-narcotic analgesics. In: *Proceedings: 1st World Congress of the International Association for the Study of Pain* (in press).

Brain Dysfunction in Infantile Febrile
Convulsions, edited by M. A. B. Brazier and
F. Coceani. Raven Press, New York © 1976.

Ontogenesis of Thermoregulation and Sensitivity to Pyrogens

W. L. Veale, K. E. Cooper, and Q. J. Pittman

Division of Medical Physiology, University of Calgary, Calgary, Alberta, Canada

Feldberg and Myers proposed their monoamine theory of thermoregulation in 1963 (10). Since that time, extensive experimentation has been carried out to elucidate further the role of norepinephrine (NE) and 5-hydroxytryptamine (5-HT) in thermoregulation. We recently reviewed the role of these substances in thermoregulation (21), and an additional review of the topic is covered in another chapter in this volume (19). In brief, in the adult mammal it appears that thermoregulation does indeed involve NE and 5-HT, and that the anterior hypothalamic-preoptic area (AH/POA) is the region of the brain in which these substances act centrally to alter body temperature. In addition to these two monoamines, perhaps others are involved in the central nervous system's (CNS) regulation of body temperature, but these are not discussed in this brief chapter.

We recently suggested that the regulation of body temperature may be considered a "normal" process, closely related to but distinctly different from the "pathological" condition called fever (5). Two lines of evidence seem to support this concept. First, ambient temperature seems to have little influence on the hyperthermic response to intravenous or central injections of pyrogens or prostaglandins (PGs), whereas it has a profound influence on the temperature response following injection of monoamines (5,23). Secondly, in mammals rendered poikilothermic because of destruction of the AH/POA, fever can still develop to intravenous pyrogen even though no apparent thermoregulatory responses are available. In short, our observations suggest that "normal" thermoregulation involves NE, 5-HT, and other potential "neurotransmitters," and the response is heavily influenced by the integration of inputs from thermosensors. Fever appears to involve another system superimposed on the thermoregulatory process and involving pyrogens and perhaps PGs. For a complete discussion of this topic the reader is referred to a contribution in a recent symposium (5).

DEVELOPMENT OF THE FEBRILE RESPONSE AND THERMOREGULATION

The work described in this chapter was carried out on the newborn lamb. One reason for selecting the lamb as an experimental animal is that, like newborn human babies, newborn lambs lack the ability to develop a fever on their first exposure to intravenous exogenous pyrogen (6,16). This lack of febrile response to exogenous pyrogen injected intravenously in an amount sufficient to produce a sharp fever in the adult sheep has been the focus of a considerable amount of research work in our laboratory. The inability to produce fever is present even though the newborn lamb can regulate its temperature quite well. For instance, if the newborn lamb is placed in a cold ambient temperature (4°C), it shivers and maintains its body temperature in much the same manner as an adult. Also, when it is placed in a hot ambient temperature, the lamb is able to maintain its body temperature at an approximately normal level. With respect to the inability to develop a fever on first exposure to exogenous pyrogen, it appears necessary for a specific interval of time to pass before a subsequent injection of the exogenous pyrogen results in fever. If, for example, newborn lambs at 4 hr of age are injected with 0.3 μg of a lipopolysaccharide extracted from *Salmonella abortus equi* (SAE), no change in body temperature is observed. If the same lambs are reinjected with the same amount of the same material at 60 hr after birth, fever results. In contrast to this, if newborn lambs are given a control injection of a sterile, pyrogen-free saline at age 4 hr, then are reinjected with SAE pyrogen at 60 hr, no temperature change occurs. In fact, lambs receiving their first injection of exogenous pyrogen, even at several days of age, often do not show the febrile response seen in adults or in lambs previously administered the SAE pyrogen.

Of additional interest, it appears that a certain interval of time must pass after birth before lambs are capable of producing a fever even on the second injection of exogenous pyrogen. That is to say, if lambs are injected with 0.3 μg SAE pyrogen intravenously at 4 hr of age, then reinjected after an additional 40 hr has passed, no fever results. It appears therefore that a time interval of more than 44–48 hr is necessary for this "sensitization" to occur. For the production of fever, it is thought that exogenous pyrogen reacts with other cells within the recipient animal and causes an endogenous pyrogen to be produced. It is believed that it is this endogenous pyrogen which actually produces the febrile response. When the endogenous pyrogen is produced *in vitro* and injected into newborn lambs, a fever develops even on first injection, providing the animals are more than 60 hr of age. If newborn lambs are less than 44–48 hr of age, they usually do not develop a fever to the endogenous pyrogen applied intravenously (16).

Thus evidence suggests that the febrile process is immature at birth even to endogenous pyrogen; superimposed on the development process is the requirement for a "sensitization" to bacterial pyrogen, which may occur independently of the maturation of the response to endogenous pyrogen. At the present time we cannot identify the component of the fever pathway that requires "sensitization." In both the newborn lamb and the foetus observed *in utero* during the last month of gestation, the leucocytes appear to recognize the injected lipopolysaccharide. Our evidence for this is that following an initial intravenous administration of bacterial pyrogen to these animals there is a considerable decrease in the number of circulating leucocytes. In the adult mammal such a phenomenon is associated with transport of the pyrogen by the leucocyte to the cells of the reticuloendothelial system. Whether such a situation would occur in the circulation of other neonatal mammals is uncertain. It is known that the chemotactic and phagocytic responses of leucocytes from human neonates are deficient when compared with those of adults (12–14).

We have no evidence as yet as to whether the leucocytes of the newborn lamb are capable of synthesizing and releasing endogenous pyrogen in response to an initial exposure to bacterial pyrogen. However, it is known that leucocytes from human neonates are capable of elaborating this substance when incubated *in vitro* with bacterial pyrogen (8). Thus in the human this part of the fever pathway appears to be functional at birth.

It is of interest to know whether the sensitization process is specific for individual pyrogens or is a process that takes place between antigenically different molecules. We have studied the sensitization phenomenon between the pyrogen from SAE and killed typhoid-paratyphoid vaccine. In four instances in which lambs were injected intravenously with one of these pyrogenic substances at 4 hr of age, and then challenged with the other one at 60 hr of age, fever occurred in all instances after the second challenge. Thus sensitization occurs between antigenically related substances. In another series of experiments, lambs were injected at 4 hr with either SAE pyrogen or a killed cell suspension of *Yersinia enterocolitica*. When the lambs were challenged at 60 hr with the substance they had not previously been exposed to, 14 of 17 lambs developed fever. Thus it appears that cross sensitization can occur between antigenically unrelated substances. We have no explanation for the fact that sensitization did not occur in three of the lambs, but we have never seen this happen when the sensitizing pyrogen and the challenging pyrogen are the same.

In the nonexperimental setting lambs must become naturally sensitized. We have evidence that lambs as old as 12 days of age still do not develop fever after intravenous bacterial pyrogen, and Blatteis (1) showed that guinea pigs up to 8 days of age do not develop fever when first exposed to intravenous bacterial pyrogen. This sensitization process may occur as a result of continual exposure to pyrogens through either the respiratory or alimentary tract. To investigate the latter possibility, four lambs at 4 hr of age were given 15–30 μg SAE pyrogen in 3 ml saline through an intragastric tube. The rectal temperature was recorded at 60 hr of age, and the lambs were given 0.3 μg SAE intravenously. None of these lambs developed fever. An additional four lambs were each given 50 μg SAE pyrogen into the colon. When these four animals were tested for their ability to develop a fever following intravenous pyrogen at 60 hr of age, one of the four developed fever while the others remained nonfebrile. These results suggest that the normal route of sensitization is not via the alimentary tract. However, a continuing exposure to pyrogen over several days, as may occur under natural conditions, may also provide the necessary exposure for the sensitization process to be initiated. Microbial activity has been found in the alimentary tract of lambs as young as 1 day of age (20).

In a number of instances, foetal animals may become exposed to pyrogens as a result of intrauterine infections. We carried out studies to determine if lambs could develop fever after birth following sensitization *in utero* (18). During the last third of pregnancy and under sterile conditions, catheters were inserted into foetal carotid and jugular vessels. Following recovery from surgery and at specific intervals before birth, each foetus was injected intravenously with SAE pyrogen (0.3 μg). The foetus was allowed to continue undisturbed until birth. At 60 hr postnatally the lambs were given a second intravenous injection of 0.3 μg SAE, and the body temperature was recorded. Four lambs that had been sensitized at either 16 days, 2 days, 18 hrs, or 5 min before birth developed fever after the second injection. Six lambs that had been sensitized at intervals of 52 days to 5 hrs before birth did not develop fever after the second injection. Thus in many cases exposure to endotoxin before birth does not sensitize the lamb so as to cause it to develop fever when challenged with pyrogen after birth.

PROSTAGLANDINS IN FEVER

As reviewed in another chapter in this volume (7), the production of fever involves several steps. Firstly, the exogenous pyrogen (SAE pyrogen in our experiments) interacts with leucocytes in the circulation or cells of other tissues to produce an endogenous pyrogen. It is thought that this pyrogen is the material which enters the AH/POA and acts on the cells there to produce fever. In 1970 Milton and Wendlandt (15) demonstrated that PGs of the E series (PGEs) are extremely pyrogenic when applied to the brain directly. A theory has been proposed, principally by Milton and Feldberg and their colleagues (9,15), suggesting that endogenous pyrogen causes the release of PGs within the hypothalamus, which in turn act on the cells to produce the febrile response. Considerable evidence has been gathered to support this theory and is reviewed elsewhere (9,22).

EXPERIMENTS ON THE NEWBORN LAMB

The inability of the newborn lamb to develop fever may be due to the immaturity of the PG synthetase system or to an inability to respond with fever to release of these substances within the AH/POA. Since the adult sheep develops fever after intraventricular infusion of PGE_1 (3,11), we thought it of interest to determine the response of the newborn lamb to PGs injected into a lateral cerebral ventricle (17). Rectal temperatures were recorded in lambs of mixed breeds of either sex at various intervals between 4 and 168 hr of age. For the injection, lambs were gently restrained; the scalp was incised under local anaesthesia and aseptic conditions, and a small hole was drilled through the skull. A needle was lowered into a lateral ventricle, and 200 μl saline containing the PGE was allowed to flow from a small reservoir. The needle was then withdrawn, and the hole and incision closed. We have used this injection procedure in more than 125 instances in our laboratory with no apparent ill effects to the lamb. Furthermore, using precautions previously described (17), we are confident that we are delivering the drug into the cerebral ventricular system and not into the tissue of the brain. In several instances dye was injected in a similar manner, and in each of these brains the walls of the entire ventricular system were stained.

The results of a series of experiments in which 40 injections of PGE_1 (2.0–200 μg) were made into 28 newborn lambs showed that fever occurred in only 15 of the 40 experiments. The remaining injections produced either temperature falls or little change at all. There did not appear to be any consistent relationship between the response and the age of the animal or the amount of PGE_1 injected. Furthermore, some of these lambs had been "sensitized" by previous intravenous injection of pyrogen and were capable of developing fever in response to intravenous bacterial pyrogen. Nevertheless, many of these lambs did not respond with fever following intraventricular PGE_1. Some of these lambs were also given bacterial pyrogen directly into the lateral ventricles in a dose 1/100 of that necessary to elicit fever following intravenous injection. This quantity of pyrogen is adequate to cause fever in other mammalian species, yet the lambs did not develop fever. PGE_1 was usually used in the present experiments, but our experience in other work of this type with PGE_2 indicates the temperature responses are identical with these two substances.

It is possible that the substances injected into the ventricles were not reaching the areas of the brain involved in thermoregulation. Since the response of the adult sheep to monoamines injected into the cerebral ventricles is well known (2,4), we undertook to inject these amines by the same ventricular approach into our newborn lambs. If the temperature changes were similar to those seen in the adult sheep, this would provide evidence that the ventricular approach was valid for the study of CNS function in the lamb and also that the neuronal pathways for thermoregulation are similar in newborn and adult sheep.

Injections of either NE, 5-HT, or saline were made into 56 different lambs on 79 separate occasions at one of three different ambient temperatures (4°, 21°, or 30°C). NE and 5-HT were given at dosages of 100 and 200 μg. The results from this series of experiments showed that newborn lambs as young as 4 hr behaved in a manner very similar to that of the adult sheep following NE and 5-HT given by the intraventricular route. In agree-

ment with the findings of others (4), the responses and physiological mechanisms which caused the temperature changes varied according to the environmental temperature. Our results did support the hypothesis that 5-HT
in both the newborn and the adult sheep is a transmitter in a heat-loss pathway. NE appears to act as an inhibitory substance on both heat-loss and
heat-gain pathways. Thus it appears that, with respect to normal thermoregulation, the CNS of the lamb is mature at birth. The response of a newborn lamb to injections of PGE$_1$, SAE pyrogen, and 5-HT into a lateral
ventricle on three separate occasions is shown in Fig. 1.

The fact that predictable, coordinated thermoregulatory responses occur
in newborn lambs following injection of putative neurotransmitters into the
cerebroventricular system suggests that the injected substances are capable
of reaching the AH/POA and exerting an effect. If injected PGE$_1$ were to
diffuse in a similar manner, the results would suggest that the newborn lamb
can develop fever without the central involvement of PGs. It may be, however, that the site of action of PG in the lamb may be at a locus in the
hypothalamus not easily accessible from the ventricles. Consequently we
undertook to investigate the responses of lambs to injections of PGs,
bacterial pyrogen, and NE directly into the tissue of the hypothalamus.

Approximately 2–4 hr after birth, lambs were anaesthetized, and under

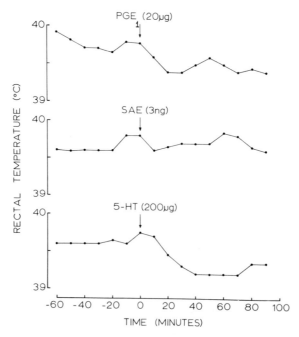

FIG. 1. Body temperatures of one lamb after injection of PGE$_1$, SAE pyrogen, and 5-HT
into a lateral ventricle on three separate occasions.

sterile conditions an assembly of four guide tubes was implanted bilaterally so the tips rested above various hypothalamic loci. Rectal temperature was recorded at 60 hr of age, and injections in a volume of 1.0 μl were made through a 27-gauge needle into the brain tissue.

PGE$_1$ (0.2 μg) or PGE$_2$ (0.2 and 2.0 μg) was injected into 23 hypothalamic sites; none of these lambs developed a fever. Injections of bacterial pyrogen (0.2 μg) caused fever in some of the sites within the AH/POA, but other injections into nearby sites did not. When lambs were placed in a 10°C environment, and NE (20 μg) was injected into the hypothalamus, seven of 16 injections were followed by falls in temperature. On subsequent histological examination of these brains, these seven injection sites were found to be within the AH/POA. The other nine sites were found to be in areas of the hypothalamus other than the AH/POA. These results support the concept that the newborn lamb does not require central involvement of PG to develop a fever after its first exposure to intravenous pyrogen.

CONCLUDING REMARKS

We have presented evidence that temperature regulation appears to occur in newborn lambs as it does in the adult. This is supported not only by the fact that the newborn lamb regulates its temperature well in both a hot and cold environment, but also that it responds as the adult to the direct application of NE either into a lateral ventricle or to the AH/POA. Even though a newborn lamb has been "sensitized" to exogenous pyrogen and can produce a fever on subsequent injection of that material, it does not respond to the central administration of PGs. In contrast to the adult in which other workers have been able to produce fevers by infusing PGs, in the newborn PGs do not cause fever even in loci in which NE produces a temperature change. It appears, therefore, that fever can develop in the newborn lamb without the involvement of PGs. This evidence, together with that presented by Cooper et al. earlier in this volume, may be an important challenge to the theory which suggests that endogenous pyrogen produces a febrile response through the release of PGs.

ACKNOWLEDGMENTS

This work was supported by the Medical Research Council of Canada. Prostaglandins were provided by Dr. J. Pike of The Upjohn Company, Kalamazoo, Michigan.

REFERENCES

1. Blatteis, C. M. (1975): Postnatal development of pyrogenic sensitivity in guinea pigs. *J. Appl. Physiol.,* 39:251–257.

2. Bligh, J., and Maskrey, M. (1969): A possible role of acetylcholine in the central control of body temperature in sheep. *J. Physiol. (Lond.)*, 203:55–57P.
3. Bligh, J., and Milton, A. S. (1973): The thermoregulatory effects of prostaglandin E_1 when infused into a lateral cerebral ventricle of the Welsh Mountain Sheep at different ambient temperatures. *J. Physiol. (Lond.)*, 229:30–31P.
4. Bligh, J., Cottle, W. H., and Maskrey, M. (1971): Influence of ambient temperature on the thermoregulatory responses to 5-hydroxytryptamine, noradrenaline and acetylcholine injected into the lateral cerebral ventricles of sheep, goats and rabbits. *J. Physiol. (Lond.)*, 212:377–392.
5. Cooper, K. E., and Veale, W. L. (1974): Fever, an abnormal drive to the heat-conserving and producing mechanisms? In: *Recent Studies of Hypothalamic Function*, edited by K. Lederis and K. E. Cooper, pp. 391–398. Karger, Basel.
6. Cooper, K. E., Pittman, Q. J., and Veale, W. L. (1975): Observations on the development of the "fever" mechanism in the fetus and newborn. In: *Temperature Regulation and Drug Action*, edited by P. Lomax, E. Schönbaum, and J. Jacob, pp. 43–50. Karger, Basel.
7. Cooper, K. E., Veale, W. L., and Pittman, Q. J. (1976): Pathogenesis of fever. *This volume.*
8. Dinarello, C. A. (1975): Personal communication.
9. Feldberg, W., and Milton, A. S. (1973): Prostaglandin fever. In: *The Pharmacology of Thermoregulation*, edited by E. Schönbaum and P. Lomax, pp. 302–310. Karger, Basel.
10. Feldberg, W., and Myers, R. D. (1963): A new concept of temperature regulation by amines in the hypothalamus. *Nature (Lond.)*, 200:1325.
11. Hales, J. R. S., Bennett, J. W., Baird, J. A., and Fawcett, A. A. (1973): Thermoregulatory effects of prostaglandins E_1, E_2, F_1 and F_2 in the sheep. *Pfluegers Arch.*, 339:125–133.
12. Matoth, Y. (1952): Phagocytic and ameboid activities of the leucocytes in the newborn infant. *Pediatrics*, 9:748–755.
13. Miller, M. E. (1969): Phagocytosis in the newborn infant: Humoral and cellular factors. *J. Pediatr.*, 74:255–259.
14. Miller, M. E. (1971): Chemotactic function in the human neonate: Humoral and cellular aspects. *Pediatr. Res.*, 5:487–492.
15. Milton, A. S., and Wendlandt, S. (1970): A possible role for prostaglandin E_1 as a modulator for temperature regulation in the central nervous system of the cat. *J. Physiol. (Lond.)*, 207:76–77P.
16. Pittman, Q. J., Cooper, K. E., Veale, W. L., and van Petten, G. R. (1974): Observations on the development of the febrile response to pyrogens in sheep. *Clin. Sci. Mol. Med.*, 46:591–602.
17. Pittman, Q. J., Veale, W. L., and Cooper, K. E. (1975): Temperature responses of lambs after centrally injected prostaglandins and pyrogens. *Am. J. Physiol.*, 228:1034–1038.
18. Pittman, Q. J., Veale, W. L., and Cooper, K. E. (1975): Studies on the maturation of the febrile response to pyrogens in newborn lambs. *Proc. Can. Fed. Biol. Soc.*, 18:103.
19. Preston, E., and Schönbaum, E. (1976): Monoaminergic mechanisms in thermoregulation. *This volume.*
20. Smith, H. W. (1965): The development of the flora of the alimentary tract in young animals. *J. Pathol.*, 90:495–513.
21. Veale, W. L., and Cooper, K. E. (1973): Species differences in the pharmacology of temperature regulation. In: *The Pharmacology of Thermoregulation*, edited by E. Schönbaum and P. Lomax, pp. 289–301. Karger, Basel.
22. Veale, W. L., and Cooper, K. E. (1974): Evidence for the involvement of prostaglandins in fever. In: *Recent Studies of Hypothalamic Function*, edited by K. Lederis and K. E. Cooper, pp. 359–370. Karger, Basel.
23. Veale, W. L., and Whishaw, I. Q. (1976): Body temperature responses at different ambient temperatures following injections of prostaglandin E_1 and noradrenaline into the brain. *Pharmacol. Biochem. Behav.*, 4:143–150.

Brain Dysfunction in Infantile Febrile
Convulsions, edited by M. A. B. Brazier and
F. Coceani. Raven Press, New York © 1976.

Developmental Assessment of Intact and Brain-Lesioned Kittens

N. A. Buchwald, C. D. Hull, M. S. Levine, and J. R. Villablanca

Mental Retardation Research Center, University of California Los Angeles, Los Angeles, California 90024

Our laboratory is interested in providing models of the kinds of neurological developmental defects that might result in permanent disabilities. We plan first to study aspects of normal development and then to assess alterations that might occur as a result of experimental manipulation of the brains of infant animals. This approach provides information concerning correlative changes in anatomical and physiological development of normal and damaged brains with changes in behavioral development. From these data we hope to be able to predict the consequences of early experimental brain damage on subsequent development and hopefully to learn how to intervene in order to alleviate the effects of this damage.

One of the principal neural systems utilized in our studies is the basal ganglia. There are increasing data to indicate that this nuclear group is of importance in cognitive development and in the carrying out of complex behaviors. In the mature brain, neurons in the basal ganglia show enhanced activity during the performance of complex tasks (28). In the developing brain, several studies indicate the relative importance of the basal ganglia (11,22). These studies show that certain behavioral deficits resulting from cerebral cortical damage are not demonstrable in the adult if the damage is incurred during infancy, while lesions to the striatum (the "head end" of the basal ganglia) during infancy result in more permanent deficits. The results cited above come from experiments using monkeys. As our research involves a large population of developing animals, the exigencies of finances and space precluded the use of a primate model. Moreover, since much of our work is based on the physiology and anatomy of the basal ganglia, the use of the less expensive rat as a model animal was eliminated. This decision was made because much of the known physiology of the basal ganglia comes from work on the cat, but more importantly the basal ganglia of rodents is relatively undifferentiated so that instead of separate nuclei (i.e., the caudate nucleus and putamen), the rat has a striatum which is composed of homologues of these structures, richly interspersed with fibers of the internal capsule. For our research we therefore established a cat breeding colony.

We were fortunate that our pharmacological collaborators, Dr. A. Heller of the University of Chicago and Dr. Donald Jenden of UCLA, were willing to undertake measurements of dopamine, acetylcholine, and their associated enzymes in cat brain tissue so that we could attempt to correlate their measures with our physiological, anatomical, and behavioral results.

THE BEHAVIORAL ASSAY

One of the endpoints of our research is the behavioral performance of the test animals. In conducting studies of the behavioral consequences of neurosurgical or pharmacological intervention on developing animals, questions arose concerning the specificity of the deficits which were observed. Had the intervention retarded or accelerated the animal with respect to particular behavioral milestones? Was the behavioral deficit attributable to an alteration in the learning domain or did it involve instead a motor or a sensory deficit?

To answer such questions, it was necessary to develop a set of measures which we called the behavioral assay. An ideal assay would provide age-graded tests that quickly and reliably sample the behavioral domain in question. The literature offers few guidelines for setting up such an assay. Fox (9) provided data regarding early postnatal development of simple reflexes in kittens, but his report did not indicate variability between kittens

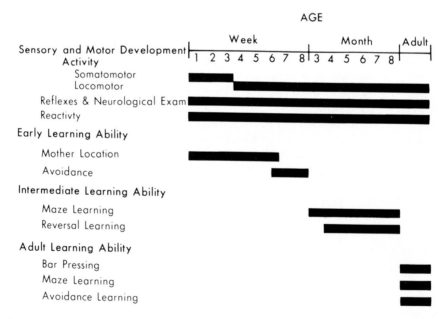

FIG. 1. Ages during which the various tests of the behavioral assay are carried out.

and across time. Smith (27) correlated development of visual acuity with eye-opening, tactile placing, and visual placing. Early studies of stability of maze learning across age and the relationship of reactivity to maze-learning ability were reviewed by Hall (12) for the rat. Again in rats, Altman (1) developed a behavioral assay for assessing the consequences of neonatal cerebellar damage.

While the reports cited provide some useful information, parametric longitudinal studies of kitten development do not exist. Therefore we have been constructing a series of tests to assess development in kittens and hopefully to predict performance of adult or juvenile cats on the basis of their scores on early measures.

Our assay is divided into four general categories: sensory and motor development, early learning ability, intermediate learning ability, and adult learning ability. The first three of these describe developmental indices, while the last provides a measure of predictive ability and of the adult consequences of early postnatal intervention. The ages at which various tests in these categories were carried out are indicated in Fig. 1.

SENSORY AND MOTOR DEVELOPMENT

Development of somatomotor and locomotor activity: Tests in this area have given us basic parametric measures of development of early motor activity and of locomotion in the kitten.

For the first 3 weeks postpartum, motor activity was quantified by recording the displacement of a sensitive force transducer. Subsequently, as locomotion developed it was measured by interruption of photocell beams in an open field. Figures 2 and 3 show the developmental changes in motor activity recorded in these tests. The bottom panel of each figure illustrates the mean activity (counts per time interval). The top panel consists of the distributions of scores making up the mean. Other measurements taken at this time included tabulation of the types of movements the kittens made at each age.

In addition to skeletal muscle activity, heart rate was also recorded during the motor activity tests during the first 3 weeks of life to determine possible relationships between cardiac and motor activity in the kitten. Figure 4 shows interbeat interval histograms recorded from a kitten when active and inactive. Interbeat intervals were smaller and less variable during activity than during periods of inactivity.

Reflexes and neurological state: These tests consisted of measurements of changes in reflexes, muscle tone, posture, gross indices of sensory capacity, and general behavior (eating, general demeanor, ability to climb) during development. Body weight was tabulated to determine the parameters of normal growth for kittens in our colony and their alterations as a result of early postnatal intervention.

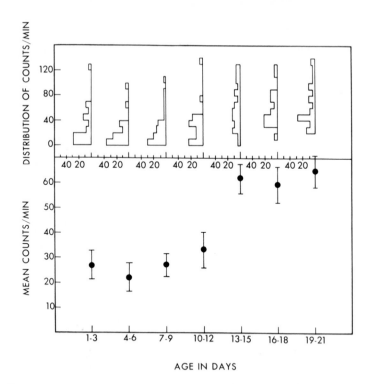

FIG. 2. Developmental changes in motor activity occurring during the first 21 postnatal days quantified by recording displacement of a force transducer. Bottom panel illustrates mean counts/minute ± standard error of mean. Top panel shows the distributions of scores for each kitten for each age period making up the mean. These values were based on means for 10-min tests administered one or two times per week per kitten.

Reactivity to stimuli: In conjunction with the measurements of development of motor activity, tests of reactivity will allow us to construct profiles of an animal's reaction to novel and familiar situations and stimuli, and to determine how such reactions are altered by early intervention. The development of these tests is just beginning, and the results provided by them are not considered in this chapter.

Early Learning Ability

Mother location test: This test has provided indications of learning ability during the first postnatal weeks. The mother was used as a reinforcer in an operant conditioning paradigm. Kittens were placed in a large enclosure containing an aperture connected to a second enclosure in which the mother was located. The task for the kitten was to find the aperture and locate its mother. When placed in the enclosure, kittens under 7 days of age rarely found the aperture on the first trial. However, after being pushed through

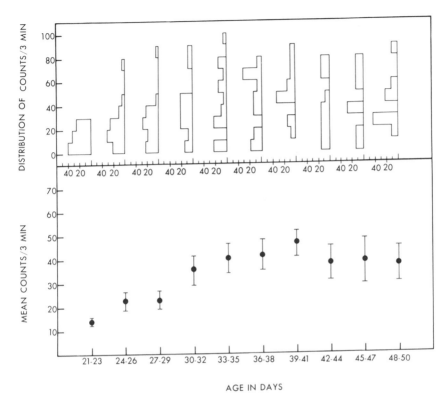

FIG. 3. Developmental changes in motor activity occurring during 21–50 postnatal days quantified by interruption of photocell beams in an open field. These values were based on means for 15-min tests administered once a week for each kitten. See legend to Fig. 2 for additional explanation. Computation of means based on 3-min epochs.

the aperture and gaining access to the mother for 5 min, most kittens were successful on second and third trials. Twenty-four hours after a first series of three trials, the kittens were given a second series. On these trials their behavior was quite similar to that on the first series. On trial one they typi-

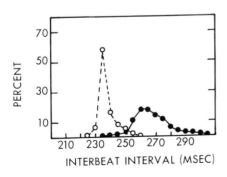

FIG. 4. Example of the differences between interbeat interval histograms in an active (open circles) and inactive (closed circles) 6-day-old kitten. During periods of motor activity, interbeat intervals are shorter and less variable than during periods of inactivity.

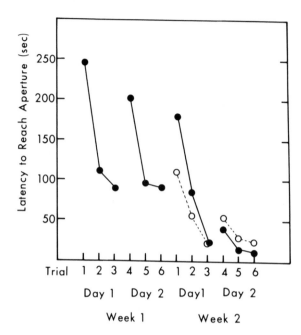

FIG. 5. Changes with repeated trials in time required (latency) to find mother in the mother location test. Values represent mean latency for a group of 8 kittens starting training during the first postnatal week (filled circles) and a group of 7 kittens (open circles) starting training during the second postnatal week. See text for further explanation.

cally did not locate their mother; on trials two and three they readily found her (Fig. 5).

The kittens were retested during the second week of life and their performances compared to those of a group of kittens receiving their first training during this time (Fig. 5, open circles). The performance of the previously experienced group and the new group were very similar, indicating that training during the first week had little effect on subsequent performance.

This test can be modified to assess additional aspects of learning in very young kittens by presenting them with two apertures, only one of which leads to the mother. Somesthetic, spatial, auditory, visual, thermal, and olfactory cues can then be used to set up discriminative situations. The earliest age at which kittens use these different cues can then be determined.

Avoidance conditioning procedures are being used to assess development of aversive behavior. One of the tasks used was the passive avoidance "step-down" procedure in which the ability of kittens to inhibit responses after negative reinforcement was tested. Results using this procedure with kittens under 2 months of age were so variable that this measure was dropped from the assay. It is being replaced with other aversive conditioning tests utilizing escape and active avoidance paradigms.

Intermediate Learning Ability

The results of performance on tests conducted on kittens 3–8 months of age have provided us with one of the first indicators of the effects of early postnatal brain damage. They may also be useful in validating our ability to predict subsequent performance on the basis of measures made during the early postnatal periods.

Maze learning and reversal: Most of our parametric learning data during this age period has been based on the ability of kittens to learn a visual discrimination and its reversal in a T-maze. Using food reinforcement, kittens were trained to make a visual discrimination in a walk-through T-maze. The stimulus consisted of a blackboard placed on the floor, just past the choice point on one side of the maze. If the kitten walked over the blackboard it was reinforced. After reaching a criterion of 80% correct for four consecutive sessions the meaning of the cue was reversed (i.e., walking over the blackboard was not reinforced), and training was continued until the same criterion level of performance was reached. This procedure allowed assessment of the animal's ability to alter its response when the significance of the discriminative stimulus was altered.

Many normal animals have been tested on this visual discrimination task. In addition, groups of animals with early caudate nucleus or frontal cortex lesions also have completed the maze. The results of these studies are summarized below, under *Testing Brain-Damaged Animals in the Behavioral Assay.*

Adult Learning Ability

The final measures made in the behavioral assay are those on adult animals. These measures will provide information on three key points. First, animals receiving lesions during infancy will be compared with their intact or sham-operated littermates. These comparisons will provide indicators of the long-lasting effects of early brain damage. Second, comparisons will be made between animals receiving lesions during infancy and littermates in which brain damage is inflicted in adulthood. These comparisons will provide indicators of the differential function of neural structures during development and in the mature animal. Finally, measures of learning in adult animals will provide us with additional indicators of our ability to make predictions about performance from measures taken at earlier ages.

The tasks used to assess learning in adults have been designed from the results of ongoing experiments on the effects of lesions of the basal ganglia or frontal cortex in cats. These include neurological examinations and tests of both motor and cognitive learning ability. These tests have been described in detail in a series of recent reports (26,29,30). Briefly, they include a bar-pressing task designed to assess motor performance and discriminative ability, a T-maze test designed to emphasize perceptual and discriminative aspects of performance, and avoidance learning tasks designed to test performance of the animals in aversive situations.

The detailed measurements achieved in the various tests of the behavioral assay will be reported elsewhere. They are already providing us with data indicating the pace of development of a variety of behaviors and the intra- and interlitter variability in these behaviors. Most of the results detail sensory and motor development and early learning ability in young kittens. In intermediate-aged animals, the maze learning and reversal tests have already produced interesting results. As yet we do not have enough data from adult animals born and raised in our kitten colony to provide information about performance on the adult learning tasks of the assay. We have preliminary indications that a positive correlation exists between certain measures achieved during infancy and performance in the maze.

TESTING BRAIN-DAMAGED ANIMALS IN THE BEHAVIORAL ASSAY

The behavioral assay is used as a baseline to test experimental animals that sustained brain damage as neonates or that underwent environmental intervention in the sense that they were reared in sensory isolation or in an artificial situation away from their mothers. A number of kittens with early postnatal brain damage have already been tested in elements of the assay.

The first groups of kittens tested had received early postnatal lesions of either the caudate nucleus or frontal cortex. Despite extensive damage to these brain areas, the operated kittens performed very well on nearly all measures in the behavioral assay. The mildness of the deficits produced by caudate and cortical lesions in kittens contrasts with the more severe deficits resulting from similar operations made in adult cats (26,29,30). However, the behavioral assay did provide us with two measures of deviant development in kittens with caudate lesions. One of the differences between kittens with caudate damage or frontal cortical damage and normal or sham-operated kittens was a statistically significant retardation in the development of placing reactions in the caudatectomized kittens as compared with those of the other two groups (2). Despite this delay in development, the caudatectomized animals did succeed in developing the placing reaction. If damage to the striatum in the neonate produces long-term deficits in motor performance, these must be sought by more subtle testing. This indicator of delayed development in caudatectomized kittens contrasts with results of experiments made in adult animals (30) in which recovery of contact placing required a longer period of time after frontal cortex lesions than after caudate ablation.

A second measure of deviant development provided by the behavioral assay was revealed by performance of the kittens on a visual discrimination task and its reversal. Intact and sham-operated animals reached criterion

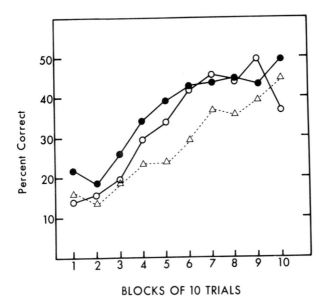

FIG. 6. Performance of 7 caudatectomized (triangles), 5 frontal-lesioned (open circles), and 14 sham-lesioned and intact kittens (closed circles) on the first 100 trials of the reversal of the T-maze discrimination. Caudatectomized kittens perseverated to the non-reinforced cue compared with the kittens in the other groups.

in the T-maze with a mean of 278 trials. Kittens with caudate and frontal cortex lesions learned this task almost as quickly (mean trials to criterion: 321 and 328 for kittens with caudate and cortical lesions, respectively). When tested on discrimination reversal, however, the kittens with caudate lesions performed more poorly than kittens with frontal lesions or than the intact or sham-operated animals. The poorer performance of the caudatectomized kittens was due to a tendency to perseverate to the previously reinforced cue (Fig. 6). Deficits in ability to perform similar tasks are characteristic of adult cats after caudate ablation as well (26). Testing of adult cats, lesioned as kittens in our series, has not as yet been completed.

ELECTROPHYSIOLOGICAL STUDIES OF NEURONAL ACTIVITY IN THE CAUDATE NUCLEUS DURING DEVELOPMENT

In parallel with the assessment of behavioral development we have been studying development of responsiveness of individual neurons in the infant brain. In a first experiment we studied neuronal responsiveness in the visual cortex (13). More recently we reported data on the electrophysiology of the developing caudate nucleus (24,25).

Much of the kitten forebrain shows a marked increase in the number of synaptic contacts per neuron during early postnatal development (7, 24).

Our recent experiments (13,25) show that all of the components of the adult synaptic response to stimuli appear prior to this period of intense synaptic growth. For example (13), both excitatory and inhibitory components of visual cortical synaptic potentials evoked by light stimuli were detected before the period of rapid synaptic growth in the visual cortex.

The electrophysiological variable which appears to correlate best with intense synaptic growth is the fidelity with which neuronal responses follow increases in stimulus repetition rate (25). This generalization comes mainly from studies of the responsiveness of caudate neurons in the developing kitten (25). Considerable information concerning the characteristics of caudate neurons has been obtained in the adult cat. Electrophysiological results (3,14) generally support anatomical data (17–20) in suggesting that the principal inputs to the striatum come from cortex, thalamus, and substantia nigra, with the bulk of the caudatopetal axons arising from cortex and thalamus. The electrophysiological evidence also suggests that the cerebral cortex is the most potent of these inputs (15). In view of the important and changing relationship between cortex and striatum mentioned at the beginning of the chapter, we decided to study the development of responsiveness of caudate neurons to cortical inputs before attempting to assess responsiveness to thalamic or nigral inputs.

Single units were recorded from the head of the caudate nucleus in a series of kittens ranging in age from 1 to 50 days. Response characteristics of each of these neurons to stimulation of the ipsilateral precruciate cortex were recorded and analyzed. Table 1 shows the number of caudate units responding to precruciate stimulation as a function of increasing age.

One finding of this research was that the synaptic effects of cortical efferents on caudate neurons in neonates were qualitatively similar to those observed in the adult (3,14,15). Even during the earliest test period following birth (5 hr), a considerable proportion of caudate neurons were excited

TABLE 1. *Changes in number of caudate units responding to stimulation of precruciate cortex as a function of increasing age*

Age (days)	No. of animals	Total No. of units	No. of resp. units
1–4[a]	5	31	16
5–8	8	41	30
9–12	7	51	35
13–16	4	29	20
17–20	4	50	38
21–30	3	22	20
31–40	2	16	13
41–50	2	20	19
Adult	2	20	18

Adapted from Lidsky et al., ref. 25.
[a] Day 1 refers to the day of birth.

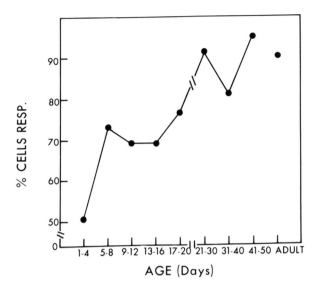

FIG. 7. Percentage of caudate units responding to stimulation of precruciate cortex as a function of increasing age. Each point represents the percentage of responsive units of all those sampled in each age group. In this and other figures, the break in the line between the 17–20 and 21–30 day groups is due to the larger age groupings used with older animals. Adapted from Lidsky et al., ref. 25.

by cortical stimulation. The most striking changes occurring during development were quantitative; i.e., the proportion of responsive units increased, response latency decreased, and the ability to follow repetitive stimuli improved (Figs. 7–9). The reasons for the increasing synaptic security of cortical efferents on caudate cells are not yet clear, although one factor may be an increase in the number of synaptic contacts in the striatum. Pre-

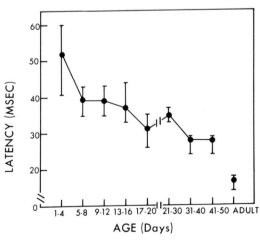

FIG. 8. Changes in response latency of caudate units to stimulation of precruciate cortex as a function of increasing age. Ranges above and below each point denote the 75th and 25th percentiles, respectively. Each point represents the median latency. Computations were based on the total sample of responsive units in each age grouping. Adapted from Lidsky et al., ref. 25.

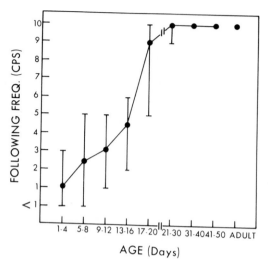

FIG. 9. Frequency following ability of caudate neurons as a function of increasing age. Computations were based on the peak following frequency of individual units pooled across the total sample of responsive units in each age grouping. Ranges and points represent interquartile ranges and median values, respectively. Adapted from Lidsky et al., ref. 25.

liminary evidence indicates that the number of synapses may increase in parallel with increases in the ability of units to respond to repetitive stimuli (24).

The results we have discussed come from extracellular recordings of caudate neuronal activity. A fuller explanation of the electrophysiological events in the neonate requires intracellular recordings as well. Synaptically induced potentials in the striatum (of the adult, at least) often are not of sufficient intensity to evoke action potentials, and the existence of subthreshold responses may easily be overlooked unless intracellular recordings are made.

NEURONAL ACTIVITY FOLLOWING NEONATAL BRAIN DAMAGE

In experiments parallel to those described with the behavioral assay, we are attempting to differentiate between the electrophysiological effects of brain damage sustained during infancy and adulthood. The first such experiments concerned measurements of spontaneous neural activity. In adult animals we measured the changes in unit activity in the caudate nucleus following selected brain damage (10,16,23). One of these studies demonstrated a slowing of spontaneous activity of caudate neurons following lesions of the frontal cortex (10). We are now completing similar experiments in adult cats which sustained cortical lesions during the neonatal period. These lesions also produced a slowing of the spontaneous activity of caudate neurons. At least in this case, measures of spontaneous activity do not seem to differentiate the effects of cortical lesions inflicted in the neonate and in the adult.

BIOCHEMICAL STUDIES DURING DEVELOPMENT

The two previous chapters in this volume (4,6) relate to neurochemical aspects of the development of the striatum in the rat brain. In an attempt to obtain neurochemical data that can be correlated with details of developing function in the basal ganglia of the cat, we have been measuring concentrations of acetylcholine and of dopamine and its associated enzymes in kittens (Fig. 10).

Acetylcholine (Fig. 10, upper panel) was measured in pieces of tissue scooped out of the exposed brain of deeply anesthetized kittens and deposited in liquid nitrogen within a few seconds. The frozen tissue was analyzed in the laboratory of Dr. Donald Jenden at UCLA. At the earliest ages measured, the acetylcholine level in the cat caudate nucleus is 40% of the adult value, compared to 20% in the rat (6). The slope of increase in concentration is also greater in the rat than in the cat. These differences may be related to species differences (e.g., the greater maturity of the newborn kitten as compared to the rat). Of more interest, however, is our finding that cortical acetylcholine content is at or near the adult value in the newborn cat cortex. In this respect, at least, the striatum lags behind the cortex.

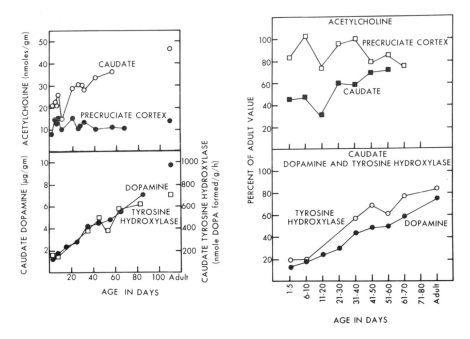

FIG. 10. Developmental changes in concentrations of acetylcholine, dopamine, and tyrosine hydroxylase in kittens. Top panels illustrate changes in acetylcholine in the caudate nucleus and precruciate cortex. Bottom panels illustrate developmental changes in striatal dopamine and tyrosine hydroxylase concentrations. Each value represents the mean concentration for the age ranges and is based on at least four or five samples.

The lower panels in Fig. 10 are measures of age-dependent increases in dopamine and tyrosine hydroxylase activity in the kitten caudate nucleus. These measures were also made on brain tissue frozen in liquid nitrogen and then analyzed in the laboratory of Dr. Alfred Heller at the University of Chicago. Our figures for dopamine and tyrosine hydroxylase concentrations in the cat caudate are comparable to those reported for the rat striatum by Coyle (6). As with acetylcholine measurements, however, the newborn kitten caudate has approximately twice as high a proportion of tyrosine hydroxylase and dopamine as does the rat pup, and the slope of increase in concentrations is less in the kitten than in the rat pup.

It is well known that the striatum contains high concentrations of acetylcholine, dopamine, γ-aminobutyric acid, and enzymes associated with these substances. Particularly during development, neurochemical studies can provide information which may in the future permit educated guesses as to the underpinnings of electrophysiological or morphological development of excitatory and inhibitory brain systems. Although we, as well as others, have been prone to speculate in this area, it is becoming increasingly apparent that many of the equations of synaptic function with pharmacological development must be considered with caution. For example, much of the hypothesizing concerning functions of the dopaminergic nigrostriatal system is based on the assumption that dopamine released by axon terminals of nigral neurons exerts an inhibitory influence on striatal cells, an assumption backed by extracellular studies of unit firing after iontophoresis of dopamine in the vicinity of striatal cells (5). More recently, however, direct intracellular measurements of synaptic responses to dopamine iontophoresis (21) suggest that, in fact, dopamine, if it acts as a transmitter, probably exerts a primary *excitatory* effect. These data are supported by results of other intracellular measurements which indicate that nigral stimulation usually evokes primary excitatory postsynaptic potentials in caudate neurons (3,14) and by data indicating that depletion of striatal dopamine after interruption of the nigrostriatal path does not result in significant increases in the firing of caudate neurons (16).

EFFECTS OF DOPAMINE-DEPLETING
LESIONS IN NEONATAL KITTENS

We have just begun developmental studies of the behavioral and electrophysiological results of neonatal manipulations of possible neurotransmitter substances in the striatum. In a first experiment we are studying the effects of dopamine-depleting lesions in neonatal kittens. Erinoff and Heller (8) demonstrated previously that lesions of the nigrostriatal tract in infant rats prevent the development of dopamine in the striatum. Since their lesions were made before any appreciable postnatal increase in striatal dopamine concentration occurred, the animals reached adulthood with a striatum whose development was minimally influenced by the presence of dopamine. We are currently assessing litters of kittens subjected to comparable lesions of the nigrostriatal pathway. With the exception of a transient retardation in body weight increase, our preliminary observations indicate that these kittens appear to be developing normally.

SUMMARY

We have constructed a behavioral assay designed to provide parametric indicators of learning and performance in cats as they mature from infancy to adulthood. The purposes of this assay include assessing the effects of brain-damage inflicted during infancy on performance as juveniles and adults, providing a means for prediction of subsequent performance on the basis of measures taken during infancy, and discovering means of intervention in young brain-damaged animals to ameliorate persisting deleterious effects of the damage.

In work completed and in progress, we have concentrated our studies on the role of the basal ganglia during development and on the contrasting effects of basal ganglionic and cerebral cortical damage in the developing animal. The behavioral assay, however, is not limited to studies of these structures; it is also being used by other members of our research group to determine the effects of brainstem lesions, early deafness, and rearing animals in a restricted environment. One of the scientists in our group has also begun to study the immediate and long-term effects of hypo- and hyperthermia induced in the neonatal kitten. With regard to the work discussed in this chapter, the behavioral assay has already allowed us to differentiate some of the consequences of neonatally inflicted cortical and caudate damage and to compare the effects of damage inflicted during infancy with lesions made in adults.

Concomitantly with the development of the behavioral assay, we have begun to study development of certain electrophysiological and biochemical events. Since most of the work discussed in this chapter is still in progress, any conclusions are tentative. Further, we can sample only a limited number of the possible physiological, behavioral, or biochemical consequences of brain damage inflicted during early postnatal periods. Nevertheless, our results indicate that the consequences of early damage to both the caudate nucleus and cortex are much less severe and persist for shorter periods than does comparable damage to these structures in adults. From previous reports in the literature we had expected to find somewhat more deleterious effects from caudate nuclear ablation than in fact occurred. Differences in animal species and/or experimental techniques may account for this outcome. With increasing refinements in our measures and our data base we hope to be able to provide information concerning additional important correlative changes in anatomical and physiological development of normal and brain-damaged animals.

ACKNOWLEDGMENTS

Supported by USPHS Grants HD-05958 and MH-7097. Biochemical determinations made with the assistance of USPHS Grant NS-12324–01 awarded to Dr. A. Heller.

REFERENCES

1. Altman, J. (1975): Effects of interference with cerebellar maturation on the development of locomotion: An experimental model of neurobehavioral retardation. In: *Brain Mechanisms in Mental Retardation,* edited by N. A. Buchwald and M. A. B. Brazier, pp. 41–92. Academic Press, New York.
2. Avery, D. L., Villablanca, J. R., Marcus, R. J., and Olmstead, C. E. (1975): Development of limb placing reactions in intact, frontal and caudate lesioned kittens. *Fed. Proc.,* 34:445.
3. Buchwald, N. A., Price, D. D., Vernon, L., and Hull, C. D. (1972): Caudate intracellular response to thalamic and cortical inputs. *Exp. Neurol.,* 38:311–321.
4. Cheney, D. L., Costa, E., Racagni, G., and Zsilla, G. (1976): Cholinergic and adenylate cyclase systems in rat brain nuclei during development. *This volume.*
5. Connor, J. D. (1970): Caudate nucleus neurons: Correlation of the effects of substantia nigra stimulation with iontophoretic dopamine. *J. Physiol. (Lond.),* 208:691–703.
6. Coyle, J. T. (1976): Neurochemical aspects of the development of dopaminergic innervation to the striatum. *This volume.*
7. Cragg, B. G. (1972): The development of synapses in cat visual cortex. *Invest. Ophthalmol.,* 11:377–385.
8. Erinoff, L., and Heller, A. (1973): Failure of catecholamine development following unilateral diencephalic lesions in the neonatal rat. *Brain Res.,* 58:489–493.
9. Fox, M. W. (1970): Reflex development and behavioral organization. In: *Developmental Neurobiology,* edited by W. A. Himwich, pp. 553–580. Charles C Thomas, Springfield, Ill.
10. Garcia-Rill, E., Levine, M. S., Hull, C. D., and Buchwald, N. A. (1975): Effects of frontal cortex lesions on spontaneous firing of caudate neurons. *Neurosci. Abstr.,* 1:190.
11. Goldman, P. S., and Rosvold, H. E. (1972): Effects of selective caudate lesions in infant and juvenile rhesus monkeys. *Brain Res.,* 43:53–66.
12. Hall, C. S. (1951): Individual differences. In: *Comparative Psychology,* 3rd ed., edited by C. P. Stone, pp. 363–387. Prentice-Hall, New York.
13. Hull, C. D., and Fuller, D. R. G. (1975): Development of PSPs recorded from immature neurons in kittens visual cortex. In: *Brain Mechanisms in Mental Retardation,* edited by N. A. Buchwald and M. A. B. Brazier, pp. 179–184. Academic Press, New York.
14. Hull, C. D., Bernardi, G., and Buchwald, N. A. (1970): Intracellular responses of caudate neurons to brain stem stimulation. *Brain Res.,* 22:163–179.
15. Hull, C. D., Bernardi, G., Price, D. D., and Buchwald, N. A. (1972): Intracellular responses of caudate neurons to temporally and spatially combined stimuli. *Exp. Neurol.,* 38:324–336.
16. Hull, C. D., Levine, M. S., Buchwald, N. A., Heller, A., and Browning, R. A. (1974): Spontaneous firing pattern of forebrain neurons. I. The effects of dopamine and nondopamine depleting lesions on caudate unit firing patterns. *Brain Res.,* 73:241–262.
17. Kemp, J., and Powell, T. P. S. (1971): The structure of the caudate nucleus of the cat: Light and electron microscopy. *Philos. Trans. R. Soc. Lond.,* 262:383–401.
18. Kemp, J., and Powell, T. P. S. (1971): The synaptic organization of the caudate nucleus. *Philos. Trans. R. Soc. Lond.,* 262:403–412.
19. Kemp, J., and Powell, T. P. S. (1971): The site of termination of afferent fibres in the caudate nucleus. *Philos. Trans. R. Soc. Lond.,* 262:413–427.

20. Kemp, J., and Powell, T. P. S. (1971): The termination of fibres from cerebral cortex and thalamus upon dendritic spines in the caudate nucleus: A study with the Golgi method. *Philos. Trans. R. Soc. Lond.,* 262:429–439.
21. Kitai, S. T., Sugimori, M., and Kocsis, J. D. (1976): Excitatory nature of dopamine in the nigro-caudate pathway. *Exp. Brain Res.,* 24:351–363.
22. Kling, A., and Tucker, T. J. (1967): Effects of combined lesions of frontal granular cortex and caudate nucleus in neonatal monkey. *Brain Res.,* 6:428–439.
23. Levine, M. S., Hull, C. D., Buchwald, N. A., and Villablanca, J. R. (1974): The spontaneous firing patterns of forebrain neurons. II. Effects of unilateral caudate nucleus ablation. *Brain Res.,* 78:411–424.
24. Lidsky, T. I., Adinolfi, A. M., and Buchwald, N. A. (1975): Development of cortico-caudate connections in kittens. *Anat. Rec.,* 181:2, 410.
25. Lidsky, T. I., Buchwald, N. A., Hull, C. D., and Levine, M. S. (1976): A neurophysiological analysis of the development of corticocaudate connections in the cat. *Exp. Neurol.,* 50:283–292.
26. Olmstead, C. E., Villablanca, J. R., Marcus, R. J., and Avery, D. L. (1976): Effects of caudate nuclei or frontal cortex ablations in cats. IV. Bar pressing and maze learning performance. *Exp. Neurol. (in press).*
27. Smith, K. U. (1951): Discriminative behavior in animals. In: *Comparative Psychology,* 3rd ed., edited by C. P. Stone, pp. 316–362. Prentice-Hall, New York.
28. Soltysik, S., Hull, C. D., Buchwald, N. A., and Fekete, T. (1975): Single unit activity in basal ganglia of monkeys during performance of a delayed response task. *Electroencephalogr. Clin. Neurophysiol.,* 39:65–78.
29. Villablanca, J. R., Marcus, R. J., and Olmstead, C. E. (1976): Effects of caudate nuclei or frontal cortical ablations in cats. I. Neurology and gross behavior. *Exp. Neurol. (in press).*
30. Villablanca, J. R., Marcus, R. J., Olmstead, C. E., and Avery, D. L. (1976): Effects of caudate nuclei or frontal cortex ablations in cats. III. Recovery of limb placing reactions, including observations in hemispherectomized animals. *Exp. Neurol. (in press).*

Brain Dysfunction in Infantile Febrile Convulsions, edited by M. A. B. Brazier and F. Coceani. Raven Press, New York © 1976.

Amygdala and Thermoregulation: Implications for Temporal Lobe Seizures

James N. Hayward

Departments of Neurology and Anatomy, Reed Neurological Research Center, School of Medicine, University of California Los Angeles, Los Angeles, California 90024

The classic studies of Barbour (1) and Isenschmid and Krehl (16) clearly established the hypothalamus as the control center and central temperature sensor in mammalian thermoregulation. Recently Simon and coworkers (22) showed that the spinal cord contains thermosensitive elements which control responses important for thermoregulation. These two areas, hypothalamus and spinal cord, are important for the "physiological" aspects of thermoregulation, whereas many other central nervous system (CNS) areas, including the thalamus (9,10) and the temporal lobes (7,12), may be involved in the "behavioral" aspects of thermoregulation (4).

We chose the unanesthetized monkey as our research subject in order to understand further the role of temporal lobe structures in the physiological and pathological regulation of behavioral and autonomic function. Under pathophysiological states such as temporal lobe seizures, disturbances in autonomic function may occur with alteration in body temperature regulation, cardiovascular function, and neuroendocrine activities (6,7,15). Some autonomic events associated with temporal lobe activity—e.g., elevation in arterial blood and brain temperature, or rises in blood hormone levels or fall in blood osmolality—may trigger temporal lobe seizures (6,7,14,17). A positive feedback perpetuation of seizure activity could result. The transient and random nature of seizure activity, however, makes such phenomena difficult to assess in man. The monkey amygdala, however, with its widespread anatomical (18) and physiological (6,7,15) connections to cortical and subcortical structures, its known activation of behavioral, respiratory, cardiovascular, thermoregulatory, and endocrine effects (6,7,15), and its unique susceptibility to seizure activity (6) is a temporal lobe structure we find very applicable to our study.

AMYGDALA AND CEREBRAL ARTERIAL BLOOD TEMPERATURE

Local temperature changes in the amygdala and other deep brain sites during various behavioral states have been attributed by some authors (5,24) to changes in cerebral blood flow; others opt for the cerebral metabolic heat production that experiments in the cat, dog, and sheep revealed. In five mammalian species — monkey, rabbit, cat, dog, and sheep — we find that the temperature of the cerebral arterial blood perfusing the amygdala and other deep sites determines shifts in brain temperature during changes in behavior (8,12,13). In the monkey, a species that has an internal carotid artery like man, the direct vascular connection between heart and brain is demonstrated when temperature changes in the central arterial blood (Figs. 1 and 2) are

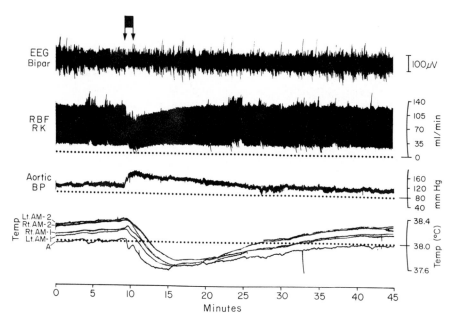

FIG. 1. Thermoregulatory, cardiovascular, and behavioral changes following amygdala stimulation in the unanesthetized monkey (*Macaca mulatta*). Air temperature 20°C. The lateral nucleus of the right amygdala was electrically excited with monophasic square wave pulses at 500 μA, 60 Hz, 1 msec pulse duration for 60 sec (between *arrows*). Stimulation produced tonic turning of the head and eyes to the left, with looking upward and smacking of the lips 1–2 min after cessation of stimulation; apnea occurred during stimulation. The monkey dozed during most of the study, with arousal during amygdala stimulation. Note the EEG low voltage during amygdala stimulation and the abrupt changes: a drop in renal blood flow, elevation in arterial blood pressure, and fall in arterial blood temperature. Sustained poststimulation effects consist of a maintained reduction of renal blood flow for 10–15 min, a 50 mm Hg elevation of arterial blood pressure with a return to normal in 15–20 min, a 0.4°C cooling of arterial blood temperature with a return to normal in 30 min, and a −0.25°C narrowing of the blood-brain gradients, suggesting increased cerebral blood flow with a return to normal in 30 min. EEG Bipar, biparietal electrocorticogram. RBF, RK, pulsatile blood flow in the right renal artery measured by a chronically implanted, noncannulating flow probe (3 mm diameter) of a pulsed-field electromagnetic flowmeter (Statham Instrument Co. model 0-5000) with electronic zero, lead wires from kidney to cranial platform. Aortic BP, silicon cannula in aortic arch. Temp, thermocouples implanted in: Lt. AM-2, left globus pallidus; Rt. AM-2, right globus pallidus; Rt. AM-1, right amygdala; Lt. AM-1, left amygdala; A, aortic arch blood.

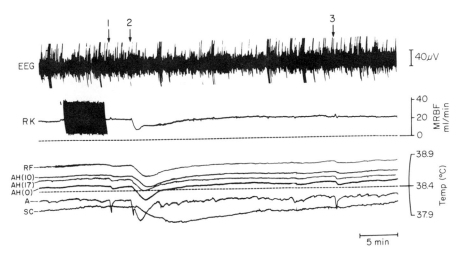

FIG. 2. Thermoregulatory, cardiovascular, and behavioral changes following intravenous infusion of lysine vasopressin in the unanesthetized monkey (*Macaca mulatta*). Air temperature 30°C. Rapid intravenous infusion of 330 mU lysine vasopressin in 3 ml isotonic saline at 20°C (2 *arrow*) produces arousal for 15 min, an abrupt reduction in mean renal blood flow of 10 ml/min for 15 min, an abrupt cooling of arterial blood temperature of −0.35°C, and parallel cooling of brain temperatures of −0.3°C, all returning to baseline within 3–5 min with more prolonged (30–35 min) cooling of subcutaneous tissues. Control injections of 3 ml isotonic saline (20°C) before (1 *arrow*) and after (3 *arrow*) hormone injection produced only a brief (30 sec) reduction (−0.2°C) in arterial blood temperature with minor but parallel reductions in brain temperature and increases in renal blood flow. LVP-induced elevation of arterial blood pressure is not shown in this experiment. Note the absence of any change in the blood-brain thermal gradients following the vasopressin injection. EEG, biparietal electrocorticogram. RK, MRBF, mean renal blood flow of right kidney. Temp, thermocouples implanted in: RF, midbrain reticular formation; AH (10), 10 mm above base of brain; AH (17), 17 mm above base of the brain; AH (0), anterior hypothalamus; A, aortic arch arterial blood; SC, subcutaneous tissues.

followed quickly by parallel shifts in blood temperature at the circle of Willis, in the amygdala, and at other brain sites (Figs. 1 and 2). Recent studies by Brundin (2,3) indicate that in man a close correlation exists between the type of exercise (dynamic versus isometric) and the oxygen uptake and arterial blood temperature.

AMYGDALA TEMPERATURE AND CEREBRAL BLOOD FLOW

In the monkey, amygdaloid temperature increases with arousal and decreases with sleep. These changes follow the earlier temperature changes of the arterial blood that circulates to the brain. Amygdaloid temperature is higher than the entering arterial blood, i.e., medial amygdala +0.27°C and lateral amygdala +0.40°C (12). Because the amygdala's metabolically produced heat is incompletely removed by the flow of cooler blood into the amygdala, the amygdala is warmer than the blood. As a result, a thermal gradient develops, perhaps owing in part to countercurrent heat exchange between arterioles and venules in the amygdala. If we manipulate the system and increase the flow of cooler arterial blood through the amygdala, we might expect the heat produced in the amygdala to be removed more efficiently and the thermal gradient between the arterial blood and amygdala to be narrowed. We induced such an accelerated amygdaloid heat exchange when experimental hypercapnia in our monkeys resulted in increased cerebral blood flow (12). Figure 1 shows that blood-brain gradients narrow from 0.3°C in the control state to 0.1°C after amygdala stimulation. Since such stimulation induces apnea, we speculate that the resultant hypoxia and hypercapnia induce increased cerebral blood flow and accelerated brain heat exchange (7,8,12,13).

AMYGDALA ELECTRICAL STIMULATION

In our unanesthetized monkeys electrical stimulation of the amygdala produced behavioral, respiratory, cardiovascular, thermoregulatory, and endocrine effects (7).

Behavioral effects of amygdala stimulation (Figs. 1 and 3) were arousal, looking around, tonic turning of head and eyes to the opposite side, lip-smacking, chewing, vocalization, retching, and occasionally vomiting (6,7,12,14,15).

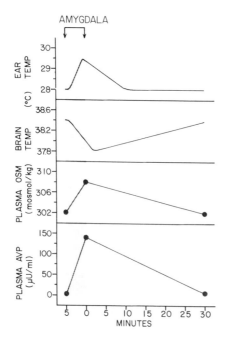

FIG. 3. Thermoregulatory, behavioral, osmotic, and endocrine effects of amygdala stimulation in the unanesthetized rhesus monkey. Air temperature 23°C. Electrical stimulation of the amygdala (*shaded bar* between *arrows*) with monophasic square wave pulses at 600 μA, 60 Hz, 3 msec pulse duration for 30 sec on/off for 5 min produced, during stimulation: arousal, lip-smacking, rotation, apnea, vocalization, retching, and (from top to bottom) a rise in ear skin temperature (+1.75°C), a fall in brain temperature (−0.65°C), a rise in plasma osmolality (+6 mosmole/kg), and a rise in plasma arginine vasopressin (+138 μU/ml) with a prompt return (within 10 min) to baseline for ear skin temperature and within 30 min for the other parameters. Ear Temp, temperature of the skin of the ear. Brain Temp, temperature of the cerebral arterial blood at the circle of Willis. Plasma Osm, plasma osmolality. Plasma AVP, plasma arginine vasopressin.

Respiratory changes induced by amygdala stimulation included apnea during stimulation and tachypnea during the poststimulation period (7,12). These amygdala-induced changes in respiration (6,7,12,15,23) may lead to hypoxia and hypercapnia (19,20) as well as increased cerebral blood flow with accelerated cerebral heat exchange and narrowing blood-brain thermal gradients (Fig. 1) (6,7,12,13).

Cardiovascular events triggered by amygdala stimulation (6,7) include an immediate (stimulus-bound) and delayed (10–30 min) (Fig. 1) elevation in arterial blood pressure with or without tachycardia, bradycardia, and cardiac arrhythmias (6,7,12,19,20). Another amygdala-induced event is an immediate (stimulus-bound) and delayed (10–30 min) (Fig. 1) reduction in renal blood flow (Fig. 1) (7).

Thermoregulatory effects of amygdala stimulation included an abrupt drop in arterial blood and brain temperatures (stimulus-bound) and a delayed (10–30 min), gradual return of these temperatures to control levels (Figs. 1 and 3) (7,12). As described above, there was narrowing of the blood-brain gradients (Fig. 1) (7,12), suggesting an increased cerebral blood flow accompanied by accelerated heat removal from deep brain sites.

Endocrine effects of amygdala stimulation included changes in several anterior pituitary hormones (6,7) and an antidiuretic response (7,14). There was a reduction in urine flow and free water clearance, and a rise in urine osmolality without changes in osmolal and inulin clearances (14). We could not determine whether such an antidiuretic response was due to the release of arginine vasopressin (AVP) from the posterior pituitary, the release of some other pituitary hormone, or an autonomic effect directly on the kidney until we measured plasma AVP levels directly. When we used the radioimmunoassay methods of Robertson et al. (21) and obtained blood before, immediately after, and 30 min after amygdala stimulation (Fig. 3), we found large increases in plasma AVP and plasma osmolality. These increases paralleled the changes—fall and return to baseline—in brain temperature that we had observed previously (Figs. 1 and 3) (7,12). In addition, there is a parallel between these changes in plasma AVP and osmolality (Figs. 1 and 3) and the prolonged elevation of arterial blood pressure and prolonged reduction of renal blood flow (Figs. 1 and 3). Infusion of lysine vasopressin produces an immediate and delayed reduction in renal blood flow (Fig. 2) and an immediate and delayed reduction in arterial blood and brain temperatures (Fig. 2).

CONCLUSIONS

In our earlier studies of amygdala stimulation in the unanesthetized monkey (7,12,14), we used a sensitive index of cutaneous, nasal, arterial blood, and brain temperature in combination with measurement of behavior (electroencephalogram, eye and body movement, and observation), renal blood flow, arterial blood pressure, respiration, urine flow and osmolality, free-water clearance, osmotic clearance, and inulin clearance.

It was readily apparent in these studies that changes in arterial blood temperature were paralleled by changes in amygdala and other deep brain temperatures (7,8,12,13). The blood-brain thermal gradient remained constant except under circumstances where there was a change in cerebral blood flow. Electrical stimulation of the amygdala induced a complex pathophysiological state with behavioral, respiratory, cardiovascular, thermoregulatory, and endocrine effects.

Our recent studies with radioimmunoassay measurements of plasma AVP indicate that the amygdala-induced antidiuretic effect (14) is indeed due to elevation of plasma AVP. In addition, these elevated levels may be responsible for prolonged arousal, prolonged reduction in renal blood flow, prolonged elevation of arterial blood pressure, and prolonged cooling of the arterial blood and brain. These conclusions are based on the observed elevations of plasma AVP over 20–30 min poststimulation and the similar effects of infused lysine vasopressin on behavior, renal blood flow, and arterial blood and brain temperature. The lack of change in the blood-brain gradients during vasopressin infusion indicates that these changes following amygdala stimulation are probably due to apnea, hypoxia, hypercapnia, and increased cerebral blood flow with accelerated heat exchange, rather than to a change in plasma AVP.

The roles such amygdala-induced vasopressin release and the subsequent behavioral, cardiovascular, thermoregulatory, osmotic, and antidiuretic effects play in temporal lobe seizures and their perpetuation remains speculative at present. It is well known that the syndrome of inappropriate release of antidiuretic hormone (SIADH) may occur in patients with seizure disorders and that hypo-osmolar states can result in a reduction in seizure threshold with increased seizure activity (11,17). Further studies are needed to connect the results of these animal studies to clinical problems of temporal lobe seizures.

ACKNOWLEDGMENTS

This review was aided in part by US Public Health Service Grants NS-05638 and NS-10129 from the National Institute of Neurological Disease and Stroke.

The author thanks Ms. R. Lawrence and S. Curtis for valuable technical and editorial assistance.

REFERENCES

1. Barbour, H. G. (1912): Die Wirkung unmittelbarer Erwärmung und Abkühlung der Warmezentra auf die Körpertemperatur. *Naunyn Schmiedebergs Arch.*, 70:1–26.
2. Brundin, T. (1974): The relationship between blood heat flow and oxygen uptake during exercise. *IRCS (Research on: Cardiovascular System; Physiology)*, 2:1044.

3. Brundin, T. (1974): Blood temperature regulation during dynamic versus isometric exercise. *IRCS (Research on: Cardiovascular System; Physiology)*, 2:1390.
4. Cabanac, M. (1972): Thermoregulatory behavior. In: *Essays on Temperature Regulation*, edited by J. Bligh and R. Moore, pp. 19–32. North-Holland Press, Amsterdam.
5. Delgado, J. M. R., and Hanai, T. (1966): Intracerebral temperatures in free moving cats. *Am. J. Physiol.*, 211:755–769.
6. Gloor, P. (1960): Amygdala. In: *Handbook of Physiology, Sect. I: Neurophysiology*, Vol. 2, pp. 1395–1420. American Physiological Society, Washington, D.C.
7. Hayward, J. N. (1972): The amygdaloid nuclear complex and mechanisms of release of vasopressin from the neurohypophysis. In: *Neurobiology of the Amygdala*, edited by B. E. Eleftheriou, pp. 685–749. Plenum Press, New York.
8. Hayward, J. N. (1973): Anatomy of heat exchange. In: *Pharmacology of Thermoregulation*, edited by E. Schönbaum and P. Lomax, pp. 22–41. Karger, Basel.
9. Hayward, J. N. (1975): The thalamus and thermoregulation. In: *Temperature Regulation and Drug Action*, edited by J. Jacob, E. Schönbaum, and P. Lomax, pp. 22–31. Karger, Basel.
10. Hayward, J. N. (1975): Response of ventrobasal thalamic cells to hair displacement on the face of the waking monkey. *J. Physiol. (Lond.)*, 250:385–407.
11. Hayward, J. N. (1975): Neural control of the posterior pituitary. *Ann. Rev. Physiol.*, 37:191–210.
12. Hayward, J. N., and Baker, M. A. (1968): The role of the cerebral arterial blood in the regulation of brain temperature in the monkey. *Am. J. Physiol.*, 215:389–493.
13. Hayward, J. N., and Baker, M. A. (1969): A comparative study of the role of cerebral arterial blood in the regulation of brain temperature in five mammals. *Brain Res.*, 16:417–440.
14 Hayward, J. N., and Smith, W. K. (1963): Influence of limbic system on neurohypophysis. *Arch. Neurol.*, 9:171–177.
15. Kaada, B. R. (1951): Somato-motor, autonomic and electrocorticographic responses to electrical stimulation of "rhinencephalic" and other structures in primates, cat and dog. *Acta Physiol. Scand. (Suppl. 83)*, 23:1–100.
16. Isenschmid, R., and Krehl, L. (1912): Über den Einfluss des Gehirns auf die Wärmeregulation. *Naunyn Schmiedebergs Arch.*, 70:109–134.
17. Millichap, J. G. (1969): Systemic electrolyte and neuroendocrine mechanisms. In: *Basic Mechanisms of the Epilepsies*, edited by H. H. Jasper, A. A. Ward, and A. Pope, pp. 709–726. Little, Brown, Boston.
18. Nauta, W. J. H. (1962): Neural associations of the amygdaloid complex in the monkey. *Brain*, 85:505–520.
19. Reis, D. J., and McHugh, P. (1968): Hypoxia as a cause of bradycardia during amygdala stimulation in monkey. *Am. J. Physiol.*, 214:601–610.
20. Reis, D. J., and Oliphant, M. C. (1964): Bradycardia and tachycardia following electrical stimulation of the amygdaloid region in the monkey. *J. Neurophysiol.*, 27:893–912.
21. Robertson, G. L., Mahr, E. A., Athar, S., and Sinha, T. (1973): Development and clinical application of a new method for the radioimmunoassay of arginine vasopressin in human plasma. *J. Clin. Invest.*, 52:2340–2352.
22. Simon, E. (1974): Temperature regulation: The spinal cord as a site of extrahypothalamic thermoregulatory functions. *Rev. Physiol. Biochem. Pharmacol.*, 71:1–76.
23. Smith, W. K. (1938): The representation of respiratory movements in the cerebral cortex. *J. Neurophysiol.*, 1:55–58.
24. Tachibana, S. (1969): Relation between hypothalamic heat production and intra- and extracranial circulatory factors. *Brain Res.*, 16:405–416.

Brain Dysfunction in Infantile Febrile Convulsions, edited by M. A. B. Brazier and F. Coceani. Raven Press, New York © 1976.

Cellular Activities in Focal Epilepsy

David A. Prince

Department of Neurology, Stanford University School of Medicine, Stanford, California 94305

Since a common consequence of disturbances in the normal patterns of brain maturation is the development of epilepsy, it seems particularly appropriate to discuss some aspects of the pathophysiology of epilepsy in this volume. If the incidence of seizure disorders is 0.5–1% of the world's population, a total of 20–40 million cases of human epilepsy must exist worldwide. Most of these probably originate during childhood or develop at a long latency after some insult to the immature brain. This should provide an overwhelming impetus for investigations of the ontogenetic aspects of epilepsy.

Experimental epilepsy research has been stimulated by observations made in patients with epilepsy which raise many important questions. What are the underlying cellular events which lead to generation of the electroencephalographic (EEG) "spike"? Are these events the same in human epilepsy and in various experimental models, or do they vary from one to the next? Are there differences in the underlying cellular mechanisms, dependent on maturation of the brain, which account for the clinical peculiarities of seizures in infants and children? To what extent do focal epileptiform discharges influence the function of connected areas of brain? This question may be relevant to the general and specific disturbances in behavior sometimes seen in clinical epilepsy. In many patients evidence of focal electrical or behavioral seizures is present, but generalized attacks either rarely or never occur. What are the control mechanisms which exist in the brain to limit the spread of seizure activity in these circumstances? Such questions are only a few of those posed by observation of even a single patient with seizures.

There are other basic questions which deal with the pathophysiology of epilepsy and its effects on the brain. For example, what accounts for the latency from the time of brain injury to the development of epileptic seizures? Do anomolous reconnections form after brain injury? To what extent does denervation supersensitivity occur in neurons of the cortex and contribute to epileptogenesis? Is epilepsy a progressive disease? To what extent does the use of circuits in the brain by abnormal (or normal) discharges influence the development and fundamental properties of those circuits? What accounts for the selective vulnerability of certain areas of the brain to damage during metabolic insult or generalized seizure activity? Most of the underlying issues posed by these questions are no different from those which form the core of modern neurobiological research. I have catalogued them here only to emphasize important areas for present and future study; unfortunately most of the answers are still unknown.

In this chapter I consider three general questions: (a) What is known about the cellular basis for focal epileptogenesis? (b) How does epileptogenesis differ in the immature versus the mature brain? (c) What are the control mechanisms in the brain which limit epileptogenesis? My review of these areas is of necessity selective, relying largely on experiments done in our own laboratories.

CELLULAR BASIS FOR FOCAL EPILEPTOGENESIS

Depolarization Shift

To date intracellular activities have been studied in at least eight varieties of experimental epileptogenic focus (see ref. 60 for review). The remarkable thing about the results of these experiments is the rather stereotyped pattern of neuronal activities encountered among those cells participating in epileptogenesis. Figure 1 illustrates this point. Intracellular recordings from four varieties of focus are shown. In each example, high-amplitude, long-duration intracellular depolarization shifts (DSs) are associated with interictal epileptiform discharges. The amplitude of these events and the frequency of associated spike discharges is highest in acute foci produced by penicillin and strychnine. Also a very high percentage of cells are involved in such acute foci. In more chronic lesions, such as alumina cream foci, uninvolved cells are more frequently found and the "intensity" of the focus is less, as judged by this, by the lower amplitudes of intracellular depolarizations and EEG discharges during epileptogenesis, and by the tendency for decreased synchronization within the involved population resulting in an epileptogenic zone where more than one electrographic focus exists (61). Such chronic foci apparently also differ from those produced by drugs in that some neurons generate rhythmic bursts of spikes with particular spike-interval patterns (11,85). It is not known whether these and other differences between acute and chronic foci indicate different underlying basic cellular abnormalities or merely variations in the intensity of epileptogenesis conditioned in part by the pathological anatomy of the chronic focus. Rhythmic burst generation is an important characteristic of neurons of human epileptogenic cortex (10), a finding which emphasizes the importance of identifying the responsible cellular mechanisms. Figure 1 also shows (right-hand column) that in and around each epileptogenic lesion numerous neurons are found in which large inhibitory postsynaptic potentials (IPSPs) are closely

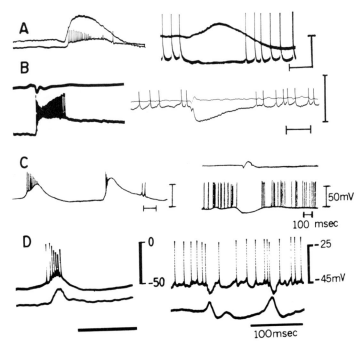

FIG. 1. Intracellular recordings and EEG traces from four types of experimental focus. First column shows neurons which generate prolonged depolarizations and repetitive spikes during each surface epileptiform transient. Second column shows cells which are predominantly inhibited during each surface event. **A:** Freeze focus (27). **B:** Penicillin focus (55). **C:** Strychnine focus (40). **D:** Alumina focus (61). Voltage and time calibrations in second segment of **A** and **B** are for both segments, and all voltage calibrations in **A–C** are 50 mV. All time calibrations: 100 msec. (From Prince, ref. 60.)

associated with interictal EEG discharges. These inhibitory events are considered below.

The characteristics of the DS in various acute foci are quite similar (for review see refs. 1,57,59,60). The depolarizations are very stereotyped and lead to generation of prolonged bursts of spike discharges with frequencies of 500/sec or more in some neurons. These cellular events are temporally coupled to large EEG potentials, which are also stereotyped in their configuration (43,44,54). Both the EEG discharges and cellular events can be evoked by stimulation of appropriate afferents at frequencies of 1–3/sec, and under these circumstances successive potentials are virtually superimposable (43,54). Over time the acute focus undergoes frequent transitions from electrographic interictal to tonic-clonic ictal activity (45).

Several lines of evidence suggest that DSs are probably giant synaptic potentials. First, although these depolarizations generate high-frequency bursts of impulses, they can occur independent of impulse generation, proving that they are not after-potentials of spike discharge (55). Secondly, DSs behave as if they were excitatory synaptic potentials when the membrane potential of the neuron is altered by applying intracellular current pulses (16,46,55). In some experiments neurons have been held long enough to see transitions between normal synaptic events and the large DSs after application of a convulsant drug (45,55). Finally, in immature neurons there are clear transitional forms between excitatory postsynaptic potentials (EPSPs) and DSs (62). These findings do not entirely rule out the possibility that other nonsynaptic mechanisms might contribute to DS generation. Recently it has become clear that large depolarizations resembling DSs can be obtained from cell bodies of invertebrate neurons isolated from possible synaptic influences and exposed to convulsant drugs (77) or to an abnormal ionic environment (5). Thus nonsynaptic alterations of neuronal membranes could play a role in epileptogenesis. The complexity of the cerebral cortex has made it difficult to determine whether abnormalities of membranes are present and contribute to the generation of DSs. Depolarizing pulses delivered through the presumably intrasomatic microelectrode do not elicit DSs (46,55), but this does not eliminate a possible membrane abnormality on distal dendrites at a location unaffected by intrasomatic depolarizing current but easily influenced by synaptic inputs (55,57).

Pathogenesis of the DS

If DSs are in fact giant EPSPs, it seems logical to propose that there must be some abnormality of synaptic function in the focus. The list of possibilities is as long as a sequence of events in synaptic transmission. Several investigators have concluded that cells of the epileptogenic focus function normally because no obvious abnormalities of impulse generation or synaptic events can be recorded from their cell bodies. Owing to the complexities of the mammalian cortex, it has generally not been possible to do the types of quantitative studies which would justify this statement. Further, as already pointed out, there are portions of the neuron (distal dendrites and axon terminals) that cannot be studied adequately with the usual intracellular recordings. Experiments in "simple systems" have shown that even a single epileptogenic agent like penicillin may produce a variety of abnormalities, e.g., depression of IPSPs due to both pre- and postsynaptic effects (47), increases in EPSPs presumably due to effects at the presynaptic terminal (4,22,23), and decreases in presynaptic inhibition (14). Any combination of these effects in an aggregate of neurons with appropriate connections could give rise to DSs and epileptogenesis.

Considerable discussion has taken place with respect to whether epileptogenic properties can reside in a single neuron (an "epileptic" neuron) or only in a group of cells (the "epileptic neuronal aggregate") (e.g., ref. 2). The significant limitations to electrophysiological investigation imposed by the complexity of the mammalian brain make this a difficult question to address with quantitative data in hand. In any case, the issue is more se-mantic than real. Altered response patterns must be present in individual units if an aggregate of neurons is to acquire the capacity for epileptogenesis. Abnormal cell responses cannot occur without leading to an "abnormal utilization of pre-existing neural circuits" (2). Certainly the summations of synaptic currents required to generate the interictal epileptiform EEG "spike" require the participation of an aggregate of neurons, as do the be-havioral changes characteristic of clinical epilepsy.

Recently two mechanisms which might contribute to the generation of DSs in epileptogenic foci—i.e., abnormalities in the function of presynaptic terminals and in the regulation of extracellular potassium ion concentration ($[K^+]_o$)—have been investigated in our laboratories.

Abnormalities of Function of Presynaptic Terminals in Epileptiform Foci

One effective mechanism for increasing the intensity of excitatory synap-tic events involved in generation of DSs would be an abnormality in axonal terminal regions, which would result in more transmitter release. It has been known since the reports of Masland and Wigton (42) and Dun and Feng (19) that certain types of drugs applied to neuromuscular junctions produce abnormalities in presynaptic terminal function that lead to generation of bursts of spikes. These spike bursts may propagate antidromically in the axon and orthodromically to release transmitter at synapses (30). Anti-dromic activity of this sort in the mammalian central nervous system (CNS) has been recorded in dorsal roots after treatment of the spinal cord with guanidine (9) or after injection of strychnine in the area of the cuneate nucleus (82). In both of these circumstances it is known that axoaxonal synapses are present on terminals, so that the antidromic discharge could be the result of synaptic depolarization of terminals. Several years ago Dr. Michael Gutnick and I investigated the possibility that repetitive activity generated in axons or terminals within the epileptic focus might contribute to the intense excitatory activities found there. We reasoned that bursts generated in depolarized terminals might propagate antidromically into cell bodies where they might be detected by means of intracellular record-ings. The experimental setup used to study this phenomenon in thalamo-cortical relay (TCR) cells is represented in Fig. 2. Sixty percent of identified TCR cells in n. ventralis posterolateralis were found to generate bursts with very regular interspike intervals, beginning 30 msec or more after the onset of the cortical interictal epileptiform event and lasting 20–50 msec. On the basis of criteria described elsewhere (32,33), it was proved that these bursts originated in cortical axons or terminals and propagated antidromic-ally into the thalamus. The antidromic burst or "backfiring" phenomenon has now also been demonstrated in relay cells of the lateral geniculate body

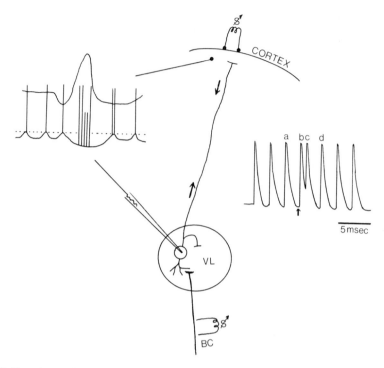

FIG. 2. Experimental setup used to study antidromic burst generation in thalamocortical relay cells. Microelectrode recording from a relay cell in the ventralis lateralis (VL) is identified by orthodromic stimulation of the brachium conjunctivum (BC) and antidromic invasion from stimulation of the cortex. **Inset at left** shows a spontaneous surface epileptiform event with an associated IPSP, and a burst without prepotentials arising below the firing level (*dotted line*). **Inset at right** shows results of a collision experiment in which an antidromic spike (c) is triggered by a stimulus to the cortex (*arrow*), invades the cell body approximately 2 msec after the onset of the preceding spontaneous spike (b), and resets the rhythm of the burst.

(25,72,76) and n. ventralis lateralis (VL) (74) whose axons project to an acute cortical epileptogenic focus. Both strychnine and penicillin were found to produce this effect on VL relay cells. Recently Schwartzkroin et al. (73) found that similar effects occur in callosal neurons whose axons project to the site of a cortical epileptogenic focus.

An example of the "backfiring" phenomena in a VL relay cell whose axon projects into a cortical penicillin focus is shown in Fig. 3. Orthodromic and antidromic stimulation serves to identify the unit as a TCR cell. Most direct cortical stimuli (Fig. 3B–D) elicit a cortical epileptiform potential and a burst of spikes with regular (4–6 msec) intervals (Fig. 3B2; C1–3; D, first stimulus). Bursts of spikes in the neuron arise during an IPSP from below the usual firing level (Fig. 3B2; D, first stimulus). Interposed antidromic spikes (dots in Fig. 3C2–3) can be elicited at a latency less than

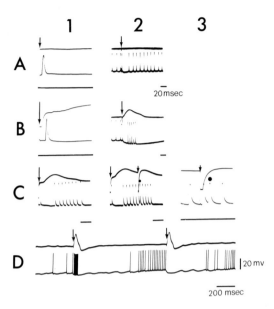

FIG. 3. Ventralis lateralis relay cell antidromically activated during cortical interictal discharges produced by penicillin application. **A1, A2:** Orthodromic activation by BC stimulation. **B1:** Antidromic activation by direct cortical stimulation. Cortical stimulation also triggered an epileptiform event, which was usually accompanied by a burst of spikes (**B2, C, D**). The burst spikes arose from a hyperpolarized membrane level (**B2, D**). **C2, C3:** Antidromic spike was interposed in the burst (spike under dot in **C2** and **C3**). The interval between the known antidromic spike and the preceding burst spike is less than two times the antidromic conduction time, and the interposed spike resets the rhythm of the following spikes in the burst. Arrows in **B–D** indicate direct cortical stimuli. Time calibrations in **A–C** are all 20 msec. Spikes in **A1, B1,** and **D** were retouched for clarity. (From Schwartz-kroin et al., ref. 74.)

twice the antidromic conduction time from the preceding spike in the burst, and these triggered antidromic spikes reset the rhythm of the burst; i.e., the interval between the two burst spikes just preceding the interposed spike was the same as the interval between the interposed spike and the following burst spike. As is seen in Fig. 3D, the phenomenon was not always elicited during interictal discharges, presumably because of blockade at a branch point in the cortical axon or failure of invasion of spikes into the hyperpolarized thalamic cell body.

There are several important implications of these findings. First, there are no known synapses on the terminals of thalamocortical relay cells or callosal neurons. This must mean that nonsynaptic depolarizations of axons or terminals occur during epileptic discharge. If the antidromic bursts originating in one terminal branch propagate orthodromically into the entire terminal arborization of the relay neuron, they may provide a potent mechanism for a large increase in transmitter release as well as synchronization of discharge of groups of neurons contacted by a single axonal arborization (probably in the order of several thousand postsynaptic cells in the case of a thalamocortical relay cell). Direct nonsynaptic depolarization of terminals removes the control of impulse generation (and subsequent transmitter resease) from the cell body; IPSPs and EPSPs no longer modulate cell activities, and the usual integrative activities of the neuron are disrupted. Since the antidromic burst always follows the onset of the cortical interictal discharge, the data to date suggest that such bursts are a consequence rather than a cause of interictal discharge, although they may contribute to the latter portions of the DSs seen in cells of the focus. Antidromic bursts that occurred in the intracortical axons of cortical neurons (e.g., excitatory interneurons) might play an important role in initiating epileptiform discharges. Antidromic burst generation becomes very prominent in some cells during the transition from interictal to ictal activity, suggesting that the phenomenon may have an important role in development of ictal episodes (34). It is not known whether such bursts occur in chronic foci or in cortical axons whose cell bodies are also within the cortex.

The mechanism by which cortical axons or terminals are depolarized is not understood. If the epileptogenic drug (penicillin or strychnine) had a direct action on terminals to produce repetitive spiking following a single orthodromic spike (e.g., ref. 30), one would expect these terminals to generate antidromic bursts unassociated with interictal discharges, e.g., during the course of spontaneous orthodromic thalamocortical spike discharge. In our experiments antidromic bursts unrelated to epilepsy were not noted. The observation that antidromic bursts may develop in a TCR cell during the course of an ictal episode, even though the neuron initially shows only inhibition of spiking with each interictal discharge (e.g., Fig. 4 in ref. 34), also suggests that backfiring may be a consequence of intense neuronal activities and not drug exposure alone. A similar conclusion was reached by Gabor and Scobey (25). A recent report that backfiring occurs in extracellularly recorded geniculocortical relay cells during evoked cortical responses unaccompanied by epileptogenesis (71) awaits confirmation. Although large transcortical currents result from synaptic activities during interictal discharge (26), their latency and time course do not coincide well with those of the antidromic bursts. Also, such currents are not cumulative during a train of "triggered" interictal discharges, whereas the antidromic bursts in TCR cells may develop progressively after a number of discharges (33).

It seems most likely that backfiring results from the depolarizing action on terminals of substances released during epileptiform discharge, e.g., ions or transmitters. For example, backfiring occurs at eserinized neuromuscular junctions, where a direct depolarizing affect of acetylcholine on terminals has been postulated (6,69). Significant changes in the extracellular microenvironment also result from epileptiform activity. Large increases in $[K^+]_0$ do occur during epileptogenesis (24,35,48,66,67, and others) and may be a potential factor in antidromic burst generation (32,33). Disorders of regulation of divalent cations such as calcium and magnesium may prove to be of importance in epileptogenesis (e.g., 5,83); however, no adequate method is yet available for *in vivo* measurement of these ions in cortex.

Potassium and Epileptogenesis

Green (28) proposed that the marked tendency for development of ictal activity in hippocampus might be due to an accumulation of potassium ions in the extracellular spaces during neuronal activity. Such an effect would result in neuronal depolarization, more potassium release, and thus a kind of positive feedback cycle which might ultimately produce an ictal episode. This suggestion received support from findings that significant K^+ was released during epileptogenesis (20,35,66,67,78,79) and reports showing that superfusion of solutions containing high potassium concentrations over the hippocampus may indeed produce epileptiform seizures (87). The potassium accumulation hypothesis was elaborated further by Pollen and Trachtenburg (53) who proposed that abnormalities of glial cell function in areas of cortical injury and gliosis might contribute to the accumulation of extracellular potassium, and by Zuckermann and Glaser (87) who suggested that focal static increases in $[K^+]_0$ might exist in areas of disturbed blood-brain barrier in epileptiform foci. Studies in invertebrates had shown that glial cells are, in effect, excellent potassium electrodes (39,50), and it had been proposed that glia serve as a spatial buffer system for $[K^+]_0$ (38,53). In order to determine whether there are abnormalities of K^+ regulation in epileptogenesis, we studied the changes which occur in $[K^+]_0$ in acute epileptiform foci and compared the kinetics of potassium movement in normal and gliotic cortex.

Figure 4 shows typical changes in $[K^+]_0$ during interictal and ictal discharge in an acute epileptiform focus in rabbit cortex (24). Essentially the same data have been obtained in the cat (48,67). At a latency of 15–60 msec from the onset of each interictal epileptiform spike there is an increase in $[K^+]_0$ from the normal baseline level of 3 mM to two to three times the resting level, followed by a slow fall back to baseline. When interictal discharges occur at frequent intervals, such changes in $[K^+]_0$ summate. During ictal episodes $[K^+]_0$ rises rapidly to a peak of 10–12 mM, plateaus, and begins to decrement slowly even though the discharge continues (Fig. 4). Levels in excess of these are seen only during the development of spreading depressions, when $[K^+]_0$ may reach 40 mM or higher (24,67,81). The onsets of ictal episodes are not related in any simple way to the $[K^+]_0$ level—i.e., there is no $[K^+]_0$ "threshold" level for ictal discharge in neocortex (24,48) or hippocampus (21) as had been proposed (17,28,79). In fact, Lux (41) showed that ictal activity may begin at times when $[K^+]_0$ is *less* than the

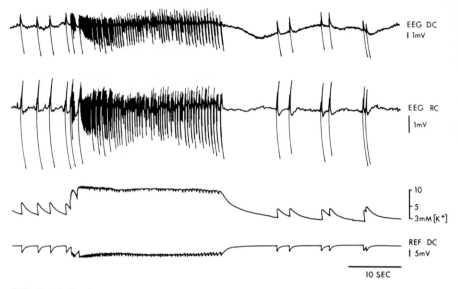

FIG. 4. Interictal and ictal events recorded from a penicillin focus in rabbit cortex. First and second traces: EEGs from cortical surface (EEG DC and EEG RC); third and fourth traces from K⁺-sensitive and reference (REF DC) microelectrodes, respectively, located approximately 1 mm below the pial surface. The ictal episode begins after the fifth interictal discharge. Surface EEG and reference positivity was up. (From Futamachi et al., ref. 24.)

normal 3 mM level. These and other data have led us to conclude that the increases in potassium concentration are always secondary to development of the interictal or ictal discharge. This does not mean that $[K^+]_0$ increases have no affect on excitability of nearby neuronal elements. An increase of $[K^+]_0$ from 3 to 9 or 12 mM would be expected to depolarize neuronal membrane (36) and have other potential effects in cortex (see discussion, ref. 48). Although $[K^+]_0$ increases do not correspond closely in time course to the generation of antidromic bursts in terminals, they could well be a contributing factor.

Our data also do not support the proposal that termination of an ictal episode results from accumulation of $[K^+]_0$ to levels which produce depolarization block in involved elements. As can be seen from Fig. 4, cessation of an ictal discharge may occur at lower than peak $[K^+]_0$ levels. Further, in immature cortex levels much higher than 10 mM $[K^+]_0$ may be reached without a resultant termination of ongoing ictal activity (49). Blockade of transmission in axons would be expected only at $[K^+]_0$ levels of around 30 mM (50). It is possible that increases of $[K^+]_0$ lead to seizure termination by activating electrogenic Na-K pumps in neural elements, which produce a hyperpolarizing block at zones of low safety factor (e.g., branch points in axons and terminals). Such a mechanism was recently demonstrated in the sensory system of the leech where repetitively evoked activity can block conduction in sensory axons (86). Indirect evidence for electrogenic pump activity in cortical neurons during ictal episodes was reported by Ayala et al. (3).

Another important feature of $[K^+]_o$ measurements during epileptogenesis is shown in Fig. 5. There is a distinct laminar profile for $[K^+]_o$ changes in the neocortex during interictal discharges, such that the largest and most rapid changes occur 1,000–1,250 μm below the pial surface. Above and below this level the increments are slower and smaller. Similar laminar analysis of K^+ release in the hippocampus is shown in Fig. 6. In Fig. 6A the site of maximal K^+ release during interictal penicillin-induced discharges in one experiment is marked (the arrow points to an extracellular dye spot). In each experiment the maximal release appeared to occur close to the stratum pyramidale where the cell bodies of pyramidal neurons are located (squares in 6B). Laminar distributions of $[K^+]_o$ changes during ictal discharge in neocortex (48) and hippocampus (21) are similar to those recorded during interictal periods. Differences in K^+ release at various depths have also been demonstrated in the spinal cord (80). When considering the potential effects of elevated $[K^+]_o$ in hippocampus or neocortex, the detailed profiles of potassium concentrations and their relation to local anatomy and physiology must be taken into account. For example, sharp vertical gradients of $[K^+]_o$ with a peak at the cell body layer might induce local current flows because of depolarization of soma relative to dendrites. However, the same distribution of $[K^+]_o$ may also affect inhibitory interneurons or proximal inhibitory synapses, etc., so that no simple relationship between $[K^+]_o$ and cortical excitability should be expected.

In an effort to explain the differences in seizure susceptibility between hippocampus and neocortex as a function of differences in K^+ regulation, we did comparative studies of interictal and ictal ($\Delta[K^+]_o$) in these two structures (21,52). The results are summarized in Table 1. The baseline $[K^+]_o$s were the same. As can be seen, the differences during interictal and ictal

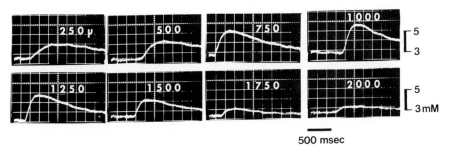

FIG. 5. Representative $[K^+]_o$ responses recorded at depths of 250–2,000 μm below the pial surface in cat pericruciate cortex penicillin focus. (From Moody et al., ref. 48.)

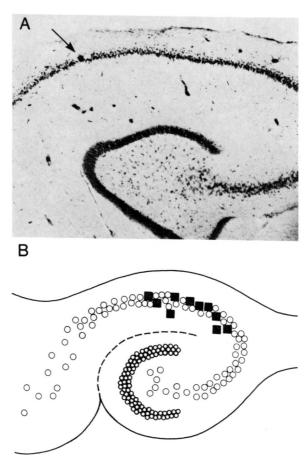

FIG. 6. A: Photomicrograph of typical hippocampal section showing fast green dye mark at the site of maximal $[K^+]_o$ response (*arrow*). **B:** Location of all marks (*black squares*) in relation to the hippocampal cross section. $[K^+]_o$s are maximal in or near pyramidal cell layer. (From Fisher et al., ref. 21.)

TABLE 1. *Comparison of baseline* $[K^+]_o$ *and changes during interictal and ictal activity in penicillin foci of hippocampus and neocortex*

$[K^+]_o$	Hippocampus	Neocortex
Baseline $[K^+]_o$ (mM)	3.7 ± 0.6	3.4 ± 0.4
Interictal $\Delta[K^+]_o$ (mM)	0.8 ± 0.7	1.8 ± 0.8
$\frac{1}{2}$ Rise time $\Delta[K^+]_o$ (sec)	0.3 ± 0.1	0.1 ± 0.1
$\frac{1}{2}$ Fall time $\Delta[K^+]_o$ (sec)	3.2 ± 1.0	0.8 ± 0.2
Rise rate $\Delta[K^+]_o$ (mM/sec)	2.9 ± 2.8	8.5 ± 8.2
Fall rate $\Delta[K^+]_o$ (mM/sec)	0.2 ± 0.1	1.1 ± 0.6
Peak ictal $[K^+]_o$ (mM)	6.9 ± 3.4	9.5 ± 1.6

From Fisher et al., ref. 21.

TABLE 2. *Comparison of baseline $[K^+]_o$, diffusion coefficient for potassium (D), and surface barrier constant (H) in normal and gliotic cortex*

Cortex	Baseline $[K^+]_o$	D (mm²/hr)	H (mm^{-1})
Normal	3.15 ± 0.15	1.03 ± 0.16	0.8 ± 0.1[a]
Gliotic	3.24 ± 0.21	0.93 ± 0.15	0.6 ± 0.2[a]

From Pedley et al., ref. 51.

[a] Difference significant at $p < 0.01$.

electrographic discharges are in a direction opposite those expected if $[K^+]_o$ changes are to account for the increased hippocampal susceptibility to seizures: The increases and peaks of $[K^+]_o$ change in hippocampus tend to be respectively slower and smaller than those in neocortex.

To explore the hypothesis that disturbances in K^+ regulation in gliotic cortex are related to epileptogenesis, we performed experiments in which potassium regulation in normal cortex and cortex made gliotic by freeze lesions was compared. The baseline $[K^+]_o$s in normal and gliotic cortex were not significantly different (Table 2). In order to obtain a measure of the functional capacity of the cortex to deal with an increased potassium load, we studied the movement of K^+ from the pial surface into the cortical depths during superfusion of artificial spinal fluid solutions containing 12 mM K^+. A lower diffusion coefficient for potassium in gliotic cortex would have the effect of favoring a local increase in $[K^+]_o$ adjacent to sites of potassium release. The diffusion coefficient (D) was approximately the same for normal and gliotic cortex. One significant difference between these two preparations was an increased surface barrier (H) to potassium in the gliotic preparation, probably owing to increased pial-glial scarring at the surface of the brain secondary to the freeze lesion. Since the freeze lesions we examined were not actively generating epileptiform activity, the possibility of a disorder in K^+ regulation in chronic epileptogenic foci remains. The results do indicate that gliosis and other changes in blood vessels and neurons in these lesions do not affect resting $[K^+]_o$ levels or $[K^+]_o$ regulation as measured by the superfusion technique.

EPILEPSY IN IMMATURE BRAIN

Clinical and laboratory observations suggest that important differences exist between epileptogenesis in immature versus mature brain. Seizures in infants or young animals tend to be fragmentary and to remain focal; there is often a poor correlation between EEG abnormalities and behavior; and behavioral seizure activity may occur without clear reflection in the EEG (7,8,12,18,29,37,84). The reasons for some of these features are seen very well in recordings from acute experimental epileptiform foci in newborn kittens and rabbits.

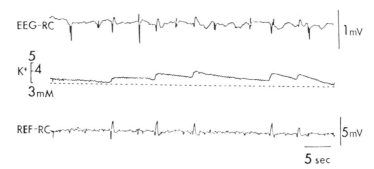

FIG. 7. EEG and $[K^+]_o$ changes during penicillin-induced interictal activity in a 6-day-old rabbit. The dashed line indicates the 3 mM $[K^+]_o$ level. Note that the $[K^+]_o$ response occurs only when interictal discharges are recorded at the reference electrode; discharges recorded only by the surface electrode are not associated with the $[K^+]_o$ increase. EEG discharges vary in amplitude and polarity. EEG-RC: positivity up. REF-RC: positivity down. (From Mutani et al., ref. 49.)

In contrast to the stereotyped synchronous EEG interictal discharges of the acute focus in mature cortex, those in immature brain tend to occur asynchronously in small subsets of the "epileptic neuronal aggregate." This is illustrated in Fig. 7, where recordings from the cortical surface and a site within cortex can be compared. A variety of epileptiform wave forms, polarities, and amplitudes are seen in the EEG, suggesting poor connectivity between different groups of cells, each of which can generate a surface event (see also below and Fig. 9). The recordings from the reference and potassium microelectrodes placed less than a millimeter below the pia show that only

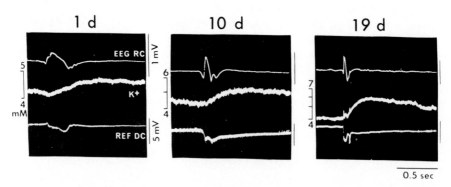

FIG. 8. Representative interictal discharges from penicillin foci in rabbits 1, 10, and 19 days old. The K^+-sensitive electrode was positioned at the cortical depth where the largest K^+ changes were recorded. Note the progressive increase in amplitude and the decrease in duration of the surface spike with age, as well as the associated increase in amplitude and decrease in rise time of the $[K^+]_o$ response. The EEG positivity is down and the reference positivity up. Time calibration is for all segments. Voltage calibrations are 1 mV for the EEG and 5 mV for the reference traces. The $[K^+]_o$ calibrations in millimoles are at the left of each segment. (From Mutani et al., ref. 49.)

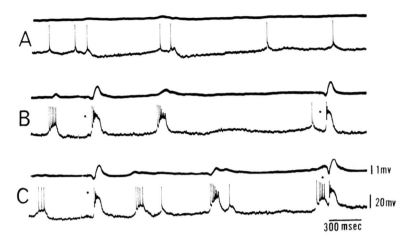

FIG. 9. Intracellular recordings of spontaneous and evoked DSs in a 6-day-old animal. **A:** "Normal" synaptic and spike electrogenesis. In **B** and **C** spontaneous DSs vary in amplitude and rise time, and in their relationship to surface epileptiform waves. The second triggered DS of **C** is evoked during the repolarization phase of a spontaneously occurring DS. Membrane potential: 43 mV. Dots indicate the forepaw stimuli. Microelectrode calibration pulses fall at the end of traces **B** and **C**. (From Prince and Gutnick, ref. 62.)

certain of the surface events are accompanied by a focal discharge in the cortical depth and potassium release at that site. This kind of uncoupling within the cortex could account for situations in which EEG and behavior are dissociated and, in part, for the lack of spread of epileptiform activity in the cortex.

The affects of maturation on interictal EEG discharges are shown in Fig. 8. The surface transient becomes progressively higher in amplitude and shorter in duration with age owing to a greater synchronization of underlying neuronal activity and certain changes in cell behavior described below. The potassium transient in the cortex undergoes a parallel change so that the rise time becomes faster and the amplitude larger. This also reflects a more synchronous discharge in a larger group of neurons.

Several features of the cellular events in immature foci which underlie the relatively low level of epileptogenesis are shown in Figs. 9–11. In contrast to the stereotyped DSs seen in the adult cortex focus, the neurons of kitten cortex show a variety of depolarizations which appear to be loosely coupled to the surface epileptiform events. For example, in Fig. 9 DSs have different amplitudes and relationships to surface epileptiform waves. At times no obvious EEG seizure discharges occur when depolarization and repetitive firing are present in the neuron (first cell discharge of line C). These characteristics of cell activity would be expected from EEG observations such as those of Fig. 7.

In addition to synchrony of discharge, two other important characteristics

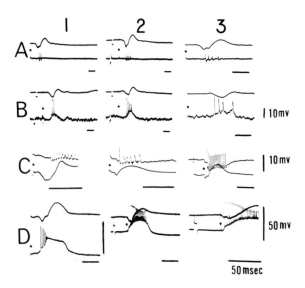

FIG. 10. Comparison of burst activity in immature (**A, B**) and mature (**C, D**) foci. Cell of **A-B** fires bursts of two to four extracellularly recorded spikes at a maximum frequency of approximately 70/sec during triggered epileptiform events in **A.** "Quasiintracellular" recordings of **B** show similar patterns of spike generation. **C1–3** show typical high-frequency extracellular spike bursts in three penicillin foci of adult cats. **D1** and **D2,3:** Intracellular recordings from neurons of two adult foci. Cell of **D2,3** is shown at two sweep speeds. Time calibration is 50 msec in all frames. Animal of **A-B** was 6 days old. EEG traces are DC coupled, positivity down. (From Prince and Gutnick, ref. 62.)

of mature neuronal activities are absent in epileptogenic foci of immature cortex: the capacity to generate (a) spikes at high frequencies and (b) repetitive EPSPs. Typical DSs of immature and mature cortex are shown in Fig. 10. In contrast to the long bursts of spikes which often occur at frequencies of 500/sec or higher in neurons of mature cortex, bursts in cells of immature foci usually contain only a few spikes with much longer interspike intervals. The lower spike frequency is in part related to longer-duration spikes, which may last 5 msec in immature cortex (68); however, even at frequencies far below 200/sec, there tends to be a failure of spike generation toward the end of a brief burst (Fig. 10B3).

The failure of cells in the immature cortex to generate repetitive EPSPs even at relatively low stimulus frequencies is illustrated in Fig. 11. In this typical example from a penicillin focus, the amplitude of EPSPs and the probability of spike firing decreases when the stimulus interval is decreased from 3.2 to 2 sec. When stimuli occur at a rate of 1/sec, the second stimulus in the train and subsequent ones fail to elicit a significant EPSP and fire the cell (Fig. 11D). Also notice in Fig. 11 that although the EPSPs are large in amplitude and of very long duration (ca. 200 msec) they are not effective in generating repetitive spike discharges. Fractionation of an EPSP into several

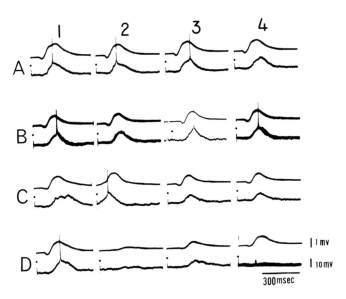

FIG. 11. Forepaw-evoked surface and intracellular responses in penicillin focus to stimulation at intervals of 3.2 (**A**), 2.4 (**B**), 2 (**C**), and 1 (**D1–3**) sec. Superimposed sweeps appear in **B1,2, B4**, and **D4**. The first few responses of a train at each frequency are shown. Frame **C2** illustrates a spontaneous epileptiform transient and corresponding cellular event (note the difference in latency and form of the surface event). **D4:** Field potential after withdrawing the electrode from the cell. Membrane potential, 40 mV; spike height, 43 mV. Rabbit age, 9 days. (From Prince and Gutnick, ref. 62.)

components can be seen in Fig. 11C1. It is probable that an asynchronous input onto the cell accounts for this fractionation and in part for the long duration of potentials seen in other traces. The consequences of these features of neuronal activity for the generation of ictal episodes in the immature cortex are illustrated in Fig. 12. Here, in a 1-day-old rabbit ictal episodes consist of an increase in the frequency of interictal spike discharges without the usual tonic-clonic electrical sequence which typifies the seizure in the adult animal.

Thus the intense synchronization of cell discharge, the tendency for stereotyped generation of prolonged bursts of high-frequency spikes, and the capacity to generate repetitive excitatory synaptic potentials are typical features of "epileptic" neuronal aggregates in the mature cortex not found in the immature brain. The electrographic and clinical features of epilepsy in the immature versus mature brain noted above result from these differences.

Although the discussion thus far has centered around focal epileptiform discharge, other data suggest that sequential changes also occur in the genesis of generalized epileptiform discharge during brain maturation (18). Figure 13 provides an example of such changes. The electrographic char-

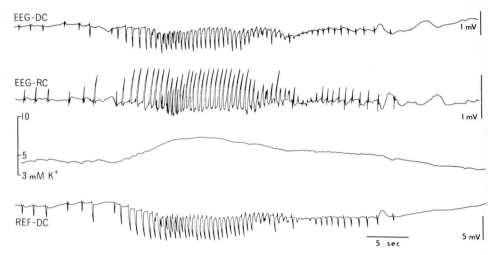

FIG. 12. EEG activities and $[K^+]_o$ increase occurring in a 1-day-old rabbit during an ictal event. Note the slow rise and decay time of the $[K^+]_o$ response, and the absence of a tonic phase during the electrographic seizure. EEG-DC and REF-DC: positivity up. EEG-RC: positivity down. (From Mutani et al., ref. 49.)

acteristics of diffuse epileptiform bursts produced in the adult cat and in kittens of various ages by intramuscular injections of penicillin (250,000 units/kg) are illustrated. In the adult these doses produce well-developed bursts of spike-wave discharges often associated with myoclonic jerks. Behavioral jerks (arrows) also occur in kittens of all ages; however, in the youngest animal (3 days) these are associated with only minimal electrographic signs. The capacity to generate rhythmic spike-wave discharge is still incomplete by 16 days and approaches the adult pattern only after 80 days in this model.

CONTROL MECHANISMS IN EPILEPTOGENESIS

As mentioned above, clinical observations suggest that there are very powerful mechanisms within the brain which limit the frequency and spread of epileptic discharges and the transition from interictal to ictal epileptogenesis. Our knowledge of these mechanisms to date involves mainly those related to synaptic inhibition, although data in experimental foci suggest that other factors may serve to regulate cortical excitability (3,58,70). Figure 14 summarizes several cellular control mechanisms in focal epileptogenesis. A typical DS in a penicillin focus neuron is shown in Fig. 14A. It is the potent high-frequency spike burst output from cells of the focus (including pyramidal tract neurons) which brings powerful and widespread inhibitory actions into play. In the focus (Fig. 14A) these bursts probably activate recurrent inhibitory circuits which in turn evoke prolonged IPSPs on the discharging

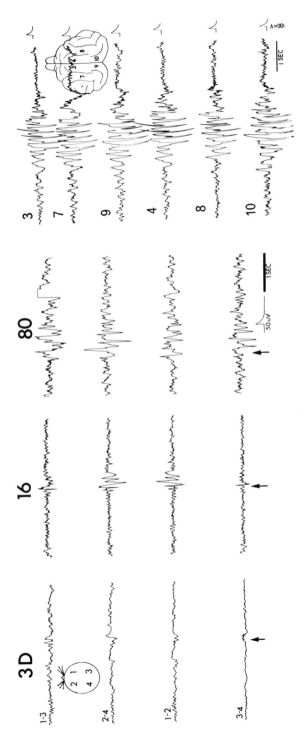

FIG. 13. Generalized epileptiform discharges produced by injecting penicillin (250,000 units/kg) in kittens aged 3, 16, and 80 days, and in an adult animal (last column). Arrows under the bottom traces indicate myoclonic jerks. Recordings in the first three columns are from electrodes as indicated. The time and voltage calibration shown beneath column 3 apply to the first three columns. (From Prince, Logan, and Farrell, *unpublished data.*)

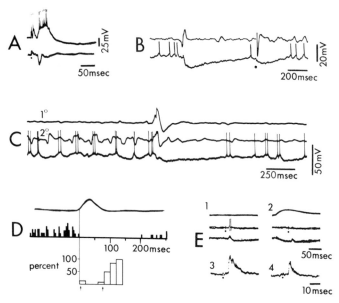

FIG. 14. Inhibition in the penicillin focus and areas of projected epileptiform activity. **A:** DS triggered by nVL stimulation (*dot*) is followed by prolonged hyperpolarization, which has characteristics of an IPSP. **B:** Brief EPSPs and prolonged IPSPs during spontaneous and nVL-triggered (*dot*) epileptiform discharges in a cell of cortex surrounding the penicillin focus. **C:** Synaptic sequence in cell (*bottom trace*) of contralateral homotopic cortex (2°) during an interictal discharge projected from the penicillin focus in the post-cruciate cortex of the cat (1°) (65). **D:** Perievent histogram (45 sweeps; second trace) showing modification of the discharge pattern in a thalamocortical relay cell in nVPL during spontaneous cortical interictal events (upper trace). Bar graph at bottom indicates the percentage of forepaw stimuli which succeeded in evoking a spike in the thalamic cell at various times after onset of the spontaneous surface epileptiform event. Bin width for histogram, 2 msec; bin width for bar graph, 20 msec. Arrows indicate one successful stimulus (31). **E:** Effect of cortical projected epileptiform discharge on relay of forepaw-evoked volleys through cuneate nucleus. **E1:** Superficial radial nerve stimulation evokes pair of spikes in cuneate relay cell (second trace) and negative-positive slow potential from the cuneate surface (bottom trace). **E2:** Surface interictal discharge (upper trace) evokes a positive wave on the cuneate surface; the same nerve stimulus falling during a positive wave fails to evoke discharges from the relay cell. **E3** and **E4:** Volleys recorded in the medial lemniscus following forepaw stimulation under conditions similar to those of **E1** and **E2,** respectively. The time calibration in **E2** is for **E1–2,** and that in **E4** for **E3–4.** (From Prince, ref. 60.)

neurons (16,56) following each DS. The post-DS hyperpolarizations may last up to 600 msec or longer and are associated with significant increases in membrane conductance. They may be reversed by intracellular injection of chloride ions, proving that they are at least in part the result of increased chloride conductance related to the effects of the inhibitory transmitter on the cell membrane (56). Data suggest that these IPSPs actually begin shortly after the onset of the surface epileptiform event, but that their early portions are masked by the concurrent DS. It is possible that other mechanisms such as activation of a sodium-potassium pump contribute to the development of the post-DS hyperpolarization. Some data suggest that prolonged hyperpolarizations which occur in cells during ictal episodes may be a consequence of such pump activities (3). Post-DS hyperpolarizations probably limit the frequency with which interictal epileptogenesis occurs. Since a buildup in the frequency of DSs is a feature of the immediate preictal period, it seems likely that this mechanism serves in part to prevent the development of ictal discharge.

In contrast to the early profound excitation in the neurons of the focus, those in the surrounding cortex show predominantly inhibitory potentials, sometimes preceded by a small excitation (Fig. 14B). "Surround" inhibition, present in both neocortex (63,64) and hippocampus (15), is a mechanism that would serve to prevent the transcortical spread of epileptiform discharges. During the transition from interictal to ictal discharge, the cells of the surround show a gradual loss of the evoked IPSPs, which are replaced by EPSPs, and eventually large DSs similar to those in the center of the focus (64). Similar patterns of brief excitation followed by prolonged IPSPs are regularly seen in neurons of cortex contralateral and homotopic to the site of penicillin application (Fig. 14C) (13,57,65,73).

IPSPs are evoked not only in surrounding and contralateral cortex but also in those subcortical structures which are synaptically connected to the area of discharge. In thalamocortical relay cells of n. ventralis posterolateralis and n. ventralis lateralis of the cat, the predominant event evoked by cortical epileptiform discharge is inhibition (33,74). A typical example of this behavior is shown in Fig. 14D, where spike discharge in a thalamic relay cell ceases for 200 msec after onset of a surface epileptiform event. The available data suggest that burst discharges in corticothalamic axons activate thalamic inhibitory circuits, resulting in IPSPs on relay cells (33). Inhibitory influences of cortical discharge extend even further downstream. When the epileptogenic focus is in sensory cortex, a blockade of transmission is seen even at the first relay station along the sensory pathway in the cuneate nucleus (Fig. 14E). Here it has been shown (75) that corticofugal volleys, probably principally in pyramidal tract axons, decrease the effectiveness of the relay of information through the cuneate as evidenced by depression in both the amplitude and duration of the relayed volley in the medial lemniscus evoked by forepaw stimulation (compare control in Fig. 14E3 with potential in Fig. 14E4, which was conditioned by cortical epileptiform discharge). Orthodromic bursts in cuneate relay cells are either blocked or shortened when they are conditioned by a preceding cortical epileptiform event (compare Fig. 14E1 and E2). This effect is mediated by postsynaptic inhibition on cuneate relay cells and presynaptic inhibition of dorsal column afferents in the cuneate nucleus, both evoked by the corticofugal epileptiform discharge.

The results of these studies on the distant effects of epileptiform activity indicate that each interictal discharge produces a widespread inhibition in populations that are presynaptic to the cortical epileptiform focus. In a sense this diffuse inhibition is deafferenting the focus and preventing the buildup of excitatory events by depressing specific afferent input. In another sense, however, the focal epileptiform discharge is producing, through this inhibition, a very widespread disorder in function throughout the brain since neurons which are inhibited are temporarily unavailable for normal activities. It is tempting to suggest that this widespread inhibitory action might produce behavioral disturbances of various sorts in situations where very active interictal epileptogenesis is ongoing.

CONCLUSION

The data presented demonstrate that the common event in neurons of various epileptogenic foci during interictal epileptogenesis is a large synaptic depolarization which generates a high-frequency burst of impulses. This intense output plus the capacity to generate repetitive synaptic potentials in an anatomically connected neuronal group forms the substrate for epileptogenesis. These elements are not present in immature cortex, where fully developed seizures do not occur. Drugs which produce large depolarization shifts have the capacity to increase excitatory synaptic potentials and decrease inhibition in simple systems and presumably in the cortex. These abnormalities plus others (e.g., repetitive firing of terminals and changes in the ionic environment) may contribute to epileptogenesis in the mammalian brain. The intense output of the epileptogenic focus activates inhibitory mechanisms locally, in adjacent cortex, and at more distant cortical and subcortical sites. This inhibition in turn decreases the input to the focus. The brain may pay a price for this type of control, which makes large aggregates of neurons at many sites unavailable for their normal activities following each interictal discharge. In a sense these remote neuronal organizations are as much a part of the process of epileptogenesis as the cells at the site of the local injury. Even in the simplest model system more than one basic cause for enhanced excitability may be present, and it is likely that human epileptogenesis is not a "single-deficit" condition but rather the result of an alteration of many types of regulatory process in various combinations.

ACKNOWLEDGMENTS

The author gratefully acknowledges the secretarial assistance of Ms. Geraldine Pickering. I am grateful to Robert Fisher, Kin Futamachi, Michael Gutnick, William Moody, Roberto Mutani, Jeffrey Noebels, Philip Schwartzkroin, and Hans van Duijn for their important contributions to this research. This work was supported by USPHS Grants NS 06477 and NS 12151 from the NINCDS, and the Morris Research Fund.

REFERENCES

1. Ajmone Marsan, C. (1969): Acute effects of topical epileptogenic agents. In: *Basic Mechanisms of the Epilepsies*, edited by H. H. Jasper, A. A. Ward, and A. Pope, pp. 299–328. Little, Brown, Boston.

2. Ayala, G. F., Dichter, M., Gumnit, R. J., Matsumoto, H., and Spencer, W. A. (1973): Genesis of epileptic interictal spikes: New knowledge of cortical feedback systems suggests a neurophysiological explanation of brief paroxysms. *Brain Res.,* 52:1–17.

3. Ayala, G. F., Matsumoto, H., and Gumnit, R. J. (1970): Excitability changes and inhibitory mechanisms in neocortical neurons during seizures. *J. Neurophysiol.,* 33:73–85.

4. Ayala, G. F., Spencer, W. A., and Gumnit, R. J. (1971): Penicillin as an epileptogenic agent: Effect on an isolated synapse. *Science,* 171:915–917.

5. Barker, J. L., and Gainer, H. (1974): Bursting pacemaker potential activity in a normally silent neuron. *Brain Res.,* 65:516–520.

6. Barstad, J. A. B. (1962): Presynaptic effect of the neuro-muscular transmitter. *Experientia,* 18:579–581.

7. Bernhard, C. G., Kaiser, I. H., and Kolmodin, G. M. (1962): On the epileptogenic properties of the fetal brain: An electrophysiological study on the electrically and chemically induced convulsive brain activity in sheep fetuses. *Acta Paediatr.* (*Uppsala*), 51:81–87.

8. Bishop, E. J. (1950): The strychnine spike as a physiological indicator of cortical maturity in the postnatal rabbit. *Electroencephalogr. Clin. Neurophysiol.,* 2:309–315.

9. Brooks, C. McC., and Koizumi, K. (1956): Origin of the dorsal root reflex. *J. Neurophysiol.,* 19:61–74.

10. Calvin, W. H., Ojemann, G. A., and Ward, A. A., Jr. (1973): Human cortical neurons in epileptogenic foci: Comparison of inter-ictal firing patterns to those of "epileptic" neurons in animals. *Electroencephalogr. Clin. Neurophysiol.,* 34:337–351.

11. Calvin, W. H., Sypert, G. W., and Ward, A. A., Jr. (1968): Structured timing patterns within bursts of epileptic neurons in undrugged monkey cortex. *Exp. Neurol.,* 21:535–549.

12. Caveness, W. F. (1969): Ontogeny of focal seizures. In: *Basic Mechanisms of the Epilepsies*, edited by H. H. Jasper, A. A. Ward, Jr., and A. Pope, pp. 517–534. Little, Brown, Boston.

13. Crowell, R. M. (1970): Distant effects of a focal epileptogenic process. *Brain Res.,* 18:137–154.

14. Davidoff, R. A. (1972): Penicillin and presynaptic inhibition in the amphibian spinal cord. *Brain Res.,* 36:218–222.

15. Dichter, M., and Spencer, W. A. (1969): Penicillin-induced interictal discharges from the cat hippocampus. I. Characteristics and topographical features. *J. Neurophysiol.,* 32:649–662.

16. Dichter, M., and Spencer, W. A. (1969): Penicillin-induced interictal discharges from the cat hippocampus. II. Mechanisms underlying origin and restriction. *J. Neurophysiol.,* 32:663–687.

17. Dichter, M. A., Herman, C. J., and Selzer, M. (1972): Silent cells during interictal discharges and seizures in hippocampal penicillin foci. Evidence for the role of extracellular K^+ in the transition from the interictal state to seizures. *Brain Res.,* 48:173–183.

18. Dreyfus-Brisac, C., and Monod, N. (1964): Electroclinical studies of status epilepticus and convulsions in the newborn. In: *Neurological and Electroencephalographic Correlative Studies in Infancy*, edited by P. Kellaway and I. Petersén, pp. 250–271. Grune & Stratton, New York.

19. Dun, F. T., and Feng, T. P. (1940): Studies on the neuromuscular junction. XIX. Retrograde discharges from motor nerve endings in veratrinized muscle. *Chin. J. Physiol.,* 15:405–432.

20. Fertziger, A. P., and Ranck, J. B., Jr. (1970): Potassium accumulation in interstitial space during epileptiform seizures. *Exp. Neurol.,* 26:571–585.

21. Fisher, R. S., Pedley, T. A., Moody, W. J., Jr., and Prince, D. A. (1976): The role of extracellular potassium in hippocampal epilepsy. *Arch. Neurol.,* 33:76–83.

22. Futamachi, K. J., and Prince, D. A. (1971): The effects of penicillin on crayfish neuromuscular junction. *Fed. Proc.,* 30:323.

23. Futamachi, K. J., and Prince, D. A. (1976): Effect of penicillin on an excitatory synapse. *Brain Res.,* 100:589–597.

24. Futamachi, K. J., Mutani, R., and Prince, D. A. (1974): Potassium activity in rabbit cortex. *Brain Res.*, 75:5–25.
25. Gabor, A. J., and Scobey, R. P. (1975): Spatial limits of epileptogenic cortex: Its relationship to ectopic spike generation. *J. Neurophysiol.*, 38:395–404.
26. Gleason, C. A. (1971): The effects of applied direct current fields on electrical activity in cat cortex. Ph.D. dissertation, Stanford University, Stanford, California.
27. Goldensohn, E. S., and Purpura, D. P. (1963): Intracellular potentials of cortical neurons during focal epileptogenic discharges. *Science*, 139:840–842.
28. Green, J. D. (1964): The hippocampus. *Physiol. Rev.*, 44:501–608.
29. Grossman, C. G. (1955): Electro-ontogenesis of cerebral activity: Forms of neonatal responses and their recurrence in epileptic discharges. *Arch. Neurol. Psychiatry*, 74:186–202.
30. Grundfest, H., and Reuben, J. P. (1961): Neuromuscular synaptic activity in lobster. In: *Nervous Inhibition*, edited by E. Florey, p. 92. Pergamon Press, London.
31. Gutnick, M. J. (1972): Effects of epileptiform discharge on neuronal activities in the ventrobasal complex of the thalamus of the cat. Ph.D. dissertation, Stanford University, Stanford, California.
32. Gutnick, M. J., and Prince, D. A. (1972): Thalamocortical relay neurons: Antidromic invasion of spikes from a cortical epileptogenic focus. *Science*, 176:424–426.
33. Gutnick, M. J., and Prince, D. A. (1974): Effects of projected cortical epileptiform discharges on neuronal activities in cat VPL. I. Interictal discharge. *J. Neurophysiol.*, 37:1310–1327.
34. Gutnick, M. J., and Prince, D. A. (1975): Effects of projected cortical epileptiform discharges on neuronal activities in ventrobasal thalamus of the cat: Ictal discharge. *Exp. Neurol.*, 46:418–431.
35. Hotson, J. R., Sypert, G. W., and Ward, A. A., Jr. (1973): Extracellular potassium concentration changes during propagated seizures in neocortex. *Exp. Neurol.*, 38:20–26.
36. Huxley, A. F., and Stampfli, R. (1951): Effect of potassium and sodium on resting and action potentials of single myelinated nerve fibers. *J. Physiol. (Lond.)*, 112:496–508.
37. Kolmodin, G. M., and Meyerson, B. A. (1966): Ontogenesis of paroxysmal cortical activity in fetal sheep. *Electroencephalogr. Clin. Neurophysiol.*, 21:589–600.
38. Kuffler, S. W., and Nicholls, J. G. (1966): The physiology of neuroglial cells. *Ergeb. Physiol.*, 57:1–90.
39. Kuffler, S. W., Nicholls, J. G., and Orkand, R. K. (1966): Physiological properties of glial cells in the central nervous system of amphibia. *J. Neurophysiol.*, 29:768–787.
40. Li, C. L. (1959): Cortical intracellular potentials and their responses to strychnine. *J. Neurophysiol.*, 22:436–450.
41. Lux, H. D. (1974): The kinetics of extracellular potassium: Relation to epileptogenesis. *Epilepsia*, 15:375–393.
42. Masland, R. L., and Wigton, R. S. (1940): Nerve activity accompanying fasciculation produced by prostigmin. *J. Neurophysiol.*, 3:269–275.
43. Matsumoto, H. (1964): Intracellular events during the activation of cortical epileptiform discharges. *Electroencephalogr. Clin. Neurophysiol.*, 17:294–307.
44. Matsumoto, H., and Ajmone Marsan, C. (1964): Cortical cellular phenomena in experimental epilepsy: Ictal manifestations. *Exp. Neurol.*, 9:305–326.
45. Matsumoto, H., and Ajmone Marsan, C. (1964): Cortical cellular phenomena in experimental epilepsy: Interictal manifestations. *Exp. Neurol.*, 9:286–304.
46. Matsumoto, H., Ayala, G. F., and Gumnit, R. J. (1969): Neuronal behavior and triggering mechanism in cortical epileptic focus. *J. Neurophysiol.*, 32:688–703.
47. Meyer, H., and Prince, D. A. (1973): Convulsant actions of penicillin effects on inhibitory mechanisms. *Brain Res.*, 53:477–482.
48. Moody, W. J., Jr., Futamachi, K. J., and Prince, D. A. (1974): Extracellular potassium activity during epileptogenesis. *Exp. Neurol.*, 42:248–263.
49. Mutani, R., Futamachi, K. J., and Prince, D. A. (1974): Potassium activity in immature cortex. *Brain Res.*, 75:27–39.
50. Orkand, R. K., Nicholls, J. G., and Kuffler, S. W. (1966): Effect of nerve impulses on the membrane potential of glial cells in the central nervous system of amphibia. *J. Neurophysiol.*, 29:788–806.

51. Pedley, T. A., Fisher, R. S., and Prince, D. A. (1976): Focal gliosis and potassium movement in mammalian cortex. *Exp. Neurol.,* 50:346–361.
52. Pedley, T. A., Fisher, R. S., Moody, W. J., Jr., Futamachi, K. J., and Prince, D. A. (1974): Extracellular potassium activity during epileptogenesis: A comparison between neocortex and hippocampus. *Trans. Am. Neurol. Assoc.,* 99:41–45.
53. Pollen, D. A., and Trachtenberg, M. C. (1970): Neuroglia: Gliosis and focal epilepsy. *Science,* 167:1252–1253.
54. Prince, D. A. (1966): Modification of focal cortical epileptogenic discharge by afferent influences. *Epilepsia,* 7:181–201.
55. Prince, D. A. (1968): The depolarization shift in "epileptic" neurons. *Exp. Neurol.,* 21:467–485.
56. Prince, D. A. (1968): Inhibition in "epileptic" neurons. *Exp. Neurol.,* 21:307–321.
57. Prince, D. A. (1969): Discussion: Microelectrode studies of penicillin foci. In: *Basic Mechanisms of the Epilepsies,* edited by H. H. Jasper, A. A. Ward, and A. Pope, pp. 320–328. Little, Brown, Boston.
58. Prince, D. A. (1971): Cortical cellular activities during cyclically occurring interictal epileptiform discharges. *Electroencephalogr. Clin. Neurophysiol.,* 31:469–484.
59. Prince, D. A. (1972): Topical convulsant drugs and metabolic antagonists. In: *Experimental Models of Epilepsy,* edited by D. P. Purpura, J. K. Penry, D. Tower, D. M. Woodbury, and R. Walter, pp. 51–83. Raven Press, New York.
60. Prince, D. A. (1974): Neuronal correlates of epileptiform discharges and cortical DC potentials. In: *Handbook of Electroencephalography and Clinical Neurophysiology,* Vol. 2, edited by O. Creutzfeldt. pp. 2C56–2C70. Elsevier, Amsterdam.
61. Prince, D. A., and Futamachi, K. J. (1970): Intracellular recordings from chronic epileptogenic foci in the monkey. *Electroencephalogr. Clin. Neurophysiol.,* 29:496–510.
62. Prince, D. A., and Gutnick, M. (1972): Neuronal activities in epileptogenic foci of immature cortex. *Brain Res.,* 45:455–468.
63. Prince, D. A., and Wilder, B. J. (1966): "Surround" inhibition in cortical epileptogenic foci. *Trans. Am. Neurol. Assoc.,* 91:14–18.
64. Prince, D. A., and Wilder, B. J. (1967): Control mechanisms in cortical epileptogenic foci: "Surround" inhibition. *Arch. Neurol.,* 16:194–202.
65. Prince, D. A., Futamachi, K. J., and Gleason, C. (1968): Cortical synaptic activities during projected epileptiform discharges. In: *Proceedings: 24th International Congress, Physiological Society,* Abstract 1065.
66. Prince, D. A., Lux, H. D., and Neher, E. (1972): Potassium activity in cat cortex measured with ion-sensitive microelectrodes. *Trans. Am. Neurol. Assoc.,* 97:24–28.
67. Prince, D. A., Lux, H. D., and Neher, E. (1973): Measurement of extracellular potassium activity in cat cortex. *Brain Res.,* 50:489–495.
68. Purpura, D. P., Shofer, R. J., and Scarff, T. (1965): Properties of synaptic activities and spike potentials of neurons in immature neocortex. *J. Neurophysiol.,* 28:925–942.
69. Randić, M., and Straughan, D. W. (1964): Antidromic activity in the rat phrenic nerve-diaphragm preparation. *J. Physiol. (Lond.),* 173:130–148.
70. Ransom, B. R. (1974): Behavior of presumed glial cells during seizure discharge in cat cerebral cortex. *Brain Res.,* 69:83–99.
71. Rosen, A. D. (1975): Antidromic activity during the evoked cortical response. In: *Neuroscience Abstracts,* Abstract 102.
72. Rosen, A. D., Vastola, E. F., and Hildebrandz, J. M. (1973): Visual radiation activity during a cortical penicillin discharge. *Exp. Neurol.,* 40:1–11.
73. Schwartzkroin, P. A., Futamachi, K. J., Noebels, J. L., and Prince, D. A. (1975): Transcallosal effects of a cortical epileptiform focus. *Brain Res.,* 99:59–68.
74. Schwartzkroin, P. A., Mutani, R., and Prince, D. A. (1975): Orthodromic and antidromic effects of a cortical epileptiform focus on ventrolateral nucleus of the cat. *J. Neurophysiol.,* 38:795–811.
75. Schwartzkroin, P. A., van Duijn, H., and Prince, D. A. (1974): Effects of projected cortical epileptiform discharges on unit activity in the cat cuneate nucleus. *Exp. Neurol.,* 43:106–123.
76. Scobey, R. P., and Gabor, A. J. (1975): Ectopic action potential generation in epileptogenic cortex. *J. Neurophysiol.,* 38:383–394.

77. Speckmann, E. J., and Caspers, H. (1973): Paroxysmal depolarization and changes in action potentials induced by pentylenetetrazol in isolated neurons of Helix pomatia. *Epilepsia,* 14:397–408.
78. Sypert, G. W., and Ward, A. A., Jr. (1971): Unidentified neuroglia potentials during propagated seizures in neocortex. *Exp. Neurol.,* 33:239–255.
79. Sypert, G. W., and Ward, A. A., Jr. (1974): Changes in extracellular potassium activity during neocortical propagated seizures. *Exp. Neurol.,* 45:19–41.
80. Vyklický, L., Syková, E., Kříž, N., and Ujec, E. (1972): Post-stimulation changes of extracellular potassium concentration in the spinal cord of the rat. *Brain Res.,* 45:608–611.
81. Vyskočil, F., Kříž, N., and Bureš, J. (1972): Potassium-selective microelectrodes used for measuring the extracellular brain potassium during spreading depression and anoxic depolarization in rats. *Brain Res.,* 39:255–259.
82. Wall, P. D., McCulloch, W. S., Lettvin, J. Y., and Pitts, W. H. (1955): Effects of strychnine with special reference to spinal afferent fibres. *Epilepsia,* 4:29–40.
83. Wilson, W. A. (1975): Postsynaptic effects of divalent cations. In: *Neuroscience Abstracts,* Abstract 1112.
84. Wright, F. S., and Bradley, W. E. (1968): Maturation of epileptiform activity. *Electroencephalogr. Clin. Neurophysiol.,* 25:259–265.
85. Wyler, A. R., Fetz, E. E., and Ward, A. A., Jr. (1973): Spontaneous firing patterns of epileptic neurons in the monkey motor cortex. *Exp. Neurol.,* 40:567–585.
86. Yau, K-W. (1975): Conduction block at branch points of sensory neurons in the leech CNS. In: *Neuroscience Abstracts,* Abstract 910.
87. Zuckermann, E. C., and Glaser, G. H. (1968): Hippocampal epileptic activity induced by localized ventricular perfusion with high-potassium cerebrospinal fluid. *Exp. Neurol.,* 20:87–110.

Brain Dysfunction in Infantile Febrile Convulsions, edited by M. A. B. Brazier and F. Coceani. Raven Press, New York © 1976.

Secondary Pathology of Febrile and Experimental Convulsions

Brian S. Meldrum

Department of Neurology, Institute of Psychiatry, London SE5 8AF, England

Febrile convulsions are usually nonlethal, so that evidence of the pathology associated with them is not normally available. In the rare cases when death occurs within a few hours or days of a febrile convulsion, the primary (and any intercurrent) illnesses are presumably severe and cerebral sequelae of such illness must be distinguished from pathology secondary to the convulsion. Although clinically it is sometimes difficult to distinguish febrile convulsions (with neurological sequelae) from convulsions secondary to bacterial or viral infection (with some degree of meningoencephalitis), this distinction is readily made at postmortem from the presence of neutrophilic leucocytes, lymphocytes, and plasma cells.

The problem that perplexes the pathologist is whether anoxic-ischaemic damage in a subject having suffered from convulsions should be attributed to the seizures or to cerebral hypoxia, oligaemia, or hypoglycaemia occurring independently. Using the microscope alone it is not possible to differentiate the cerebral pathology in a child dying after a prolonged febrile convulsion from that due to cerebral hypoxia.

PATHOLOGY OF FEBRILE CONVULSIONS/STATUS EPILEPTICUS

There have been numerous descriptions (8,12,34,36,37,40,47) of the cerebral pathology in children dying after prolonged febrile convulsions. The following case history may serve as a representative example.

A 5-month-old boy was admitted to the hospital with a diagnosis of bronchopneumonia; his rectal temperature was 105.5°F (40.8°C), and he convulsed during the initial clinical examination. He had frequent rigid episodes and convulsions throughout the following 24 hr and died 5 days later. At autopsy there was no evidence of meningitis or encephalitis. Microscopic examination revealed ischaemic nerve cell change in all areas of the cerebral cortex, associated with reactive astrocytosis. This commonly took the form of a laminar necrosis involving especially the third layer (Fig. 1); the frontal and occipital areas were more severely affected than the temporal lobes. Bilaterally, acute Ammon's horn necrosis was characterised by loss of

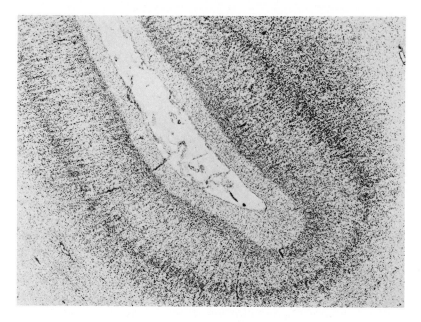

FIG. 1. Laminar necrosis in depth of a sulcus in the neocortex of a 5-month-old boy dying 5 days after prolonged febrile convulsions. Nissl stain. ×25.

neurones of the pyramidal cell layer in the h_1 or Sommer sector, with a proliferation of glia in this layer and in the subjacent white matter (Fig. 2). In the cerebellum there was a widespread loss of Purkinje cells, leaving "empty baskets" (Fig. 3) with a proliferation of Bergmann glia (astrocytes).

This picture of ischaemic nerve cell change, neuronal loss, and glial proliferation involving the brain areas that are selectively vulnerable to all types of hypoxia is typical of children dying a few days after prolonged convulsions.

With very short survivals, a glial reaction is absent and classic ischaemic neuronal changes as described by Spielmeyer (42) are the predominant finding. These histological appearances are seen after any severe disturbance of cerebral energy metabolism, e.g., profound arterial hypotension, cardiac arrest, cerebral ischaemia, or severe hypoglycaemia (5). With survivals of a week or so, neuronophagia is evident and subsequently later stages of the gliomesodermal reaction are seen with the ultimate appearance of lipid phagocytes. These histological changes are of course the accompaniment of the macroscopic atrophy of the neocortex and cerebellum that may be radiographically apparent (1). Other brain areas that sometimes show neuronal loss and a glial reaction include the thalamus (especially the anterior nuclei), the amygdala and uncus, the basal ganglia, and inferior olives.

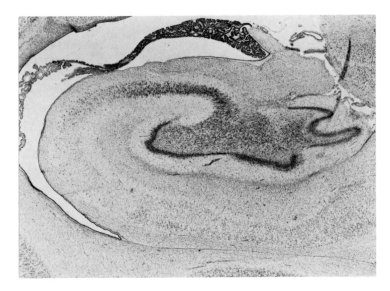

FIG. 2. Hippocampus from same case as Fig. 1, showing preservation of pyramidal neurones in the h_2 sector and their almost total loss in the Sommer sector. Glial proliferation is very marked in the white matter lying between the dentate fascia and the h_1 sector. Nissl stain. ×16.

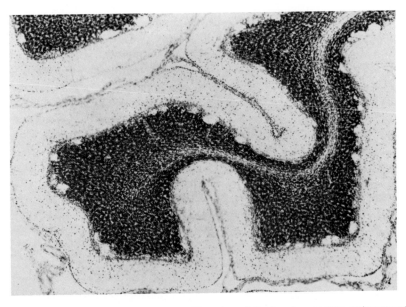

FIG. 3. Cerebellum from same case as Figs. 1 and 2, showing spaces subsequent to Purkinje cell loss ("empty baskets") and the appearance of clusters of Bergmann glia in the overlying molecular layer. Nissl stain. ×70.

PATHOGENESIS OF BRAIN DAMAGE–EXPERIMENTAL STUDIES

As clearly stated by Spielmeyer (43,44), the lesions, both in their cellular type and their distribution, are typical of cerebral hypoxia. Evidently one might conclude, as did Spielmeyer and Scholz (40,41), that cerebral hypoxia occurring in relation to the status epilepticus is responsible for the brain damage. However, there are two difficulties about this attractively simple view. Clinical studies have not provided the quantitative data necessary to permit evaluation of the contribution due to events early and late in status or during the postictal period. Animal experimental studies in which the oxygenation of cerebral venous blood or of the cortex was measured during seizures have frequently shown that the venous oxygen tension or cortical redox potential rises rather than falls (35,38). However, recent experimental studies in subhuman primates have clarified this situation (22,25,26,29).

Physiological changes were monitored during and after prolonged seizures induced by the alkaloid bicuculline and their severity correlated with the ultimate cerebral pathology. In adolescent baboons undergoing seizures lasting 1.5–5 hr, early ictal events (which included marked rises in arterial and cerebral venous pressure, and mild systemic hypoxia) showed no correlation with the ultimate incidence of ischaemic neuronal changes (but might have contributed to the occurrence of petechial haemorrhages).

Events occurring late in the seizures (30–300 min) did correlate with neuronal damage. Most significant were the duration of electroencephalographic (EEG) seizure activity, the degree and duration of hyperpyrexia, the severity and duration of arterial hypotension, and the severity of hypoglycaemia. The hyperpyrexia and arterial hypotension appeared to be most relevant to the cerebellar damage, especially as this was accentuated at the boundary zone between the two major arterial territories in the cerebellum.

Hyperpyrexia, which can raise the cerebral metabolic rate by as much as 25% (32) is itself capable of inducing cerebellar lesions (15), and profound arterial hypotension can induce arterial boundary zone lesions in the cerebellum (5). In such generalised seizures, direct effects of the abnormal cerebral activity cannot be separated from secondary consequences of the autonomic and motor disturbances associated with the seizures. However, if animals are paralysed and artificially ventilated, the secondary consequences of prolonged cerebral seizure discharges are largely prevented. In such circumstances cerebellar pathology is no longer found. However, provided the seizures are sufficiently sustained (3.5–7.5 hr in adolescent baboons), ischaemic neuronal changes still occur in the neocortex, thalamus, and hippocampus.

The increased energy demand of the epileptic discharges themselves thus appears to be making an important contribution to the pathogenesis of the lesions. Although this concept has been frequently referred to by previous authors–e.g., "consumptive hypoxia" of Scholz (40,41)–accurate measurements of the enhanced metabolic rate due to seizure activity have not so far been available. However, in recent experiments (6,27) we determined cerebral blood flow in rats during status epilepticus induced by bicuculline, and from measurements of cerebral arteriovenous difference in total oxygen content we calculated the cerebral metabolic rate for oxygen (Table 1).

After seizure activity is sustained for 20–120 min, cerebral blood flow is three to four times normal, although it can be as high as nine times normal during the first few minutes of seizure activity. The cerebral arteriovenous difference for oxygen is lower than normal throughout the seizure, so the proportional increase in cerebral metabolic rate is less than that in cerebral blood flow. However, a two- to threefold increase in metabolic rate for oxygen was sustained throughout the 2-hr seizure period. Previous reports that indicated an increase of less than 100% during shorter seizure periods (38,39) apparently underestimated the increase, probably because of inadequate maintainance of physiological state of the experimental animals.

During the first few minutes of seizure activity there is a greater percentage increase in the rate of glycolysis than in the rate of oxygen consumption, and lactate accumulates in the brain (7,18). Subsequently the rate of glycolysis matches that of oxidative metabolism (i.e., two to three times normal) (4,7).

The concentration of high-energy phosphate compounds in the brain shows a transient fall during the first minute of seizures (7,18). However, provided arterial pressure, arterial oxygenation, and blood glucose are kept within normal limits, the concentrations of creatine phosphate and adenosine triphosphate return nearly to normal and can remain stable throughout 2 hr of seizure activity. However, the more than doubled requirement for oxygen and glucose means that the brain is extremely vulnerable to hypoglycaemia

TABLE 1. *Cerebral blood flow and metabolic rate for oxygen during sustained seizures in rats*

Time[a]	No. of rats	Mean BP (torr)	Cerebral blood flow (ml $\cdot 100_g^{-1} \cdot$ min^{-1})	Metabolic rate (ml $O_2 \cdot 100_g^{-1} \cdot$ min^{-1})
Control	6	145 ± 2	100 ± 3	10.2 ± 0.3
20 min	5	136 ± 2	411 ± 56	28.7 ± 4.4
60 min	6	125 ± 3	357 ± 44	23.0 ± 2.3
120 min	6	132 ± 6	274 ± 44	22.7 ± 2.6

Measurements were made in adult Wistar rats that had been curarized and under N_2O anesthesia (numbers in parentheses).

Data are from Norberg and Siesjo (33), Chapman et al (6), and Meldrum and Nilsson (27). Further experimental details are given in these references.

[a] Times refer to the interval between seizure induction with bicuculline (1.2 mg/kg i.v.) and cerebral blood flow and metabolic rate determinations.

or to any fall in arterial blood pressure or arterial oxygenation, and is also of course vulnerable to any regional reduction in cerebral blood flow.

The importance of the increased energy demand of the epileptic discharge is most evident in the hemiatrophy of the brain that follows unilateral seizures (1,2,14,17). Although the primary pathological event (i.e., a virus infection or a venous thrombosis) may sometimes contribute to the atrophy, it is evident that in many cases the seizure activity itself must be the major factor.

HIPPOCAMPUS AND MESIAL TEMPORAL SCLEROSIS

The hippocampus provides us with a special problem in that there is clinical and experimental evidence that it may be particularly vulnerable under certain circumstances. It should be appreciated that in children dying after prolonged status epilepticus (or in experimental status epilepticus in baboons) the hippocampus is not in general more vulnerable than the neocortex. However, there are patterns or types of seizures which put the hippocampus particularly at risk. Two experimental situations deserve comment.

Allylglycine, which inhibits the cerebral enzyme glutamate decarboxylase (16), induces sequences of brief repetitive seizures in baboons. The systemic changes associated with a sequence of 30–60 brief seizures within 8–11 hr are relatively mild (22,28), although late in the sequence behavioural and EEG recovery between seizures is partial or absent. Neurological recovery is complete 24–48 hr later, and neuropathological examination 1–6 weeks afterward reveals no cerebellar or neocortical neuronal damage (24,28).

However, the hippocampus contains lesions corresponding closely to the Ammon's horn sclerosis found in chronic epileptic patients (20,23). Thus there is neuronal loss and gliosis symmetrically in the endfolium (especially in h_3 at its junction with h_2) but asymmetrically in the Sommer sector (28).

It also appears that purely hippocampal seizures can lead to hippocampal sclerosis. Thus prolonged rhinencephalic seizures induced by the injection of ouabain into the septal region in the cat are followed by hippocampal lesions with neuronal loss and glial reaction (3).

PATHOGENESIS OF HIPPOCAMPAL SCLEROSIS

The immediate cause of hippocampal pathology has been and still is the subject of much controversy. There are undoubtedly several mechanisms that can give rise to a similar final pathology. Systemic factors (e.g., hypoxia, arterial hypotension, and hypoglycaemia) clearly can play a contributing or even dominant role but are not essential. The importance of sustained excessive neuronal activity is clearly seen when lesions follow focal status epilepticus. However, local vascular factors have been invoked repeatedly to explain the pathogenesis of hippocampal sclerosis (with or without concurrent status epilepticus) (10,21,31,41).

There are three mechanisms requiring consideration. Arterial obstruction might arise if the anterior choroidal artery or the posterior cerebral artery are compressed at the tentorial edge when an increased supratentorial pressure leads to herniation of the uncus or medial aspect of the hippocampal gyrus.

This mechanism was supposed by Earle et al. (10) to allow ischaemic sclerosis of the hippocampus and medial aspect of the temporal lobe to result from moulding of the head during birth. Postmortem studies conducted in infants have provided little support for this concept (46). Scholz considered that raised supratentorial pressure associated with cerebral oedema late in seizures or postictally might similarly cause herniation at the tentorial edge and ischaemia from arterial compression. As pointed out by Norman (34,36), the anatomy of the lesions is not consistent, with obstruction of the anterior choroidal artery or posterior cerebral artery being responsible, and another explanation must be sought for the hippocampal lesions. Nevertheless the uncal pathology might itself be a direct result of uncal herniation in some cases.

The small vessels within the vulnerable part of the hippocampus are more tortuous than those in the resistant zone (31) so that a local increase in tissue pressure would be particularly apt, by locally impaired cerebral perfusion, to produce selective damage. Astrocytic end feet have been observed to swell during experimentally induced seizures (9,30), and this type of focal oedema could readily impede capillary flow.

An additional possibility is that an element of venous obstruction contributes to the focally inadequate perfusion of the hippocampus. This could arise from systemic causes, local herniation, or local anatomical abnormalities (21,30).

INCIDENCE AND SIGNIFICANCE OF CEREBRAL PATHOLOGY FOLLOWING FEBRILE CONVULSIONS

It is unfortunately impossible to give precise answers to such basic questions as: How often and under what circumstances do febrile convulsions cause cerebral pathology? What are the clinical consequences of such pathology?

It is clear that the majority of the 1 in 20 children who experience febrile convulsions in temperate climates suffer no sequelae (19). Equally clear is the high incidence of neurological deficits in the large hospital series of prolonged febrile convulsions described by Aicardi (1,2).

What is in doubt is the incidence and significance of cerebral lesions following febrile convulsions that are neither brief nor excessively prolonged.

There is presumably a continuous gradation from the severe generalised or hemi-atrophies described by Aicardi to very mild pathology involving the loss of a small number of neurones in the hippocampus and not associated with any neurological disorder.

The incidence of asymmetrical EEG abnormalities 1 week after febrile convulsions lasting 30 min or more (19) may give an indication of the group at risk for minimal pathology. It has also been suggested that behavioural and learning disabilities are common in this group (13), although the evidence for this is not decisive.

A proportion of children or adolescents or adults submitted to anterior temporal lobectomy for temporal lobe epilepsy have both mesial temporal sclerosis and a history of febrile convulsions. (11,45). The presumption is very strong that this lesion is a result of the febrile convulsions. What other pathology the brains of such patients may contain is largely unknown.

It is clear that long-term prospective studies of large groups of children having had febrile convulsions are needed to elucidate the secondary pathology and ultimate prognosis of this syndrome.

SUMMARY

Prolonged febrile convulsions in children and sustained drug-induced seizures in adolescent baboons give rise to "anoxic ischaemic" pathology involving the neocortex, thalamus, cerebellum, and hippocampus. Among causal factors contributing to this pathology are an increased metabolic demand arising from the seizure activity (100–300%), as well as from the hyperpyrexia (25%) and systemic disturbances including hypoxia, hypoglycaemia and arterial hypotension.

Local impairment of vascular perfusion probably contributes to hippocampal lesions. The prevention of such secondary pathology would avoid substantial neurological disability, including some cases of temporal lobe epilepsy.

ACKNOWLEDGMENTS

The author's research is supported by the Wellcome Trust, the National Fund for Research into Crippling Diseases, the British Epilepsy Association, and the Medical Research Council. The histological illustrations and case history were kindly supplied by Dr. J. A. N. Corsellis.

REFERENCES

1. Aicardi, J., and Baraton, J. (1971): A pneumoencephalographic demonstration of brain atrophy following status epilepticus. *Dev. Med. Child Neurol.*, 13:660–667.
2. Aicardi, J., and Chevrie, J. J. (1970): Convulsive status epilepticus in infants and children: A study of 239 cases. *Epilepsia*, 11:187–197.

3. Baldy-Moulinier, M., Arias, L. P., and Passouant, P. (1973): Hippocampal epilepsy produced by ouabain. *Eur. Neurol.*, 9:333–348.
4. Borgström, L., Chapman, A. G., and Siesjö, B. K. (1976): Glucose consumption in the cerebral cortex of rat during bicuculline-induced status epilepticus. *J. Neurochem. (in press).*
5. Brierley, J. B., Meldrum, B. S., and Brown, A. W. (1973): The threshold and neuropathology of cerebral "anoxic-ischemic" cell change. *Arch. Neurol.*, 29:367–374.
6. Chapman, A. G., Meldrum, B. S., and Siesjö, B. K. (1976): Cerebral blood flow and cerebral metabolic rate during prolonged epileptic seizures in rats. *J. Physiol.*, 254:61–62P.
7. Chapman, A. G., Meldrum, B. S., and Siesjö, B. K. (1976): Cerebral energy metabolic changes during prolonged epileptic seizures in rats. *J. Neurochem. (in press).*
8. Corsellis, J. A. N., and Meldrum, B. S. (1976): The pathology of epilepsy. In: *Greenfield's Neuropathology,* 3rd edition, edited by W. Blackwood and J. A. N. Corsellis, pp. 771–795. Arnold, London.
9. De Robertis, E., Alberici, M., and De Lores Arnaiz, G. R. (1969): Astroglial swelling and phosphohydrolases in cerebral cortex of metrazol convulsant rats. *Brain Res.*, 12:461–466.
10. Earle, K. M., Baldwin, M., and Penfield, W. (1953): Incisural sclerosis and temporal lobe seizures produced by hippocampal herniation at birth. *Arch. Neurol. Psychiatry,* 69:27–42.
11. Falconer, M. A. (1974): Mesial temporal (Ammon's horn) sclerosis as a common cause of epilepsy: Aetiology, treatment and prevention. *Lancet,* 2:767–770.
12. Fowler, M. (1957): Brain damage after febrile convulsions. *Arch. Dis. Child.,* 32:67–76.
13. Frantzen, E. (1971): In roundtable discussion. *Epilepsia,* 12:192 pp.
14. Gastaut, H., Poirier, F., Payan, H., Salamon, G., Toga, M., and Vigoroux, M. (1960): H. H. E. syndrome: Hemiconvulsions, hemiplegia, epilepsy. *Epilepsia,* 1:418–447.
15. Hartman, F. W. (1937): Lesions of the brain following fever therapy. *JAMA,* 109:2116–2120.
16. Horton, R. W., and Meldrum, B. S. (1973): Seizures induced by allyglycine, 3-mercaptopropionic acid and 4-deoxypyridoxine in mice and photosensitive baboons, and different modes of inhibition of cerebral glutamic acid decarboxylase. *Br. J. Pharmacol.,* 49:52–63.
17. Isler, W. (1969): *Akute Hemiplegien und Hemisyndrome in Kindersalter.* Thieme, Stuttgart.
18. King, L. J., Lowry, O. H., Passonneau, J. V., and Venson, V. (1967): Effects of convulsants on energy reserves in the cerebral cortex. *J. Neurochem.,* 14:599–611.
19. Lennox-Buchthal, M. A. (1973): *Febrile Convulsions.* Elsevier, Amsterdam.
20. Margerison, J. H., and Corsellis, J. A. N. (1966): Epilepsy and the temporal lobes—a clinical electroencephalographic and neuropathological study of the brain in epilepsy with particular reference to the temporal lobes. *Brain,* 89:499–530.
21. McLardy, T. (1974): Pathogenesis of epileptic-hypoxic Ammon's horn sclerosis: Contribution of basal vein contriction by looped posterior cerebral artery. *IRCS,* 2:1574.
22. Meldrum, B. S. (1973): The physiological mechanisms leading to epileptic brain damage: an animal model of status epilepticus. In: *Prevention of Epilepsy and its Consequences,* edited by M. J. Parsonage, pp. 73–79. International Bureau for Epilepsy, London.
23. Meldrum, B. S. (1975): Present views on hippocampal sclerosis and epilepsy. In: *Modern Trends in Neurology,* 6th edition, edited by D. Williams, pp. 223–239. Butterworths, London.
24. Meldrum, B. S., and Brierley, J. B. (1972): Neuronal loss and gliosis in the hippocampus following repetitive epileptic seizures induced in adolescent baboons by allylglycine. *Brain Res.,* 48:361–365.
25. Meldrum, B. S., and Brierley, J. B. (1973): Prolonged epileptic seizures in primates. *Arch. Neurol.,* 28:10–17.
26. Meldrum, B. S., and Horton, R. W. (1973): Physiology of status epilepticus in primates. *Arch. Neurol.,* 28:1–9.
27. Meldrum, B. S., and Nilsson, B. (1976): Cerebral blood flow and metabolic rate early and late in prolonged epileptic seizures induced in rats by bicuculline. *Brain (in press).*
28. Meldrum, B. S., Horton, R. W., and Brierley, J. B. (1974): Epileptic brain damage in adolescent baboons following seizures induced by allylglycine. *Brain,* 97:407–418.
29. Meldrum, B. S., Papy, J. J., Touré, M. F., and Brierley, J. B. (1975): Four models for studying cerebral lesions secondary to epileptic seizures. *Adv. Neurol.,* 10:147–161.

30. Meldrum, B. S., Vigouroux, R. A., and Brierley, J. B. (1937): Systemic factors and epileptic brain damage. *Arch. Neurol.*, 29:82–87.
31. Morel, F., and Wildi, E. (1956): Sclerose ammonienne et epilepsies. *Acta Med. Belg.*, 61–74.
32. Nemoto, E. M., and Frankel, H. M. (1970): Cerebral oxygenation and metabolism during progressive hyperthemia. *Am. J. Physiol.*, 219:1784–1788.
33. Norber, K., and Siesjö, B. K. (1974): Quantitative measurement of blood flow and oxygen consumption in the rat brain. *Acta Physiol. Scand.*, 91:154–164.
34. Norman, R. M. (1964): The neuropathology of status epilepticus. *Med. Sci. Law*, 4:46–57.
35. O'Connor, M. J., Herman, C. J., Rosenthal, M., and Jöbsis, F. F. (1972): Intracellular redox changes preceding onset of epileptiform activity in intact cat hippocampus. *J. Neurophysiol.*, 35:471–483.
36. Ounsted, C., Lindsay, J., and Norman, R. (1966): *Biological Factors in Temporal Lobe Epilepsy.* Heinemann, London.
37. Peiffer, J. (1963): *Morphologische Aspekte der Epilepsie.* Springer, Berlin.
38. Plum, F., Posner, J. B., and Troy, B. (1968): Cerebral metabolic and circulatory responses to drug-induced convulsions in animals. *Arch. Neurol.*, 18:1–13.
39. Schmidt, C. F., Kety, S. S., and Pennes, H. H. (1945): The gaseous metabolism of the brain of the monkey. *Am. J. Physiol.*, 143:33–52.
40. Scholz, W. (1951): *Die Krampfschädigungen des Gehirns.* Springer, Berlin.
41. Scholz, W. (1959): The contribution of pathoanatomical research to the problem of epilepsy. *Epilepsia*, 1:36–55.
42. Spielmeyer, W. (1922): *Histopathologie des Nervensystems*, pp. 74–79. Springer, Berlin.
43. Spielmeyer, W. (1925): Zur Pathogenese ortlich elektiven Gehirnveranderungen. *Z. Neurol. Psychiatr.*, 99:756–776.
44. Spielmeyer, W. (1927): Die Pathogenese des epileptischen Krämpfes. *Z. Gesamte Neurol. Psychiatr.*, 109:501–520.
45. Van Buren, J. M., Ajmone Marsan, C., Mutsuga, N., and Sadowsky, D. (1975): Surgery of temporal lobe epilepsy. *Adv. Neurol.*, 8:155–196.
46. Veith, G. (1970): Anatomische Studie uber die Ammonhornsklerose in Epiletikegehirn. *Dtsh. Z. Nervenheilk.* 197:293–314.
47. Zimmerman, H. M. (1938): The histopathology of convulsive disorders in children. *J. Pediatr.*, 13:859–890.

Brain Dysfunction in Infantile Febrile Convulsions, edited by M. A. B. Brazier and F. Coceani. Raven Press, New York © 1976.

Structure-Dysfunction Relations in the Visual Cortex of Preterm Infants

Dominick P. Purpura

Department of Neuroscience and the Rose F. Kennedy Center for Research in Mental Retardation and Human Development, Albert Einstein College of Medicine, Bronx, New York 10461

There is an urgent need for information on the normal and abnormal morphological development of the cerebral cortex from the earliest period of postnatal viability in the preterm infant, as well as a need for reliable methods to assess the functional integrity of the immature brain throughout infancy and early childhood. Until such morphophysiological data are available, it is unlikely that there will be an adequate understanding of the pathophysiological basis of febrile convulsions and their sequelae. One approach to the problem of evaluating cortical activity in preterm infants has made use of visual evoked potentials (VEPs) since it is known that VEPs exhibit systematic changes in electrographic characteristics with advancing conceptional age (5,14,17). However, if these electrophysiological data are to provide clues to the maturational status of the cerebral cortex, they must be related to specific morphogenetic features of cortical neuronal development. It will also be necessary to determine whether perturbations in cortical maturational processes are reflected in developmental changes in VEPs and vice versa.

In a previous study developmental aspects of immature human cerebral cortex (9,11) were examined to define the most impressive normal morphogenetic events in primary visual cortex of the preterm infant during the period when VEPs undergo major maturational changes (10). The present report extends this line of inquiry by considering the extent to which developmental alterations in VEPs are associated with significantly different structural features of primary visual cortex neurons. A summary of earlier findings in preterm infants with apparently normal age-related VEPs (10) serves as a prelude to the analysis of pathophysiological processes affecting the cerebral cortex of the preterm infant.

"NORMAL" STRUCTURE-FUNCTION RELATIONS IN VISUAL CORTEX OF THE PRETERM INFANT

Seven preterm infants (gestational age 25–33 weeks) who survived for 2–29 days in the neonatal intensive care unit at our institution represent the "normal" developmental series in which consistent morphogenetic features have been observed in rapid Golgi preparations of primary visual cortex (10). Figure 1 summarizes the electrographic characteristics of the averaged VEPs recorded from three infants in this series as well as the appearance of different types of neurons in the primary visual cortex. In all cases noted here and below, the rapid Golgi method was applied to small blocks of calcarine cortex from fresh or formalin-fixed (5–18 hr) brain tissue removed at the time of postmortem examination.

The youngest infant studied (*V1*) was 25 weeks estimated gestational age (g.a.) and survived 2 days prior to intraventricular hemorrhage. Averaged VEPs recorded the day after birth consisted of a prominent initial negative component followed by a large positive-negative-positive sequence (Fig. 1A).

The primary visual cortex in this infant exhibits a well-developed molecular layer characterized by an extensive system of Cajal-Retzius elements. Pyramidal neurons at all depths have thin, unbranched apical dendritic shafts with limited vertical extent. Only small and medium-sized pyramidal neurons in superficial regions have apical dendritic terminals in the molecular layer. Basilar dendrites are absent on small and medium pyramids and are represented by thin, short perisomatic processes in large pyramidal neurons. Small, ovoid and round cells with a few wisps of radiate processes are found in regions corresponding to the distribution of large obliquely coursing axons typical of geniculocalcarine radiation fibers (1). Most of the nonpyramidal cells in midcortical locations are devoid of perisomatic processes, although a small axonal segment was usually revealed. Dendritic spines are not present on any of the neurons in the primary visual cortex at this age. However, apical dendritic shafts of large pyramidal cells exhibit an occasional fine filopodium-like process.

VEPs in an infant 27 weeks g.a. (*Co*) who survived for 3 days exhibited a small but consistent positive wave which preceded the early negative component (Fig. 1B). Later waves were less prominent than in the 25-week-old infant. Golgi studies of visual cortex in infant *Co* show that by 27 weeks large and medium pyramidal neurons possess short basilar dendrites, and several apical dendrites have a few short tangential branches. Nonpyramidal neurons have more prominent dendrites, and some pyramidal neurons with cell bodies at midcortical sites have apical dendrites that extend to superficial regions. Dendritic spines were not observed on any elements of the visual cortex in this infant or in three other preterm infants of 26–28 weeks conceptional age (c.a.).

VEPs from a 32-week-old infant (*Sb*) are shown in Fig. 1C. This infant was born at 29 weeks g.a. and survived 4 weeks. VEPs exhibited an initial positivity that was followed by a negative wave. All of the VEP components are substantially smaller than in younger infants.

Striking morphogenetic changes are evident in visual cortex neurons of

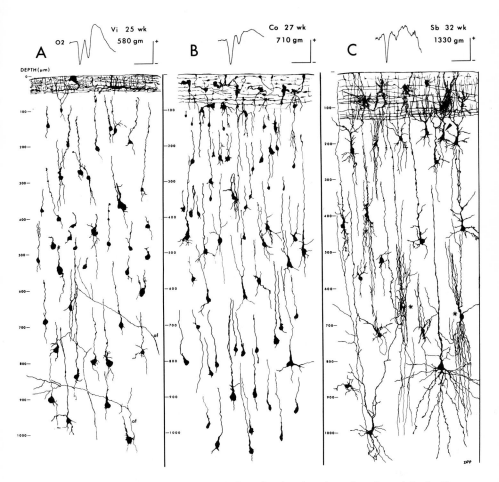

FIG. 1. "Normal" structure-function relations in visual cortex of preterm infants. **Top:** Averaged VEPs to stroboscopic flash, 8-sec interstimulus interval, 50 responses. Occipital lead (02) referred to ipsilateral ear. Gestational ages and birth weights of preterm infants are as indicated. Amplitude bar, 24 μV for **A** and **B**, 3 μV for **C**. Time bar 0.5 sec. **Bottom:** Composite camera lucida drawings of neurons in primary visual (calcarine) cortex of preterm infants whose VEPs are shown above. Neurons were identified at different depths from the pial surface and drawn at ×400 magnification. **A:** (*Vi,* 25 weeks g.a.). Note obliquely coursing large axons (af) in midcortical regions corresponding to layer IV. Most pyramidal cells have poorly developed basilar dendrites and relatively short apical dendrites. Dendritic spines are absent. **B:** (*Co,* 27 weeks g.a.) Basilar dendrites are short, and some tangential branches of apical dendrites are evident. Dendritic spines are absent. **C.** (*Sb,* 33 weeks g.a.) Primary visual cortex in this preterm infant (VEP recorded at 32 weeks) is 1.8 mm in thickness (compared to 1.0 mm in **A** and **B**). Neurons in the upper two-thirds of the cortex are illustrated. Note the development of superficial small pyramids. Asterisks identify Cajal's *cellules à double bouquet dendritique.* Dendritic spines are abundant but not illustrated at this magnification. (VEPs from Vaughan, Kurtzberg, Kreuzer, and Eisengart, *unpublished data.* Camera lucida panels modified from Purpura, ref. 10.)

infant *Sb* at 33 weeks c.a. (Fig. 1C). All varieties of pyramidal neurons have extensive basilar dendritic systems. The apical dendritic shafts are long and have side branches in different laminae. The dendrites of stellate cells are also well differentiated, and a wide variety of nonpyramidal neurons are evident. Several types of Cajal's (1) *cellules à double bouquet dendritique* are frequently encountered in superficial and midcortical regions (Fig. 1C, asterisks). Dendritic spines are prominent on all types of pyramidal neurons, from small superficial pyramids to large Meynert cells (10). Dendritic spines are also observed on many forms of stellate and other nonpyramidal cells, including double-tufted cells. Dendritic development and dendritic spine formation were prominent in the visual cortex of another infant 33 weeks g.a. who survived 2 days.

STRUCTURE-DYSFUNCTION RELATIONS: MATURATIONAL DELAY IN VISUAL CORTEX DEVELOPMENT

Evoked potential studies carried out on preterm infants admitted for intensive neonatal care have disclosed a variety of abnormal electrographic patterns in infants with a number of severe cardiorespiratory metabolic and genetic abnormalities. Three infants from this series, all of whom were 34 weeks c.a. when they succumbed, illustrate relationships between alterations or abnormalities in VEPs and neuronal morphology that emphasize the impact of high-risk factors on cortical maturation processes in the preterm infant.

The first infant in this series (*Ne*) was born after 28 weeks' gestation with a birth weight of 1,000 g. The clinical course included respiratory distress syndrome, bilateral pneumothoraces, hyperbilirubinemia, hypocalcemia, anemia, necrotizing enterocolitis, coagulopathy, and heart murmur. VEPs recorded 9 days before expiration, at 5–6 weeks of age (34 weeks c.a.), are shown in Fig. 2.

The occipital VEP consisted of a large initial negativity followed by several smaller components. Similar potentials were recorded from the parietal electrode, but the temporal lead response had a different morphology. The evoked potential configuration and distribution at 33 weeks in this infant are characteristic of VEPs in younger infants (27–30 weeks).

Examples of rapid Golgi preparations of primary visual cortex neurons in *Ne* are shown in Fig. 3. Figure 4 is a composite of camera lucida drawings of elements at different depths in the calcarine cortex. Superficial small and medium pyramidal neurons (Figs. 3A and C) had thin apical dendrites but were virtually devoid of basilar dendrites. Basilar dendrites were occasionally seen on deeper-lying medium pyramids (Fig. 3D) and some large pyramidal cells (Fig. 3F). Double-tufted cells were seen in superficial cortex (Fig. 3B), but these lacked the extensive dendritic plumes characteristic of such elements in normal cortex at 33 weeks (cf. Fig. 1C). Apical dendrites frequently

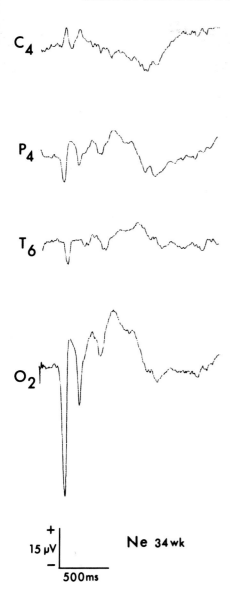

FIG. 2. Averaged VEPs recorded from infant *Ne,* at 33 weeks c.a. Recordings from occipital (O), temporal (T), parietal (P), and central (C) regions of scalp referred to ipsilateral ear. Latency of occipital VEP is approximately 200 msec and consists of a prominent negativity succeeded by several smaller components. Note that the activity recorded from the temporal region of the scalp is different from the occipital or parietal configurations. Morphological characteristics of visual cortex neurons in infant *Ne* are shown in Figs. 3 and 4. (From Vaughan, Kurtzberg, and Kreuzer, *unpublished data.*)

exhibited lumpy enlargements along the main shaft (Fig. 3C) or in distal segments (Fig. 3F). Few thin tangential or oblique branches were present on apical dendrites (Fig. 3E and 3F). Although filopodium-like processes were occasionally detectable on some apical dendritic shafts, *dendritic spines were not observed on any element.*

It is instructive to compare the general characteristics of various types of neurons at different depths in *Ne* (Fig. 4) with the elements observed in the "normal" visual cortex of *Sb* at 33 weeks (Fig. 1C). The molecular layer in

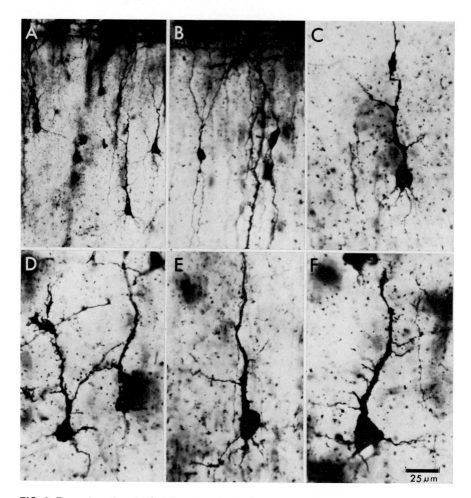

FIG. 3. Examples of rapid Golgi preparations of neurons in the primary visual cortex of a preterm infant (*Ne*, 34 weeks c.a.). Averaged VEPs recorded from this infant are shown in Fig. 2. **A–C:** Cells in superficial cortical regions lack basilar dendrites. Note lumpy enlargement of apical dendrite shaft in **C. D–F:** Medium and large pyramidal neurons of the cortical depths. Apical dendrites have a few tangential or oblique branches but lack prominent basilar dendrites. Magnification bar in **F** applies to **C–F;** for **A** and **B** the bar is 50 μm.

DEPTH (μm)

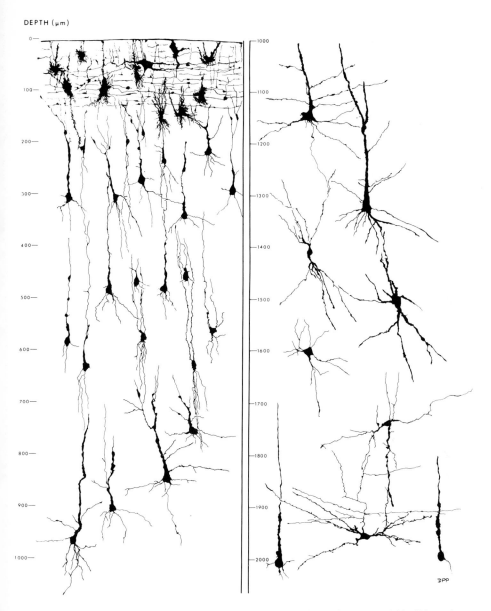

FIG. 4. Camera lucida drawings of neurons in calcarine (visual) cortex of *Ne* (34 weeks c.a.). Rapid Golgi preparations. The molecular layer contains large numbers of glia. Superficial pyramids have poorly developed basilar dendrites and thin apical shafts. None of the dendrites have spines. Stellate cells in the cortical depths (1,400–1,800 μm) are relatively well developed in contrast to most medium and large pyramidal neurons. Double-tufted Cajal cells are present but do not have elaborate dendritic plumes. Cortical neurons are not as well developed for 34 weeks as in the 34-week-old preterm infant (*Sb*) considered in the normal series (Fig. 1C).

Ne is less well organized and contains large numbers of glia. Overall, apical dendrites of medium and large pyramids are shorter and thinner, and contain fewer tangential branches in *Ne* than *Sb*. It is of interest that large stellate cells in the cortical depths are among the most mature-appearing elements in *Ne*. Giant pyramids have few prominent basilar dendrites.

In general, the morphological development of cortical neurons in *Ne* at 34 weeks c.a. has attained a stage similar to that of normal cortex at about 28 weeks c.a., or perhaps slightly more developed than the visual cortex at 27 weeks (Fig. 1B). Maturational "delay" is thus suggested by three morphological features: minimal basilar dendritic growth, thin poorly branched apical dendritic shafts, and an absence of dendritic spines. It is especially noteworthy that the initial component of the occipital VEP in *Ne* is a prominent negativity, which is characteristic of VEPs in infants less than 33 weeks c.a. (5,14,17). Thus there is good agreement between the electrographic features of VEPs and the developmental status of visual cortex in this preterm infant with multiple cardiorespiratory and metabolic disorders, all of which undoubtedly influenced the temporal patterns of dendritic development and differentiation. The data suggest that dendritic development attained at the time of birth (28 weeks c.a.) remained essentially unchanged during the subsequent 5–6 weeks postnatally.

ARREST AND FAILURE OF VISUAL CORTEX MORPHOGENESIS

Two preterm infants illustrate the marked abnormalities in VEPs observed in association with dramatic disruption and disorganization of cortical maturational events.

Infant *Gl* was born after 34 weeks' gestation with a birth weight of 2,040 g. Premature rupture of membranes occurred 3 weeks prior to delivery. The infant was febrile at birth and icteric at day 1. Abnormal posturing was noted and continued into the second day along with bleeding diathesis, abnormal distention, and apneic spells. At 3 days the infant was cyanotic, had a decreased blood pressure, and continued to pass blood clots. Death occurred on the fifth day as a result of intracranial hemorrhage.

VEPs recorded at 4 days of age in *Gl* consisted of biphasic broad positive-negative potentials widely distributed over the scalp (Fig. 5). The prolonged latency, biphasic wave shape, and diffuse distribution are grossly pathological.

Rapid Golgi preparations of medium and large pyramidal neurons from the primary visual cortex in *Gl* are shown in Fig. 6. A composite of camera lucida drawings of elements at different depths in the calcarine cortex is illustrated in Fig. 7. Most pyramidal neurons in this case were completely devoid of basilar dendrites. In a large proportion of medium and large pyramids, apical dendrites were foreshortened or absent (Figs. 6C–E). In these elements cell bodies were considerably longer than usual and were

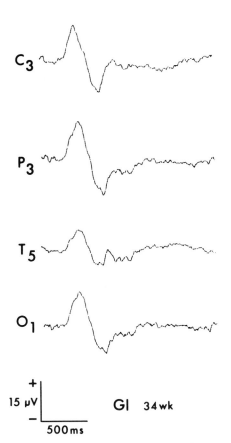

FIG. 5. Averaged VEPs recorded from infant *Gl* at 34 weeks c.a. The VEP consists of a biphasic prolonged positive-negative deflection widely distributed over the scalp. Latency of the occipital VEP is 250 msec. The prolonged latency, wave shape, and diffuse distribution of VEPs are grossly abnormal electrographic characteristics for 34 weeks c.a. Morphological features of visual cortex neurons in this infant are shown in Figs. 6 and 7. (From Vaughan, Kurtzberg, and Kreuzer, *unpublished data*.)

smooth in contour, lacking perisomatic processes. Large, lumpy excrescences were noted in apical dendritic shafts of some medium pyramidal neurons (Fig. 6A and B).

Examination of the camera lucida composite drawing in *Gl* reveals a markedly disorganized molecular layer with poorly developed small and medium superficial pyramidal cells. Curiously, many pyramidal neurons at different depths exhibit trailing processes that resemble the primitive trailing processes of postmigratory elements (6,7). It is as if these processes have not been resorbed after the neuron has attained its position in cortex. Such primitive trailing processes are not encountered in the human visual cortex after 28–29 weeks c.a. (10).

A small proportion of pyramidal neurons with apical dendrites exhibit dendritic varicosities and pleomorphic lumpy enlargements. Dendrites appear shrunken and atrophic in deep-lying pyramidal neurons. An occasional double-tufted cell is noted, but most cells in midcortical locations are large, round or ovoid elements with a few neurites. Some of the morphological

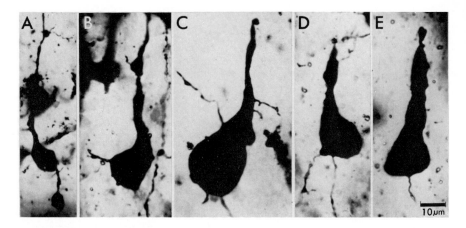

FIG. 6. Examples of rapid Golgi preparations of neurons in the primary visual cortex of preterm infant *Gl* (34 weeks c.a.). Averaged VEPs recorded from this infant are shown in Fig. 5. **A:** A medium pyramidal neuron exhibits a trailing process emerging from the base of the cell body. No basilar dendrites are observed. The apical dendrite is present but short, as in the superficial medium pyramidal neuron in **B. C–E:** Large pyramidal neurons without distal apical dendritic shafts and an absence of perisomatic dendritic processes. Magnification bar in **E** applies to **B–E** and is 20 μm for **A.**

features of visual cortex neurons resemble those observed at 24–25 weeks c.a., not 34 weeks (cf. Fig. 1A). However, the persistence of trailing processes of neurons and general lack of cortical organization is suggestive of a failure of cortical neuronal maturation with minimal synaptogenesis. It is doubtful on the basis of the morphological findings if the VEP in this case (Fig. 5) reflects significant activity generated postsynaptically in cortical neurons.

The third infant in this series (*Gr*) was born after 34 weeks' gestation with a birth weight of 1,880 g. Congestive heart failure with respiratory distress was evident shortly after birth. Episodes of seizures developed with extension of extremities and upward rolling of eyes. Death occurred on the third day. Multiple congenital anomalies suggested the clinical picture of trisomy 18. VEPs recorded on the day of death are shown in Fig. 8. An initial negative deflection with an onset latency exceeding 250 msec is present in the occipital VEP. It is remarkable that there was a total absence of evoked activity rostral to the occipital region in this infant.

Rapid Golgi preparations of visual cortex neurons in infant *Gr* are shown in Fig. 9. With the possible exception of some deep pyramidal neurons (Fig. 9D), most of the superficial small and medium pyramidal neurons (Fig. 9A and B) were devoid of basilar dendritic systems. Apical dendritic shafts did not possess spines (Fig. 9C), although a few large pyramidal neurons with relatively normal basilar dendritic branching patterns (Fig.

PTH (μm)

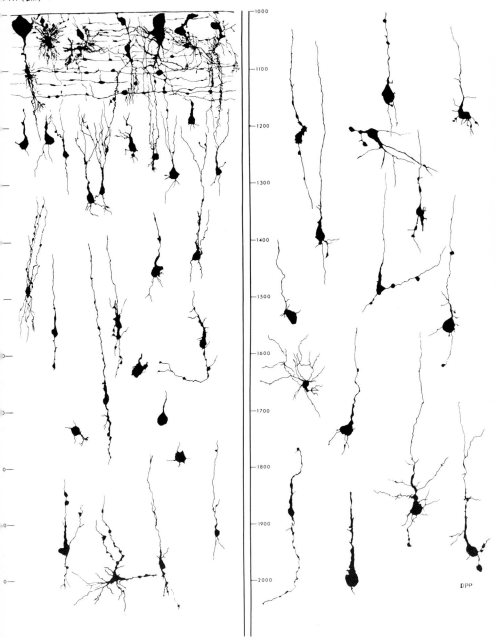

FIG. 7. Camera lucida drawings of neurons in calcarine cortex of *GI* (34 weeks c.a.). Rapid Golgi preparations. Some of the small and medium pyramidal neurons of the superficial cortex have features shown in Fig. 6A,B. Apical dendrites of medium and large pyramidal neurons are generally short and thin. A number of cells are shown with primitive trailing processes. Basilar dendrites are generally absent, and no cells exhibit dendritic spines. A double-tufted Cajal cell is shown at 500 μm.

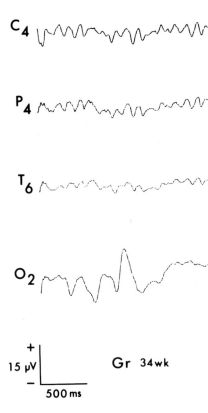

FIG. 8. Averaged VEPs recorded from *Gr* at 34 weeks c.a. The occipital (O) VEP consists of an initial negative deflection with a latency exceeding 250 msec (normal, 175–200 msec). The initial "W-shaped" negativities are characteristic for VEPs at 34 weeks, but the rhythmicity of the later components is distinctly unusual as is the absence of evoked activity rostral to the occipital region. Morphological characteristics of visual cortex neurons in this infant are shown in Figs. 9 and 10. (From Vaughan, Kurtzberg, and Kreuzer, *unpublished data*.)

9D) had dendritic spines on distal oblique and tangential branches of apical dendrites (Fig. 9E).

The composite of camera lucida drawings in this case (*Gr*) emphasizes the minimal organization of the molecular layer and the marked atrophy of apical dendrites of pyramidal neurons (Fig. 10). The characteristics of a large cell with thin basilar dendrites at a depth of 1,200 μm illustrate the most advanced features of the pyramidal neurons in this preterm infant with suspected trisomy 18. Several cells possess primitive trailing processes, as in infant *Gl*.

The presence of dendritic spines on some apical dendritic branches of midcortical pyramidal neurons (Fig. 9D and E) indicates that some degree of synaptogenesis has occurred in this otherwise grossly abnormal immature visual cortex. It is possible that the presence of initial negative components in the occipital VEP reflects the activity of a limited number of dendritic synapses that have developed in a restricted part of the visual cortex. Failure to detect evoked activity in other than occipital leads is suggestive of the lack of cortical synaptogenesis and dendritic differentiation in extrastriate cortex in this case of suspected genetic disorder.

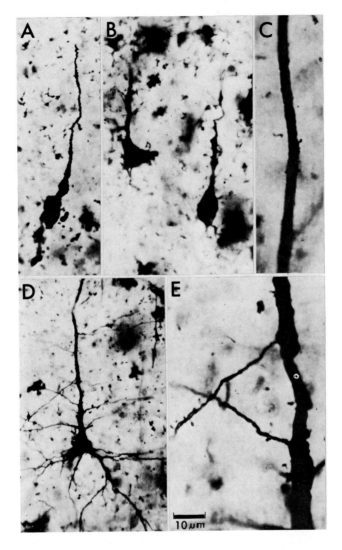

FIG. 9. Examples of rapid Golgi preparations of neurons in primary visual cortex of pre-term infant *Gr* (34 weeks c.a.). Averaged VEPs recorded from this infant are shown in Fig. 8. **A** and **B**: Superficial pyramidal neurons are atrophic and devoid of basilar dendrites. **C**: Apical dendritic shaft of a medium pyramid is devoid of spines. **D**: A large pyramidal neuron in the cortical depth has thin basilar dendrites and oblique and tangential branches of apical dendrites. **E**: Higher magnification of oblique branch of apical dendrite in **D** to show presence of dendritic spines. Magnification bar applies to **C** and **E** only. Bar is 20 μm for **A, B,** and **D.**

DEPTH (µm)

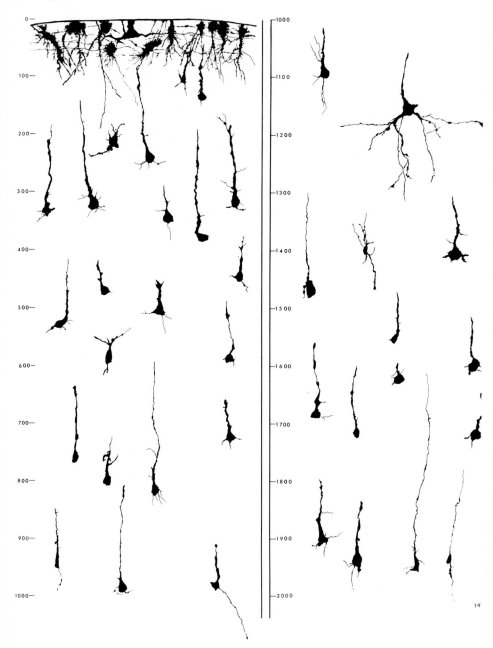

FIG. 10. Camera lucida drawings of neurons in calcarine cortex of *Gr* (34 weeks c.a.).
Rapid Golgi preparations. The molecular layer is grossly disorganized and is virtually
completely occupied by glia. Rarely a pyramidal neuron is encountered that has an array
of basilar dendrites. Apical shafts of most pyramidal neurons are grossly abnormal
throughout. A few cells have retained trailing processes.

DISCUSSION

The foregoing observations on VEPs and Golgi preparations of visual cortex neurons in preterm infants address several issues.

1. *Do visual evoked potentials in human infants provide information on the normal structural development of the primary visual cortex?*

The answer to this question is provided by the extraordinary morphogenetic changes observed in visual cortex neurons in the preterm infant (10) during the period when VEPs undergo significant electrographic changes (5,14,17) (Fig. 1). In very young preterm infants (25–27 weeks c.a.) the characteristic early negative wave of the occipital VEP reflects the activity of grossly immature pyramidal and nonpyramidal neurons. Evidently thin spine-free apical dendrites of pyramidal neurons and rare dendritic processes of nonpyramidal cells are the only postsynaptic targets for geniculocortical afferents at this developmental stage: By 34 weeks dendritic development is prominent in all elements and the basic structural pattern of the primary visual cortex is established. The most impressive morphogenetic event that parallels electrographic changes in VEPs is the extensive development of dendritic spines (10). Since dendritic spines receive the vast majority of geniculocortical afferents in adult animals (2–4,13,15), it seems likely that the development of an axospinodendritic mode of synaptic engagement of visual cortex neurons is related to the VEP changes observed around 33–34 weeks. In terms of the emphasis on dendritic differentiation and dendritic spine development, the findings in human preterm infants parallel those reported previously in morphophysiological studies of cortical ontogenesis in the feline brain (12,16).

2. *Are VEPs in preterm infants "sensitive" to minor perturbations in the temporal pattern of cortical maturation?*

The availability of several postmortem specimens of visual cortex of preterm infants permits a tentative but by no means unequivocal answer to this question. The morphophysiological observations summarized in Fig. 1 and elsewhere (10) provide a "normal" reference of developmental events. Three preterm infants were selected in the present study as examples of the effects of varying degrees of potential insult to the developing brain on VEPs and neuronal structure. The infants were approximately the same conceptional age (34 weeks) as the oldest preterm infants in the "normal" series.

Preterm infant *Ne* exhibited VEPs similar to the pattern of responses characteristic of an earlier phase of electro-ontogenesis. Remarkably, the morphological features of the major types of neurons in the primary visual cortex in this infant resemble the features observed prior to 32–33 weeks c.a. This may be coincidental, or it may simply indicate the normal range of variation in the tempo of cortical maturation. On the other hand, the discrepancy between conceptional age and "cortical maturation age" may reflect delay in or interference with the biosynthetic events required for the elaboration of dendrites and axodendritic synapses during the critical phase of cortical dendritic differentiation (27–33 weeks) (9,10). In the case of infant *Ne,* the hemorrhagic diathesis and repeated episodes of cardio-respiratory arrest during the 5–6 postnatal weeks prior to death are sufficient to explain the postnatal maturational "delay" in cortical neuronal develop-ment and the "immature" nature of the VEP.

3. *What significance can be attached to finding grossly abnormal VEPs in neonatal preterm infants?*

In contrast to the relatively subtle differences in maturational status in infants *Ne* (Fig. 4) and *Sb* (Fig. 1C) at 34 weeks c.a., the two preterm infants with grossly abnormal VEPs had overtly abnormal immature cortical neu-rons. It is unlikely that the absence of basilar dendrites and a lack of dendri-tic spines and paucity of branches of apical dendrites in infant *Gl* resulted from the fetal distress at birth or the subsequent bleeding diathesis. Infant *Gl* survived 5 days and had cortical neurons almost completely devoid of secondary (including basilar) dendritic systems. On the other hand, it should be recalled that infant *Ne* survived for 5 weeks with major cardiorespiratory and metabolic insults. Yet cortical neurons in *Ne* showed evidence only of delay or interference with *continuing postnatal* maturation. Further it should be noted that although VEPs in infant *Ne* were "immature for age" they were nevertheless well organized. In view of this, it follows that the very immature appearance of cortical neurons and the grossly abnormal VEP in infant *Gl* attest to a prolonged *antenatal* interruption of metabolic processes required for dendritic development and differentiation. Antenatal sepsis of 3 weeks' duration and its ensuing complications may have been major factors contributing to the interruption of neuronal maturation in this case.

Even more dramatic is the picture of abnormal neuronal development in infant *Gr* (34 weeks c.a.) who survived 3 days after an elective caesarean section and uneventful prenatal history. Congestive failure was noted on the day of birth, and seizures developed thereafter with cardiac arrest on the third (last) day. Again, this brief but stormy postnatal course does not account for the bizarre appearance of the cortical neurons in infant *Gr.* Rather, the diffusely abnormal VEP and the failure of cortical neuronal de-velopment beyond approximately 18–20 weeks c.a. – as judged by dendritic features (9–11) – are reasonably explained by the devastating impact of multiple congenital anomalies probably associated with a chromosomal abnormality.

A curious observation common to infants *Gl* and *Gr* was the finding of persisting primitive trailing processes characteristic of postmigratory neuroblasts (6,7). Such embryonic remnants are detectable in deep-lying large stellate cells in the "normal" 34-week-old preterm infant (10), but they are generally not present in more superficial pyramidal neurons after the 28th week. The persistence of embryonic trailing processes in cortical neurons in infant *Gl* (Fig. 7) and to a lesser extent in infant *Gr* (Fig. 10) lends support to the view that the diffusely abnormal VEPs in these preterm infants are attributable primarily to longstanding *antenatal* disturbances in the cortical maturation process.

The tentative conclusion that may be drawn from morphophysiological observations on infants *Gl* and *Gr* is that diffusely abnormal VEPs recorded during the neonatal period in preterm infants are indicative of profound neuronal developmental retardation secondary to antenatal insults to the developing brain. However, it is conceivable that short-term interruption of synaptic interactions in the developing brain could result in marked functional disorganization of VEPs in the absence of overt morphogenetic abnormalities. Thus abnormal VEPs may occur in normal immature brain, but well-organized "normal-for-age" VEPs cannot be expected in conditions in which cortical neurons exhibit maturational "arrest" of *antenatal* origin.

The foregoing results encourage the expectation that the continuing pursuit of structure-dysfunction relations in the immature human brain will yield information relevant to the problem of susceptibility to febrile convulsions during infancy. This expectation is rooted in the premise that functional disturbances of the immature brain have their counterpart in alterations in morphophysiological developmental processes. Viewed in this fashion it can be anticipated that factors influencing the appearance of febrile convulsions influence developmental events as well. The problem is to define the level of organization of neuronal operations most likely to bear the major impact of these factors. This approach has already been productive in recent Golgi studies of dendritic spine abnormalities in unclassified mental retardation (8). It will be of interest to determine whether further refinements in morphophysiological techniques will permit elucidation of more subtle developmental disturbances that may be reflected in susceptibility to febrile convulsions.

ACKNOWLEDGMENTS

The author wishes to thank Dr. Herbert G. Vaughan, Dr. Diane Kurtzberg, and Ms. Judith Kreuzer for permission to publish visual evoked potential data obtained in collaborative studies. This research was supported in part by NIH Grant NS-07512 and NICHD Grant HD-01799. Mrs. M. Buschke's technical assistance in the preparation of the histologic material and Mr. S. Brown's assistance with the photographic reproductions are greatly appreciated.

REFERENCES

1. Cajal, S. R. (1911): *Histologie du Système Nerveax de l'Homme et des Vertébrés,* Vol. II. Maloine, Paris. (Reimpresse: Madrid Instito Cajal, 1955.)

2. Colonnier, M. L., and Rossignol, S. (1969): Heterogeneity of the cerebral cortex. In: *Basic Mechanisms of the Epilepsies,* edited by H. H. Jasper, A. A. Ward, and A. Pope, pp. 29–40. Little, Brown, Boston.
3. Garey, L. J., and Powell, T. P. S. (1971): An experimental study of the termination of the lateral geniculo-cortical pathway in the cat and monkey. *Proc. R. Soc. Lond. [Biol.],* 179:41–63.
4. Globus, A., and Scheibel, A. B. (1967): Synaptic loci on visual cortical neurons of the rabbit: The specific afferent radiation. *Exp. Neurol.,* 18:116–131.
5. Hrbek, A., Karlberg, P., and Olsson, T. (1973): Development of visual and somatosensory evoked responses in preterm newborn infants. *Electroencephalogr. Clin. Neurophysiol.,* 34:225–232.
6. Morest, K. (1969): The differentiation of cerebral dendrites: A study of the post-migratory neuroblast in the medial nucleus of the trapezoid body. *Z. Anat. Entwicklungsgesch.,* 128:271–289.
7. Morest, K. (1970): A study of neurogenesis in the forebrain of the opossum pouch young. *Z. Anat. Entwicklungsgesch.,* 130:265–305.
8. Purpura, D. P. (1974): Dendritic spine dysgenesis and mental retardation. *Science,* 186:1126–1128.
9. Purpura, D. P. (1975): Dendritic differentiation in human cerebral cortex: Normal and aberrant developmental patterns. *Adv. Neurol.,* 12:91–116.
10. Purpura, D. P. (1975): Morphogenesis of visual cortex in the preterm infant. In: *Growth and Development of the Brain,* edited by M. A. B. Brazier, pp. 33–49. Raven Press, New York.
11. Purpura, D. P. (1975): Normal and aberrant development in the human cerebral cortex of human fetus and young infant. In: *Brain Mechanisms in Mental Retardation,* edited by N. A. Buchwald and M. A. B. Brazier, pp. 141–169. Academic Press, New York.
12. Purpura, D. P., Shofer, R. J., Housepian, E. M., and Noback, C. R. (1964): Comparative ontogenesis of structure-function relations in cerebral and cerebellar cortex. *Prog. Brain Res.,* 4:187–221.
13. Szentágothai, J. (1973): Synaptology of the visual cortex. In: *Handbook of Sensory Physiology,* Vol. VII, 3B, edited by R. Jung, pp. 269–324. Springer Verlag, New York.
14. Umezaki, H., and Morell, F. (1970): Development study of photic evoked responses in premature infants. *Electroencephalogr. Clin. Neurophysiol.,* 28:55–63.
15. Valverde, F. (1968): Structural changes in the area striata of the mouse after enucleation. *Exp. Brain Res.,* 5:274–292.
16. Voeller, K., Pappas, G. D., and Purpura, D. P. (1963): Electron microscope study of development of cat superficial neocortex. *Exp. Neurol.,* 7:107–130.
17. Watanabe, K., Iwase, K., and Hara, K. (1973): Visual evoked responses during sleep and wakefulness in preterm infants. *Electroencephalogr. Clin. Neurophysiol.,* 34:571–577.

Brain Dysfunction in Infantile Febrile
Convulsions, edited by M. A. B. Brazier and
F. Coceani. Raven Press, New York © 1976.

Bridges Joining the Basic Sciences and Clinical Practice

Christopher Ounsted

Human Development Research Unit, The Park Hospital for Children, Old Road, Headington, Oxford OX3 7LQ, England

In other chapters in this volume the authors devoted their reports to the sciences basic to the main topic. The following is an attempt to form a bridge between these basic mechanisms and the problems we see in the clinic.

Rabinowicz (*this volume*) stressed three points in developmental anatomy. The central portion of the neural plate develops earlier than those above and below it. Those concerned with the epidemiology, aetiology, and (hopefully soon) the prevention of meningomyocoele will be alert to this. Timing is central to developmental medicine. Ammon's horn develops early and shows a growth spurt between 3 months and 3 years. This system is the one that is lesioned, in this age range, in 50% of the drug-resistant epilepsies. It is the active tissue at any moment which bears the brunt of developmental disaster. Brain growth rates are systems-specific; e.g., the geniculate body and its associated cortex are synchronized. Our neuropathologists, finding a congenital lesion in one section of a functional system, should search in other parts of the same system for further evidence of developmental anomalies. I doubt whether hamartomata, hamartia — those strange focal dysplasias (14) — angiomata, and the like are isolated phenomena in all our epileptic patients. Mesial temporal sclerosis is not (11).

Purpura (*this volume*) linked the visual evoked potentials (VEPs) of neonates with the maturity of their dendritic arborizations. In trisomy 18 with early seizures, both VEPs and dendrites were bizarre. In trisomy 21, *per contra,* both dendrites and VEPs were natural. One's thoughts fly to the remarkable studies by the Scheibels: Brain removed for the relief of epilepsy shows, by modified Golgi staining and electron microscopy, progressive dendritic disorganization, which may well be acquired through repeated seizures. Childhood epilepsy may be a progressive disease, cryptically afflicting dendritic anatomy (13).

Buchwald's work on maze-learning and mother-location in kittens parallels work in human developmental psychology in three fields. Early and mutual interactions and recognition are fundamental to the establishment of affectional bonds: Paediatricians who, perforce, separate premature and sick infants from their mothers may impair that bonding and, as Margaret Lynch has shown (5), add a crucial factor to those developmental trajectories which culminate in child abuse. Brain injury and seizures may follow.

There were two predictors of later skills in Buchwald's animals: weight and activity level. The correlates of weight at birth and later development are under intense paediatric scrutiny (9). Self-regulatory mechanisms in human infants regulate both milk intake and weight gain per kilogram such that postnatal growth is inversely related to birth weight: large-for-dates neonates grow slowly, and small-for-dates fast. Their trajectories draw them away from the extremes towards the safer median of size. Does this happen in any other mammal? Hammond showed it did not in the horse (8).

Activity levels, both high and low, bring toddlers to our clinics, and all too often the literature persuades us to medicate with drugs such as amphetamine which interact with brain transmitters. However, intense activity may be intense exploratory learning, the necessary precursor of later intellectual aptitudes (6). Chemical intervention could be perilous.

Yet the brain-injured child is overactive and does show learning deficits. Buchwald's animals, lesioned in the caudate, had trouble only with reversal learning, specifically because of perseveration. It is the perseveration of the damaged child which disrupts his strategy of exploratory learning, and it is this that we clinicians must learn to measure and modify (4).

From Prince's work (*this volume*) we learned that potassium is regional in its distribution and effects. The fluxes of potassium, sodium, and calcium figure largely in our thoughts on the ionic factors in neonatal, febrile, and (later) limbic seizures (1). His discourse on the widespread effects of a discharging lesion interlocks with clinical studies showing that the electroencephalographic (EEG) paroxysm—the so-called subclinical paroxysm—is not subclinical at all when the brain is performing skilled tasks rapidly. Channel capacity is reduced by a mere 150 μV of spike-and-wave, and a transient impairment of information-processing occurs (7).

Anticonvulsant drugs, psychotropic drugs, and stimulants if they work at all do so by selective poisoning, usually of one of the normal transmitter systems in the brain. These actions, as Coyle showed for fluphenazine, are always age-dependent. Drugs standardized on adults can and often do have different and even paradoxical effects on the immature brain. The drugs we give can interfere with excitatory and inhibitory transmitters, but these are not independent. Coyle showed that, developmentally, dopamine, γ-aminobutyric acid, and acetylcholine rise exactly in parallel. I interpret that to mean that there are servolinks between their systems. When our drugs block or enhance one transmitter system, they may alter all of them.

We were told there are five processes in every synapse: synthesis, storage, release, reception, and reuptake. We need the basic scientists to study where and how our common drugs—phenobarbitone, diphenylhydantoinate, and the rest—actually operate. At the moment we clinicians, like St. Paul, "see through a glass darkly."

Costa and his colleagues fixed their animals' brains instantly with a mag-netron and examined acetylcholine and cyclic nucleotides developmentally at many brain sites. I think that the most important of these sites for epi-leptologists is the locus coeruleus—that blue patch in the ventricular floor. (It is really brown inside, is it not?) Choline acetyltransferase and acetyl-choline seem somewhat out of phase here in early development. Now Gray (2), in Oxford, has shown a specific effect of minor tranquillizers on those neural processes which arise from the locus coeruleus. The drugs he uses, however, are diazepam and amylobarbitone (Amytal®)—the very drugs we find most effective in the arrest of status epilepticus, both febrile and non-febrile, in our young patients. Paediatricians must learn more about this blue patch and its processes. These may be central to our most important activ-ity: saving the immature brain from death or partial destruction during long febrile fits.

By definition fever is present in the phenomenon we are concerned with. The relationship between fever, the infective agent (if any), and convulsions is not simple. Those who have not yet learned Lennox-Buchthal's (3) classic work by heart should do so straightaway if you wish to grasp the complexity of the facts.

How is temperature regulated? How is fever generated? Our basic scien-tists claimed not to know—and then expounded in profuse detail. Schön-baum and Lomax conspired and created a scholarly historical account and a coherent theory. They follow Claude Bernard who wrote: "An hypothesis is the obligatory starting point of all experimental reasoning. Without it no investigation would be possible, and one would learn nothing. . . ." How-ever, all the theories we heard were instantly, and with proper modesty, qualified. There were age differences; there were species differences within the mammalia; the phylogeny of the prostaglandins was puzzling; different neurochemical sequences led to the same hyper- or hypothermia. Therefore all would agree with Claude Bernard's second dictum (less often quoted): "When propounding a general theory in science, the one thing one can be sure of is that, in the strict sense, such theories are mistaken."

Our scientists' theories are surely very nearly right. Temperature is regu-lated centrally, mainly in the anterior hypothalamus. Sensors on either side of a set point (which may simply be the balance of gains in the feedback loops) respond to neural and chemical changes. They can anticipate the need to conserve or dissipate heat. They can heed the psyche. In a warm theatre I shivered uncontrollably and cowered in my seat during the opening scene of Shakespeare's *Tempest;* but regulation is normally efficient and continues, as Liebermeister argued 90 years ago, during fever. The nature of that regu-lation may vary. Sellers (12) established that rats in a cold room shiver to gain heat, but after 30 days they have acclimated and learned nonshivering heat production. Our neonates do not shiver: They have available brown fat richly adrenergically innervated as a heat source; yet weak ones, exposed to infection and cold, may come to us in hypothermia, which is worse than its opposite, the febrile convulsion, in its effects on the brain. The Creator took note of this (may I remind the scientists?) when He arranged that all regulators, including that for temperature, should be *un*evenly sensitive on either side of their set points.

Lomax, Schönbaum, Cooper, Veale, Ziel, and Milton—each in his own idiosyncratic but equally elegant researches—built up a body of evidence linking the invasion by an alien agent and the febrile response. Wolff and his colleagues argue that exogenous pyrogens enter. White cells, other than lymphocytes, release endogenous pyrogens, one of large and the other of small molecular weight. White cell interactions are central to febrile convulsions. Lennox-Buchthal (3) showed that nearly half of all children with febrile convulsions have neutropenia below 2,000 mm^3. She showed that these convulsing children with febrile neutropenia had other features in common. They were younger than others convulsing to fever; the convulsions were more severe; often the virus was that of exanthem subitum (or, if we follow Zahorsky, roseola infantum); the patients often came from all-male single-sexed sibships. Here is a challenge to basic scientists to help us. Recall Veale's observation that the first injection of exogenous pyrogen did not cause fever, but it did cause neutropenia.

The two endogenous pyrogens are released from white cells and they home (both of them? why two of them?) on the hypothalamic preoptic regions. Prostagladin E_1 (PGE_1) or others of this ubiquitous species, are released. Prostaglandins were central to everyone's discourse. Ziel convinced us that antipyretics are also anti-inflammatory, analgesic, and inhibitory to platelet aggregation. These four properties are due to one fact. They block the synthesis of PGE_1, whether this occurs in the brain or in the seminal vesicles (organs geographically removed, but, if we believe the early paediatric neurologist S. Freud, psychiatrically linked). Paediatricians are concerned with PGE_1 not only in fever and convulsion but also during labour. Parturition is now regularly induced in women with unripe cervices by PGE_2 either by the intravenous or the extra-amniotic route. What is the effect on the neonate and its subsequent development? A woman who shares my surname is currently investigating this, and the early results are hopeful. PGE has a mercifully short half-life.

Prostaglandins, Coceani reported, are probably not transmitters; rather they are modulators or messengers or both within the central nervous system. The paths of prostaglandin formation and degradation, he showed, were branching, controlled, and lawful. Veale demonstrated that PGE_1 release of fever is dose-dependent. Cooper, filling the ventricles with oil, produced sustained PGE_1-based fever. He showed also (and this we clinicians must be alert to) that transmitter depletion by reserpine lagged PGE_1 fever to a slow rise. We know that the sharply rising high fever is that which triggers convulsion in our patients.

We are deeply concerned with the limbic ictus (11), and Hayward's work on vasopressin release by amygdala stimulation is directly relevant: vasopressin release, temperature fluctuation, water retention, apnoea. Compare the limbic ictus: blanch-blush sequence; paroxysmal hypertension with tachycardia; borborygmus; the rising abdominal aura; respiration arrested in expiratory apnoea.

What happens when a long seizure occurs? Most convulsions are brief. They serve, I believe, a homeostatic function, perhaps to deplete the brain of an excess of both excitatory and inhibitory transmitters brought about by sudden fever and driving transmitter production beyond a safe limit. (A grotesque guess but testable by the delicate methods available.)

Runaway seizure into febrile status is what we all fear. Positive feedback has taken over. Could Veale's vasopressin play a part?

We repeatedly considered acetylcholine as a unitary chemical, but Tangri neatly showed us that, in relation to fever, this compound is, as always, Janus-faced. Its nicotinic actions, controlled by norepinephrine neurons, may serve to raise temperature. Its muscarinic actions, controlled by serotonin neurons, subserve heat loss.

Finally some questions from us to the basic scientists. Why do you speak of "the brain?" In our species, at least, there are four brains (10). The left female, the left male, the right female, and the right male. They differ in their anatomy, development, and functional capacities. Pray attend to the gender difference. Please tell us the sex of your animals. You have told us much about transmitters and fever but what about convulsions? Why do they afflict the immature brain? Why are they ubiquitous?

I have oversimplified these impressive researches. I plead in mitigation Isaac Newton, in whose third volume of the *Principia Mathematica* — issued under the imprimatur of Samuel Pepys himself — we read: "Nature is pleased with simplicity and affects not the pomp of superfluous causes." At the same time we discern within the immense complexity of the basic work a rigorous lawfulness expressed by Albert Einstein when he said of the general theory of relativity: *"Raffiniert ist der Herrgott, aber boshaft ist Er nicht."* The Lord God is subtle but He does not cheat.

REFERENCES

1. Glaser, G. (1975): Epilepsy. In: *Recent Advances in Clinical Neurology,* edited by W. B. Matthews, pp. 23–66. Churchill, Livingstone, London.
2. Gray, J. Personal communication.
3. Lennox-Buchthal, M. (1973): Febrile convulsions: A reappraisal. *Electroencephalogr. Clin. Neurophysiol. (Suppl. 32).*
4. Lindsay, J. (1972): The difficult epileptic child. *Br. Med. J.,* 3:283–285.
5. Lynch, M. (1975): Ill-health and child abuse. *Lancet,* 2:317–319.
6. Ounsted, C. (1970): A biological approach to autistic and hyperkinetic syndromes. In: *Modern Trends in Paediatrics,* edited by J. Apley, pp. 286–316. Butterworths, London.
7. Ounsted, C. (1971): Some aspects of seizure disorders. In: *Recent Advances in Paediatrics,* 4th edition, edited by D. Gairdner and D. Hull, pp. 371–374. Churchill, London.

8. Ounsted, C., and Ounsted, M. (1973): On fetal growth rate. In: *Developmental Medicine,* No. 46, pp. 32–38. Heinemann, London.
9. Ounsted, M., and Sleigh, G. (1975): The infant's self-regulation of food intake and weight gain. *Lancet,* 1:1393–1396.
10. Ounsted, C., and Taylor, D. C., editors. (1972): The Y chromosome message: a point of view. In: *Gender Differences: Their Ontogeny and Significance,* pp. 241–262. Churchill, Livingstone, London.
11. Ounsted, C., Lindsay, J., and Norman, R. (1966): The pathogenesis of temporal lobe epilepsy. In: *Biological Factors in Temporal Lobe Epilepsy,* pp. 32–49. Heinemann, London.
12. Preston, E., and Schönbaum, E. (1976): Monoaminergic mechanisms in thermoregulation. *This volume.*
13. Scheibel, M. E., and Scheibel, A. B. (1973): Hippocampal pathology in temporal lobe epilepsy: a Golgi survey. In: *Epilepsy: Its Phenomena in Man,* edited by M. A. B. Brazier, pp. 315–337. Academic Press, New York.
14. Taylor, D. C., Falconer, M. A., Bruton, C. J., and Corsellis, J. A. N. (1971): Focal dysplasia of the cerebral cortex in epilepsy. *Neurol. Neurosurg. Psychiatry,* 34:369–387.

Brain Dysfunction in Infantile Febrile Convulsions, edited by M. A. B. Brazier and F. Coceani. Raven Press, New York © 1976.

Febrile Convulsions: Neurological Sequelae and Mental Retardation

Jean Aicardi and Jean-Jacques Chevrie

Hôpital Saint Vincent de Paul, 75674 Paris Cedex 14; and Institut National de la Santé et de la Recherche Medicale, Paris, France

The sequelae of febrile convulsions has long been a subject of interest. Some of these sequelae have received particular attention, i.e., epilepsy, especially temporal lobe epilepsy (e.g., 5,8,9,15,23) and hemiplegia subsequent to prolonged unilateral febrile seizures (3,11,13,21). However, to our knowledge no work has been concerned specifically with sequelae in general of febrile convulsions or with the factors which might favour their appearance.

We are reporting here a retrospective study of a series of 402 patients with febrile convulsions (a) to describe in general the epileptic, mental, and neurological complications as observed in this series; and (b) to try to determine, by comparing patients whose febrile convulsions had sequelae with those that did not, whether the occurrence of sequelae is associated with certain characteristics of the febrile seizures themselves or of the population affected.

PATIENTS AND METHODS

Febrile convulsions were defined as convulsions occurring with a fever of 38°C or more. When the fever was due to infection of the central nervous system (e.g., meningitis or encephalitis), the patient was excluded from the study, as were patients with fever and acute dehydration and those with an abnormal cerebrospinal fluid. When the fever was due to one of the common infectious diseases of childhood, only those patients who had a convulsion during the initial phase of the disease were included.

A series of 402 patients with febrile convulsions, hospitalized or seen as outpatients at our hospital between January 1963 and December 1971 who fulfilled the above criteria were studied retrospectively. The composition of the series is shown in Table 1.

All patients in whom epilepsy (defined as one afebrile seizure or more), mental retardation (IQ $\leq$ 80), or neurological deficit was present after the febrile seizure were considered to have sequelae when there was no evidence of antecedent mental retardation or neurological abnormality; 18 infants

TABLE 1. *Composition of the series of 402 patients*

Convulsions	Male	Female	Total
Bilateral < 30 min	137	119	256
Bilateral ≥ 30 min			
First FC[a]	14	22	36
Later FC	6	0	6
Unilateral < 30 min			
First FC	16	12	28
Later FC	0	0	0
Unilateral ≥ 30 min			
First FC	25	34	59
Later FC	7	10	17
Total	205	197	402

[a] FC, febrile convulsion.

with such evidence were not considered to have sequelae. Minor psychological or behavioral abnormalities were not studied.

The children with sequelae were then compared with a group of 86 patients selected from the total series because they had been followed for 3 years or more (mean 5.2, median 4.75, range 3–12 years) and had had no sequelae when last seen. This "control" group was in turn compared with the remaining patients who had had febrile convulsions but no known sequelae who were followed for less than 3 years. This was to check whether a long follow-up found characteristics different from those in patients with no sequelae but who were followed for a shorter period; no difference between the two groups was found.

The following factors were compared in the group with sequelae and the controls: age at the time of the first febrile convulsion; incidence of long convulsions (30 min or more); incidence of unilateral convulsions, including convulsions predominating on one side of the body or followed by transient or permanent hemiparesis; sex; abnormal pregnancy; abnormal delivery (for details see ref. 6); birth weight; family history of febrile convulsions or epilepsy in parents, grandparents, siblings, aunts, and uncles; recurrence of febrile convulsions one or more times.

Comparisons were made by usual statistical methods. Because of their log-normal distribution, ages were compared using a log transformation. The mean and standard deviation (SD) are given without log transformation in the text and tables. When it was necessary to take a third factor into account, the method of adjustment by summation of the expected number for each cell was used (4,25).

RESULTS

Clinical Features

A total of 131 patients, 67 girls and 64 boys, had one or more sequelae (Table 2). Epilepsy was the most frequent one, being present in 114 children.

TABLE 2. *Neurological and mental sequelae of febrile convulsions*

Sequelae	No.
Epilepsy	114
Frequency of seizures	
Rare or infrequent	65
Frequent to daily	49
Type of seizure	
Partial and secondarily generalized	81
Lennox	9[a]
Partial motor	19[a]
Psychomotor	51[a]
Generalized	28
Unclassified	5
Neurological abnormalities	37
Hemiplegia	24
Right	12
Left	12
Other	13
Mental retardation	54
Severe	15
Moderate	39
Total	131[b]

[a] More than one type of seizures in some patients.

[b] More than one type of sequela in several patients.

It varied in severity from rare or infrequent seizures (65 patients) to repeated and sometimes daily fits (49 patients). Two distinct patterns emerged; in 81 patients the seizures were of a type usually associated with brain pathology (partial motor seizures, partial seizures with complex symptomatology, Lennox syndrome); in 28 patients seizures were primarily generalized, including 3 cases of pure petit mal and 12 of myoclonic epilepsy. Partial motor seizures were equally distributed between the right and the left side (24 right, 25 left); and in patients with partial complex epilepsy without associated partial motor seizures, paroxysmal electroencephalographic (EEG) abnormalities affected the left hemisphere in 6 and the right hemisphere in 4. In 40% of our patients the first afebrile seizure occurred within 1 year after the first febrile convulsion, within 3 years in 67%, and within 4 years in 85% (Fig. 1). Epilepsy during the first year after the onset of febrile convulsion was much more often of the partial or secondarily generalized type (83%, $p < 0.05$), whereas epilepsy of late onset (after 5 years) was usually primarily generalized.

In 64 patients who developed epilepsy the involved hemisphere could be identified, from either the side of partial motor seizures (49 cases), a pronounced EEG focus (15 cases), or both. One febrile convulsion or more had been lateralized in 42 of these 64 patients. In all but 2 cases the hemi-

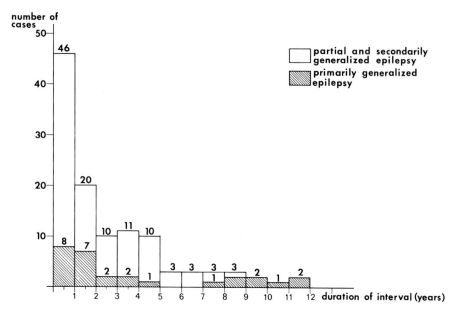

FIG. 1. Interval between the first febrile convulsion and the first epileptic seizure.

sphere that was the site of the epileptic process was the same as that pre-dominantly involved in the lateralized febrile convulsion. In 2 more patients no conclusion was possible since unilateral febrile seizures had involved first one and then the other side. The mean age when the febrile convulsions occurred in patients who developed partial epilepsy was 16.2 months for those with left-sided lesions (boys 16.5 months, girls 16.1 months) and 19.8 months for those with right-sided lesions (boys 21.5 months, girls 18.2 months). The differences are not significant. Epilepsy was the sole sequela in 58 patients. In 30 children it was associated with mental retardation, in 8 with neurological sequelae, and in 18 with both.

Mental retardation was a sequela of the febrile convulsion in 54 patients. It was severe in 15 and moderate in 39. Mental deficiency was seldom the sole residuum. In all but 6 patients it was associated with epilepsy, and in 18 children with both epilepsy and neurological deficit.

Neurological sequelae were seen in 37 children, associated with epilepsy in 26 and with mental retardation in 18. Hemiplegia was the most common deficit, being present in 24 patients (12 right-sided and 12 left-sided); 75% of hemiplegias were in girls. The mean age of the lateralized febrile convulsions followed by hemiplegia was 15.9 months and did not differ between boys (15 months) and girls (16.2 months). Other neurological sequelae included diplegia, bilateral pyramidal and cerebellar syndromes, and micro-cephaly in various combinations. Pneumoencephalography performed in

23 patients disclosed dilatation of one or both lateral ventricles in 21. In 3 of these the ventricular dilatation was present only on a pneumoencephalogram repeated 1–5 months after the first one (1). No vascular abnormality was found by any of the nine carotid angiographies performed in hemiplegic patients.

Although two or more sequelae were present in 56 patients, the three main sequelae were statistically independent of each other. For example, the incidence of epilepsy was not different in patients with or without mental retardation or neurological sequelae. This was true, however, only when all cases of epilepsy were combined, for a significant relation was evident only when partial and secondarily generalized epilepsies were considered (see below).

Patients with Sequelae Compared with Controls

The occurrence of sequelae was related significantly with four factors: age at the first febrile convulsion; duration and lateralization of at least one of the febrile seizures; and occurrence of febrile recurrences. The mean age of patients at the time of the first febrile convulsion was significantly younger for those in each category of sequela and in the whole group with sequelae than in the control group (Table 3). The incidence of long-lasting and of one-sided febrile seizures in children with sequelae was much higher than in the controls. Since there was a strong relation between long duration and unilateral localization of the febrile convulsions ($p < 0.001$), each factor was compared. After adjustment for lateralization, only duration remained significantly linked with the occurrence of sequelae ($p < 0.05$). Febrile recurrences, on the other hand, were more common in children without sequelae than in those with residua, but significantly so only when all sequelae were combined.

No significant differences were found between the two groups for the other factors studied. Girls outnumbered boys in those with neurological sequelae but not significantly so except in the subgroup of hemiplegias ($p < 0.05$). There was a trend towards a higher incidence of abnormal deliveries among the controls. No relation with positive family history was apparent in any category of sequelae.

Since patients with residual epilepsy seemed to belong in two categories, this group was analyzed by comparing the 28 patients with generalized epilepsy with 81 children with partial or secondarily generalized seizures (Table 4). Patients in the former subgroup were significantly older at the time of the first febrile seizure ($p < 0.001$) and only exceptionally had their febrile seizures been localized or of long duration. Furthermore, boys outnumbered girls ($p < 0.05$); also the incidence of associated mental retardation (14%) and of neurological deficit (4%) was lower than in children with partial epilepsy, of whom 52% had mental deficiency and 31% had neuro-

TABLE 3. *Comparison between patients with sequelae and control*

Factor studied	Controls N = 86	Epilepsy N = 114	p	Mental retardation N = 54	p	Neurological sequelae N = 37	p	All sequelae N = 37	p
Age at first febrile convulsion (months)	20.3	16.3	<0.05[a]	13.8	<0.001[b]	14.0	<0.001[b]	16.2	<0.05[a]
Seizure ≥ 30 min	15 (17.4)	53 (46.5)	<0.001[b]	36 (66.8)	<0.001[b]	33 (89.2)	<0.001[b]	66 (50.4)	<0.001[b]
Lateralized seizure	15 (17.4)	50 (43.9)	<0.001[b]	28 (51.8)	<0.001[b]	31 (83.8)	<0.001[b]	57 (43.5)	<0.001[b]
Female sex	40 (46.5)	60 (52.6)	<0.20	26 (48.1)	>0.40	24 (64.9)	<0.10	67 (51.1)	<0.30
Abnormal pregnancy	5 (5.8)	11 (9.6)	<0.20	6 (11.1)	<0.30	6 (16.2)	<0.30	15 (11.4)	<0.20
Abnormal delivery	19 (22.1)	15 (13.2)	<0.10	7 (12.9)	<0.20	6 (16.2)	<0.30	19 (14.5)	<0.20
Birth weight (g)	3,195	3,205	>0.40	3,104	>0.50	3,179	>0.80	3,178	>0.80
Positive family history	29 (33.7)	40 (35.1)	>0.40	15 (27.8)	<0.30	8 (21.6)	<0.20	44 (33.6)	>0.50
Febrile recurrences	51 (59.3)	52 (45.6)	<0.10	25 (46.3)	<0.20	14 (41.2)	<0.10	58 (44.3)	<0.05[a]

See text for details.

In each column, the first figure indicates the number of cases with the factor, the second figure (in parentheses) the percentage of patients with the factor.

[a] Significant.

[b] Very highly significant.

TABLE 4. *Comparison between 81 partial and 28 generalized epilepsies*

Factor studied	Partial epilepsy[a]	Generalized epilepsy[b]	p
Age at first febrile convulsion (months)	14.2	20.7	<0.001[c]
Seizure ≥ 30 min	49 (60.5)	1 (3.6)	<0.001[c]
Lateralized seizure	46 (56.8)	1 (3.6)	<0.001[c]
Female sex	44 (54.3)	8 (28.6)	<0.05[d]
Positive family history	30 (37.0)	8 (28.6)	>0.40
Frequency of mental retardation	42 (51.8)	4 (14.3)	<0.001[c]
Frequency of neurological sequelae	25 (30.9)	1 (3.6)	<0.001[c]
Febrile recurrences	33 (40.7)	16 (57.1)	<0.10

[a] Partial or secondarily generalized.
[b] Five cases were excluded because of uncertainty of type.
[c] Very highly significant.
[d] Significant.

logical sequelae. Children with generalized epilepsy did not differ from patients without sequelae except for the higher incidence of boys ($p < 0.05$).

DISCUSSION

Although the high incidence of sequelae in our series attests to the potential seriousness of febrile convulsions, it cannot be taken to indicate the incidence in febrile seizures in general. Severe cases from a large population are referred to our hospital, while less severe cases are treated locally. Likewise, the proportions of the various types of sequela may reflect preferential referral of a particular category of patients. This study is therefore especially concerned with the relation of certain characteristics of the febrile convulsion with the outcome. As ours is a retrospective series, only simple criteria defining relatively clear-cut categories were used to limit the number of misclassifications. The unequal duration of the follow-up introduces a special problem since sequelae may first appear late and since many patients without known sequelae were followed for only brief periods. Mental and neurological sequelae, however, are usually rapidly evident and therefore unlikely to be missed, even when the follow-up is short. Epileptic sequelae, on the other hand, may emerge at any time. In this series, as in previous ones (2,11,24) however, a great majority of the epilepsies had their onset within 3 years of the first febrile convulsion, so that selection of the "control" group on the basis of a 3-year follow-up is probably reasonable. Moreover, no difference was found, for the factors studied, between those patients without known residua observed for 3 years or more and those with shorter follow-up periods, which suggests that our "controls" constitute a valid sample of our population of uncomplicated febrile convulsions.

Our results support the previously expressed opinion that a young age at onset of febrile convulsions, a long duration or a unilateral localization of the febrile seizures, or both significantly increase the likelihood of sequelae. In addition, they bring out more information on the respective roles of the duration and lateralization of the convulsions in the genesis of sequelae and on certain aspects of some of the complications of febrile convulsions, especially epilepsy and hemiplegia.

There is considerable evidence—clinical (1,5,9,23), pathological (16, 22,27), and experimental (17–19)—that long-lasting, often unilateral convulsions can produce brain damage, so that both one-sided and prolonged seizures are usually regarded as severe (14,20). The relative importance of the two factors—lateralization and duration—known to be strongly associated with each other (12) has not been previously studied. When an appropriate method is used, however, it can be shown that duration of the convulsion is the important factor and that lateralization acts only through its usual association with long-lasting seizures. Short, unilateral convulsions do not seem to be particularly dangerous.

On the other hand, lateralization of sequelae, whether neurological or epileptic, is closely related with lateralization of the febrile convulsion, as shown by the almost invariable concordance between the side affected by the unilateral febrile convulsion and the site of the later epileptic focus or neurological deficit. It is thus probable that the frequent unilateral location of brain lesions believed to be the result of prolonged convulsions—i.e., Ammon's horn sclerosis (16,26) or mesial temporal sclerosis (7,9)—is mainly due to the fact that most long-lasting febrile convulsions are predominantly unilateral and that lateralized seizures induce ipsilateral brain damage.

Since in our series the right and left side are affected equally often, and since there is no difference between boys and girls or between sides in the age when the insult occurred, our data do not support the hypothesis of Taylor and Ounsted (28,29). They suggested that convulsions during the first 2 years are apt to involve the left hemisphere, whereas convulsions after age 2 years are more apt to damage the right hemisphere and the differential rate of cerebral maturation is responsible. Our patients, however, may not be directly comparable with theirs since they included patients with febrile convulsions due to central nervous system infection (14).

Epilepsy following febrile convulsions has been extensively studied (for references see ref. 14), some authors focusing on its incidence in series known to have had febrile convulsions while others were especially interested in the mechanism, especially of temporal lobe epilepsy. It has seldom been mentioned, however, that epileptic seizures complicating febrile convulsions are of two distinct types with differing mechanisms, and that they affect different populations of patients. Some are of the generalized variety and are apparently not due to brain lesions, as shown by the rarity of mental retardation and neurological deficit. They probably represent the persisting expression of a genetic propensity to seizures previously manifested by the febrile convulsion. The others are of the partial or secondarily generalized types and seem to result from brain damage incurred during a severe febrile convulsion. They are commonly accompanied by mental and neurological abnormalities. Thus epilepsy occupies a unique place among the complications of febrile convulsions as only the lesional epilepsies have the same significance as the other sequelae. In those cases the same factors which are at play in the genesis of the other residua are found, e.g., long duration and early age of onset of the febrile seizures. Girls are affected slightly more frequently in this group. In nonlesional cases, on the other hand, the age of onset and the characteristics of the antecedent febrile convulsions are not different from uncomplicated febrile seizures. The remarkably excessive number of boys in this group has not previously been mentioned and is not readily explainable.

Hemiplegia is the commonest neurological sequela and, curiously enough, affects far more girls than boys, a fact previously reported (3,14). A possible explanation could be that hemiplegia is a complication of the longest seizures and that these are more apt to occur in girls than in boys. In fact, the proportion of girls increases with the severity of febrile seizures, being lower in the case of brief convulsions and higher in the case of unilateral, prolonged seizures. Our impression is that convulsions leading to hemiplegia are even longer than those associated with other complications. They would thus constitute the severest form of sequelae, and their preponderance in girls would be in conformity with the tendency for severe febrile convulsions to predominate in the female sex.

Finally, the lack of relation of some of the factors studied in this work with the occurrence of sequelae deserves some comment. Contrary to previous reports (10), we did not find that a positive family history of convulsions or epilepsy was more common in febrile convulsions followed by epilepsy than in the remaining cases, regardless of whether the epilepsy was of the lesional or nonlesional type. The higher incidence of recurrence of febrile convulsions in patients without sequelae may also seem surprising. It is perhaps due to the fact that once a brain lesion has occurred as a consequence of a severe convulsion the following seizures are more apt to be true epileptic ones, rather than recurring febrile seizures. This interpretation is supported by the fact that febrile recurrences were much more common in the group of patients with generalized epilepsies than in the lesional cases.

SUMMARY

In a series of 402 patients with febrile convulsions, 131 had one or more sequelae: 114 had epilepsy, 54 mental retardation, and 37 neurological sequelae including 24 with hemiplegia.

The incidence of these sequelae was significantly higher when the first febrile convulsion had occurred at an early age and when one or more of the febrile seizures had lasted more than 30 min or had been unilateral than when febrile convulsions were brief and bilateral (controls). Hemiplegia was significantly more common in girls and could not be explained by an earlier age at onset than in boys.

Residual epilepsy was either the primary generalized type (28 cases) or the partial or secondarily generalized types (81 cases). In patients with primary generalized epilepsy the antecedent febrile seizures did not differ from those in the controls, whereas the same factors associated with the other sequelae were found in patients with other types of epilepsy.

REFERENCES

1. Aicardi, J., and Baraton, J. (1971): A pneumoencephalographic demonstration of brain atrophy following status epilepticus. *Dev. Med. Child Neurol.,* 13:660–667.
2. Aicardi, J., and Chevrie, J. J. (1971): Convulsive status epilepticus in infants and children: A study of 239 cases. *Epilepsia,* 11:187–197.
3. Aicardi, J., Amsilie, J., and Chevrie, J. J. (1969): Acute hemiplegia in infancy and childhood. *Dev. Med. Child Neurol.,* 11:162–173.
4. Boyd, J. T., and Doll, R. (1954): Gastrointestinal cancer and the use of liquid paraffin. *Br. J. Cancer,* 8:231–237.
5. Cavanagh, J. B., and Meyer, A. (1956): Aetiological aspects of Ammon's horn sclerosis associated with temporal lobe epilepsy. *Br. Med. J.,* 2:1403–1405.
6. Chevrie, J. J., and Aicardi, J. (1975): Duration and lateralization of febrile convulsions: Relations with etiological factors. *Epilepsia,* 16:781–789.
7. Corsellis, J. A. N. (1970): The pathological anatomy of the temporal lobe with special reference to the limbic areas. In: *Modern Trends in Psychological Medicine,* Vol. 2, edited by J. H. Price. Butterworths, London.
8. Falconer, M. A. (1971): Genetic and related aetiological factors in temporal lobe epilepsy: A review. *Epilepsia,* 13:279–285.
9. Falconer, M. A., Serafetinides, E. A., and Corsellis, J. A. N. (1964): Etiology and pathogenesis of temporal lobe epilepsy. *Arch. Neurol.,* 10:232–248.
10. Frantzen, E., Lennox-Buchthal, M., Nygaard, A., and Stene, J. A. (1970): A genetic study of febrile convulsions. *Neurology (Minneap.),* 20:909–917.
11. Gastaut, H., Poirier, F., Payan, H., Salamon, G., Toga, M., and Vigouroux, M. (1960): H. H. E. syndrome: Hemiconvulsions, hemiplegia, epilepsy. *Epilepsia,* 1:418–447.
12. Herlitz, G. (1941): Studien über die sogennanten initialen Fieberkrämpfe bei Kindern. *Acta Paediatr. (Uppsala) (Suppl. 1),* 29:1–142.
13. Isler, W. (1971): *Acute Hemiplegias and Hemisyndromes in Childhood.* Heinemann, London.
14. Lennox-Buchthal, M. A. (1973): *Febrile Convulsions. A Reappraisal.* Elsevier, Amsterdam.
15. Lindsay, J. M. M. (1971): Genetics and epilepsy: A model from critical path analysis. *Epilepsia,* 12:47–54.
16. Margerison, J. H., and Corsellis, J. A. N. (1966): Epilepsy and the temporal lobe: A clinical, electroencephalographic and neuropathological study of the brain in epilepsy, with particular reference to the temporal lobes. *Brain,* 89:499–530.
17. Meldrum, B. S., and Brierley, J. B. (1973): Prolonged epileptic seizures in primates: Ischemic cell change and its relation to ictal physiological events. *Arch. Neurol.,* 28:10–17.
18. Meldrum, B. S., and Horton, R. W. (1973): Physiology of status epilepticus in primates. *Arch. Neurol.,* 28:1–9.
19. Meldrum, B. S., Vigouroux, R. A., and Brierley, J. B. (1973): Systemic factors and epileptic brain damage: Prolonged seizures in paralyzed, artificially ventilated baboons. *Arch. Neurol.,* 29:82–87.
20. Millichap, J. G. (1968): *Febrile Convulsions.* Macmillan, New York.

21. Norman, R. M. (1962): Neuropathological findings in acute hemiplegia in childhood, with special reference to epilepsy as a pathogenic factor. In: *Acute hemiplegia in Childhood. Clinics in Developmental Medicine No. 6,* edited by M. Bax and R. G. Mitchell. Heinemann, London.
22. Norman, R. M. (1964): The neuropathology of status epilepticus. *Med. Sci. Law,* 4:46–51.
23. Ounsted, C., Lindsay, J., and Norman, R. (1966): *Biological Factors in Temporal Lobe Epilepsy.* Heinemann, London.
24. Roger, J., Bureau, M., Dravet, C., Dalla Bernadina, B., Tassinari, C. A., Revol, M., Challamel, M. J., and Taillandier, P. (1972): Les données EEG, et manifestations épileptiques en relation avec l'hémiplégie cérébrale infantile. *Rev. Electroencephalogr. Neurophysiol. Clin.,* 2:5–28.
25. Rouquette, C., and Schwartz, D. (1970): *Methodes en Épidémiologie.* Flammarion, Paris.
26. Sano, K., and Malamud, N. (1953): Clinical significance of sclerosis of the cornu ammonis: Ictal psychic phenomena. *Arch. Neurol. Psychiatry,* 70:40–53.
27. Scholz, W. (1951): *Die Krampfschädigungen des Gehirns.* Springer, Berlin.
28. Taylor, D. C. (1969): Differential rates of cerebral maturation between sexes and between hemispheres: Evidence from epilepsy. *Lancet,* 2:140–142.
29. Taylor, D. C., and Ounsted, C. (1971): Biological mechanisms influencing the outcome of seizures in response to fever. *Epilepsia,* 12:33–45.

*Brain Dysfunction in Infantile Febrile
Convulsions*, edited by M. A. B. Brazier and
F. Coceani. Raven Press, New York © 1976.

Neurological and Intellectual Deficits: Convulsions with Fever Viewed as Acute Indications of Life-Long Developmental Defects

Sheila J. Wallace

*Department of Child Health, University Hospital of Wales, Heath Park,
Cardiff CF4 4XW, Wales*

"No fit can be studied outside the context of developmental medicine" (36). It has been suggested that a febrile convulsion is a symptom of an organic cerebral lesion precipitated by a raised body temperature, and that such a convulsion is not the response of a normal child (38). Further substance is given to these statements by the finding that only 11% of children admitted to hospital with fever have a seizure (13).

I propose to examine the concept that a convulsion with fever is a symptom of developmental aberration. Special reference is made to a prospective series of 134 children with a convulsion admitted consecutively to the Royal Hospital for Sick Children, Edinburgh, between December 1964 and August 1966. All were more than 2 months and less than 7 years of age at the time of admission and were febrile or had definite evidence of active infection; 124 were seen at the time of their first convulsion, and 10 with their second or third convulsion with fever. Their fits are considered in the context of their development prior and subsequent to their seizures.

INCIDENCE OF FACTORS ASSOCIATED WITH SUBOPTIMAL NEUROLOGICAL DEVELOPMENT

Inherited Factors

Although the exact neurophysiological mechanism involved in the production of a convulsion in response to a febrile illness has not been elucidated, it is well documented that children who convulse with fevers have a high incidence of convulsive disorders amongst relatives (24). Inheritance of a convulsion trait must therefore be considered one of the neurological deficits in these children. Lennox-Buchthal (24), reviewing reports from many authors, found widely differing incidences of positive family history. In the Edinburgh series family histories were available for 131 of the 134 children;

50 (38%) had a positive history of convulsive disorder in siblings or parents. Conversely, detailed questioning in a small series of 35 control children admitted to the Royal Hospital for Sick Children, Edinburgh, febrile but without fits, revealed a positive family history for convulsive disorders in only 6 (17%) (χ^2 5.45, df 1, p 0.02).

At least one neurological deficit of a more obviously anatomical nature which also has an increased familial incidence is associated with an enhanced risk of convulsions when the child becomes febrile. A group of 70 children with spina bifida with or without clinical hydrocephalus were studied in Cardiff Royal Infirmary between 1968 and 1971 (52); 10 (14%) had convulsions with a feverish illness in the absence of evidence of raised intracranial pressure. This compares with the usual maximal incidence of 5–6% for the general population. It seems possible that less gross but equally important anatomical deficits may be inherited more commonly than is generally appreciated and may contribute to familial propensities to convulsions with fever.

Preconceptual Environmental Factors

A number of chronic disorders in mothers have been identified as associated with increased fetal wastage and a high incidence of suboptimal neurological development in those children who survive (5,8,12,14,16,21, 27,28,33,39,44,45). Nonspecific chronic ill health has been reported often in mothers of children with congenital diplegia (20) and epilepsy (25). The common factor is probably undernourishment of the fetal brain at a critical period in its development, as described by Dobbing (6).

The parents of 108 of the 134 Edinburgh children, and those of 33 of the 35 controls satisfied criteria for a study of reproductive efficiency (49). A significant excess of mothers whose children convulsed suffered from chronic illnesses (χ^2 5.95, df 1, $p < 0.02$). Examination of the reproductive histories of the mothers of the 71 males showed significant lengthening of the intervals between conceptions adjacent to those involving a patient when these were compared with intervals between other members of a sibship (χ^2 4.2, df 1, p 0.05). A multiplicity of pregnancy and perinatal abnormalities was also significantly more likely in those males whose mothers were subfertile according to criteria defined by Ingram and Russell (20). There is evidence therefore that mothers who have chronic illnesses and those who are delivered of a male during a period of relative infertility have an increased risk of producing a child liable to convulse when febrile.

Of 65 children of either sex born to subfertile mothers, 32 (49%) had convulsed compared with 68 (36%) of 188 offspring of fertile mothers (χ^2 3.19, not significant). After correction for sex and positive history of convulsions in parents, when compared with those born to subfertile mothers, convulsing children born to fertile mothers had a significant excess of siblings who also convulsed (χ^2 4.98, df 1, $p < 0.05$). It is suggested that the inherited convulsion trait and parental subfertility act independently in the production of neurological deficits.

Postconceptual and Perinatal Factors

Incidents likely to affect the brain during the ante- or perinatal periods have been reported by many authors. Millichap (31), reviewing previous papers, gives the average frequency of "birth injury" in children with febrile convulsions as 17%, with a variation of 3–34%. The implications of such percentages are doubtful in the absence of reference to comparable children who have not convulsed.

In the Edinburgh series the baby and maternal records of 132 children who had had convulsions were compared with those of 180 of their nonconvulsing siblings (48). Eighty patients (61%) had at least one adverse factor during the pre- or perinatal periods significantly more often than their siblings. For both sexes these factors were threatened abortion (χ^2 8.6, df 1, p 0.005), caesarean section (χ^2 7, df 2, p 0.02), moderately low birth weight (χ^2 6.4, df 1, p 0.02), and maternal medication with substances other than iron (χ^2 14, df 1, p 0.005). Of the 48 mothers who were medicated, 27 were given drugs such as barbiturates, antiemetics, and antidepressives, which are known to affect the central nervous system. At birth 24 (18%) of the patients weighed less than those in the tenth percentile for sex, gestation, maternal height, and birth order, suggesting some degree of intrauterine malnutrition. The male patients suffered significantly more often from fetal distress (χ^2 6.2, df 1, p 0.02) and more frequently fed poorly during the neonatal period (χ^2 4.3, df 1, p 0.05). By the end of the neonatal period, therefore, at least 61% of the Edinburgh patients either had suffered an insult that could predispose to anatomical neurological deficit, or already had a symptom (i.e., poor feeding) which could be neurologically determined.

DEVELOPMENTAL HISTORY PRIOR TO CONVULSIONS

The first convulsion with fever usually occurs so early in a child's life that sophisticated motor and intellectual performance are not expected, and it is probable that minor degrees of developmental aberration pass unremarked by parents. However, many authors comment on the presence of conditions that must have predated the first seizure. Aicardi and Chevrie (1) report neurological abnormality before status epilepticus in 41 of 88 who were abnormal after the episode, and mental retardation before status in 26 of 114 children who were retarded afterwards. Approximately half of their series had raised temperatures during the status, but the exact number of febrile children with preceding neurological abnormality or mental retardation is unclear. Degen and Goller (4) found that 14 of 133 had delayed milestones, and that 6 of the 14 were abnormal before the first fit. Doose et al. (7) also include children with previous brain damage in their series of 525 patients, 63 (12%) of whom had had disturbances of development prior to their first fit. Two of 208 children were mentally retarded prior to their first fit in the group reported by Frantzen et al. (11). Herlitz (17) performed a retrospective study of 776 cases; 17 were abnormal before the first convulsion with fever. Of these, 14 were mentally retarded, 2 hemiplegic, and 1 hydrocephalic. These children were no different in age or temperature from others in the series. Horstmann and Schinnerling (18) also included children with a previous abnormality in their series, but the exact number of those with delayed milestones as a separate entity from those with birth injury is not stated. Although Hrbek (19) felt children with brain damage should be excluded from a treatise on febrile convulsions, he has alluded to some with birth injury and lowered intelligence amongst his patients. It is not clear, however, whether the latter patients were abnormal before their first seizure. Bamberger and Matthes (2) report that 61 (9.6%) of 634 children had neurological damage prior to their first febrile convulsion. These included disorders of pregnancy 28, birth injury 43, "debility" 12, hemiplegia 2, hydrocephalus 1, and kernicterus 1. One-third of the children in their series who died in a febrile convulsion had had neurological abnormality preceding the fit. Lennox (22) found IQs of less than 80 in 22% of her series of 240 cases, but the ages and states at which these were measured is not obvious. Melekian et al. (30) examined 24 children in whom episodes of acute dehydration occurring with fever were complicated by fits; 7 of the 9 who were neurologically abnormal had been so prior to the dehydrating event. Cerebral dysgenesis was reported in 5 of 302 patients by Peterman (38). Zellweger (54) examined the preictal state of his patients in more detail than most authors. His series consists of 151 children who had fits when febrile and 27 who had febrile and other convulsions; 12 had neurological disorders including "mild debility," hydrocephalus, microcephaly, infantile hemiplegia, diplegia, hemispheric damage, lowered intelligence, and previous head injury prior to their first fits. Three of the 7 patients who had their first fit with fever during the first 6 months of life had other abnormalities. Seven children are reported as high-grade mental defectives, but it is unclear whether these included some who were also neurologically abnormal. Anthropomorphic measurements were performed on some of the patients at the time of the first fit. Head circumferences were more than 1 cm above the mean for age in 32, and more than 1 cm below the mean for age in 7 of 58 children measured. Of 38 children whose heights were measured, 27 were taller and 8 shorter than expected. Apart from mentioning that the heads of 4 children were larger than expected and that there was 1 microcephalic, correlation of height and head circumference measurements is not made. Although only gross neurological changes have been described, in virtually all the foregoing series the incidence of neurological abnormality antedating the first fit with fever is higher than would be expected in the general population.

At the time of admission to hospital, detailed developmental histories were taken from the parents or guardians of the 134 Edinburgh patients. These are compared with the histories of those of the patients' siblings who had not themselves had convulsions (51). Although many of the patients were subsequently thought to have been neurologically disadvantaged prior to their first fit, in no case had the parents felt any symptom to have been of sufficient moment for medical advice to have been sought.

The age at independent walking was available in 82 male patients and 81 male siblings. Compared with the siblings, a nonsignificant trend towards later independent walking was observed in the patients. Of the 81 male siblings, 60 walked before the age of 14 months, whereas only 44 of 66 male patients whose first fit occurred after they had started to walk achieved this milestone before 14 months. As expected, male patients who were not walking at the time of the first fit had fits significantly earlier than those who walked before the first seizure ($p < 0.005$). However, those who had had a fit before starting to walk walked after 14 months significantly more often than those who had walked before their first fit (χ^2 4.72, df 1, p 0.05). This may be interpreted either as showing that damaged male children have fits earlier, or that early fits predispose to delay in independent walking. Age at walking was available for 48 female patients and 82 female siblings; 39 of the 48 patients walked before their first fit. The proportion of these walking before 13 months was exactly comparable with the female siblings. The 9 females who had fits before walking were more likely than the others to walk later than 13 months, but the small numbers involved preclude further useful statistical analysis.

Disordered speech development is defined here as failure to make two-word phrases by the age of 2 years, or as defective articulation for age. Those 121 (M63, F58) siblings who were personally examined are compared with the 50 (M34, F16) patients who had their first fit after age 2 years. In contrast to the usual male preponderance, speech disorders were equally common in male and female patients; 34% of patients (12 male and 5 female) and 13% of siblings (10 male and 6 female) had delayed or disturbed speech development (χ^2 9.96, df 1, $p < 0.005$).

Other indications that neurological disorder had preceded convulsions were obtained in 38 (28%) of the 134 children; there were 25 males and 13 females. Favouring of one side of the body or dwarfing of one side were present in 12 (M6, F6); neurological signs found on admission which remained static in severity throughout the illness and follow-up occurred in 18 (M12, F6); the parents of 3 males thought their sons excessively messy or clumsy; and 5 (M4, F1) children had motor milestones delayed by more than 2 SD from the means given by Neligan and Prudham (34). The clinical diagnoses in these patients were: left hemiplegia (M9, F8); right hemiplegia

(M4, F4); bilateral ataxia (M1, F3); left-sided ataxia (M3); diplegia (M3); ataxic diplegia (M3); ataxia and pes cavus (M1); choreoid syndrome (M1). (One female had mild bilateral hemiplegias and ataxia.) A total of 121 siblings (M63, F58) who had not had fits were neurologically examined. Excluding isolated speech problems, 16% (M12, F7) were thought mildly abnormal neurologically. Comparing this with the 28% of patients who had histories or examinations suggesting neurological disorder prior to their first fit, a significant excess of patients had abnormal neurological states which it could be presumed were not due to damage caused by a fit (χ^2 5.8, df 1, p 0.02).

Evidence of possible disproportionate growth of the brain or other skull contents was sought by comparison of occipitofrontal circumference and height measurements. Within a month of the first fit, both of these had been measured in 127 patients (M80, F47). Eight males had disproportionately small and 13 disproportionately large heads; 3 of the 8 and 6 of the 13 had other evidence suggesting prior neurological disorder. Of the 10 females with disproportionately small heads, 5 were otherwise suspected of abnormality prior to the first fit, as was 1 of the 5 females with disproportionately large heads.

It would be unjustifiable to suggest on the rather slender evidence of delay in walking, increase in speech disorders, or disproportionate head size that children who convulse with fever are frequently seriously neurologically disordered prior to their first fit. However, the evidence presented allows the suggestion that a cerebral state may often exist which could respond at a critical age to a feverish illness by having a convulsion. More concrete evidence of pre-existing cerebral disorder is given in the 28% of patients whose history or unchanging signs indicated abnormality before the first fit.

NEUROLOGICAL DEFICITS IN ASSOCIATION WITH THE FIRST AND SUBSEQUENT CONVULSIONS

Relationship of Pre-existing Neurological Disorder to Type of Fit

Because most children who convulse with fever are not seriously disturbed neurologically, the relationship between pre-existing neurological disorder and the type of initial fit has rarely been examined. Nevertheless, it has been noted that unilateral convulsions frequently arise as a result of brain damage regardless of its aetiology (2).

In the Edinburgh children only the females who had evidence of pre-existing neurological disorder had a significant excess of initial fits which lasted over 30 min or were unilateral or repeated during the same illness (χ^2 4.52, df 1, $p < 0.05$) (50). In addition, the presence of a significant disorder of the perinatal period appeared to enhance the effect of a positive family history of convulsive disorders, and patients of either sex with both these factors present had a significant risk of having a complicated initial fit (χ^2 4.72, df 1, $p < 0.05$).

Neurological Deficits During the Immediate Postictal Period

Even considering that most large series of febrile seizures are retrospective, it is surprising that very few reports of early postictal findings appear in the literature. In any case, the defects found depend on the skill of the examiners, as well as on the time after the fit that the examination takes place (2). Temporary pareses are not uncommon (4,17,32,43,54), and their frequent association with unilateral fits is emphasised (15,17,54). Temporary hypertonicity (4) and extrapyramidal signs (17) have also been observed. Bamberger and Matthes (2) comment that it is clinically more useful to record asymmetry than generalised postictal states. The most comprehensive report of hemiconvulsions and hemiplegia is that of Gastaut et al. (15). They comment also that the hemiplegia may remain unnoticed, disappear after a few hours or days, slowly regress and leave a slight motor deficit, or persist indefinitely.

An attempt was made to see the Edinburgh children as soon after the initial fit as possible. Most were seen within 6 hr, and all 124 admitted with an initial convulsion were examined within 24 hr. Excluding those who were thought to have definitely had pre-existing neurological disorder, the findings for 90 children were available (51). They were as follows: normal 28 (M15, F13); hemiplegia: right 14 (M9, F5), left 18 (M14, F4); cerebellar ataxia 25 (M17, F8); upper motor neurone (UMN) facial weakness 7 (M4, F3). (One child of each sex had a unilateral facial weakness and cerebellar ataxia.) The higher proportion of females who were normal during the 24 hr after the initial fit is not significant. In conclusion, where children were examined in detail after their initial convulsion, as many as 69% were found to have abnormalities that had not been previously suspected. The majority of these abnormalities were mild or minimal and might not have been noted during a cursory routine examination.

Neurological Deficits 1 Week to 6 Months After the Initial Fit

Although it is usually unclear from their reports, it is assumed that those authors (4,15,17,32,43,54) referring to transient neurological states would expect the signs to have disappeared within 6 months of the seizure. Of the 124 Edinburgh children seen with their first convulsion, 119 were re-examined 1 week to 6 months later. The children are considered in four groups. Firstly, diagnoses in those 34 who had had definite evidence suggesting that neurological disorder had been present before the first fit were: right hemiplegia 7 (M3, F4); left hemiplegia 15 (M9, F6); diplegia M3; ataxic diplegia M3; left-sided ataxia M2; bilateral ataxia 4 (M1, F3); ataxia with pes cavus M1; choreoid syndrome M1. (One female had multiple disorders, as noted in a previous section.) Secondly, a group of 6 children who definitely acquired abnormal signs (which persisted) in association with the illness in which a fit occurred is considered. Five developed their abnormal signs at the first fit, and the sixth had a subsequent attack and was noted to have a change in his neurological status thereafter. In all 6 cases parents commented on a change in their child's motor abilities. The diagnoses were: right hemiplegia 4 (M2, F2); left hemiplegia F1; bilateral ataxia M1. The third group comprises 58 children who had no recurrence of fits within 6 months. Of the 58, 35 were consistently normal on examination. Diagnoses in the other 23 were: left hemiplegia 5 (M2, F3); generalised brisk tendon reflexes and extensor plantar responses F1; bilateral cerebellar ataxia 4 (M3, F1); left-sided ataxia M2; UMN facial weakness: right 7 (M5, F2), left 5 (M4, F1). (Two males had facial paresis and ataxia.) In the fourth group are 21 children who had a subsequent fit within 6 months; 10 (M4, F6) were neurologically normal. Diagnoses in the remaining 11 were: left hemiplegia 5 (M3, F2); bilateral cerebellar ataxia 3 (M2, F1); right-sided ataxia M2; UMN facial weakness left, M1. No parent of any child in the third or fourth groups commented that there was any change in their child's abilities as a result of the initial or subsequent convulsions. It is suggested that parents scrutinise their children very carefully after a fit. The absence of comment in 34 children whose neurological abnormalities persisted might be interpreted as a return by the child to a preseizure state which was not entirely normal. Table 1 summarises the findings in the four groups of children.

Where positive evidence of viral infection as a cause of the original illness had been obtained, there was a significant excess of persisting neurological disorder (χ^2 4.1, df 1, p 0.05) (53). This finding is not necessarily incompatible with the proposal that many children were abnormal before their first fit. Worsening of preexisting neurological abnormalities was observed in control children, and viral illness may merely highlight a previous state. However, 4 of the 6 children with signs definitely acquired at the time of a fit had positive viral findings. There was one case each of infection with respiratory syncytial virus, mumps, parainfluenza 2, and *Mycoplasma pneumoniae*.

Despite these findings, evidence for the production of brain damage by the fit itself should not be ignored (10,29,37,42). Taylor and Ounsted (46), in their discussion on differential cerebral maturation, feel that the age at onset of fits and the sex of the child are crucially related to the outcome for epilepsy and intellectual prowess. In only 6 of 119 Edinburgh children seen after the immediate postictal period had new signs definitely been acquired. Of the 4 with right hemiplegias, the illness was at 15 and 23 months in the 2 girls and at 10 and 22 months in the boys. The left hemiplegia appeared at 33 months in a girl. These findings are at variance with those of Taylor

TABLE 1. *Neurological status of 119 children examined 1 week to 6 months after their first convulsion with fever*

Neurological findings	Evidence suggesting CNS abnormality prior to first fit	Parents made no comment on change in child's abilities		Parents commented on change in child's abilities
		No further fit within 6 months	Further fit within 6 months	
Right pyramidal tract signs	7[a]	7[a,b]	—	4
Left pyramidal tract signs	15[a]	10[a]	6	1
Bilateral pyramidal tract signs	3	1	—	—
Right-sided ataxia	—	—	2	—
Left-sided ataxia	2	2	—	—
Bilateral ataxia	4[a]	4[a]	3	1
Ataxic diplegia	3	—	—	—
Choreoid syndrome	1	—	—	—
Ataxia + pes cavus	1	—	—	—
Brachial plexus injury	1[a]	—	—	—
Normal	—	35	10	—
Total children in each group	34	58	21	6

[a] Includes children with more than one type of disorder.
[b] No hemiplegias; all cases UMN facial weakness.

and Ounsted (46) where damage to girls occurred earlier than damage to boys and the left side of the brain tended to be vulnerable later than the right. However, on referring to Table 1 it becomes apparent that the proportion of children with presumed longstanding left-sided signs far outweighs the one left hemiplegia in five of those definitely acquired. The opposite appears to hold for children with right-sided pyramidal tract signs. These findings are compatible with the theory of differential cerebral maturation (46) in that damage to the right hemisphere might have occurred very early, before the first fit, whereas the left hemisphere was vulnerable later, at the time of a severe fit. Four of the 5 children with definitely acquired hemiplegias had prolonged fits in association with proved viral infections. Therefore despite the findings of Meldrum et al. (29), the infecting agent may be as important in determining the long-term outlook as the duration of the fit itself.

CONTINUING NEUROLOGICAL DEFICITS

In order to give a total statement on the outlook for children who convulse with fever, the incidence and types of neurological deficit considered permanent are stated without reference to the timing of their acquisition. Although when Millichap reviewed information on long-term neurological findings he commented on the paucity of details, many reports of gross deficits exist (31). The possibility that minor deviations from normal are common has rarely been considered (51,54). The enthusiasm with which children have been examined must bear a relationship to the reported incidence of continuing disability. Where authors cite series collected as a result of referral to a specialist clinic, there is an inevitable bias to more disabled patients. Attention has been drawn to pareses which appear transient but which may reappear weeks or months later (2,15). It seems possible that ill-founded complacency may lead the casual paediatrician to assume complete recovery has taken place soon after a convulsion, whereas re-examination at a later date might reveal persisting signs.

The incidences of neurological abnormalities reported, being dependent on the source of material and definitions of abnormality, have varied from 1.3% to 80% (1,2,4,7,15,18,23,26,30,32,38,40,51,54).

Cases were selected by at least one criterion of severity in some series (1,15,23,26,30). Fifty-seven percent of 239 children with status, approximately half of whom were febrile, were permanently disabled (1). Hemiparesis persisted in 80% where the fit had been unilateral (15). In discussing cases where febrile seizures had recurred, 33% were described as "brain damaged" (23) and 10% as having organic brain damage (26). Where dehydration and convulsions had complicated a febrile illness, 37.5% of 24 children were abnormal on review (30). Other authors group perinatal abnormalities, neurological findings, electroencephalographic (EEG) changes, and continuing fits together (18,38,40). Horstmann and Schinnerling (18) found 29% of the children were epileptic or had neurological or EEG abnormalities. Roseman (40) suggested 40% of cases had EEG or clinical evidence of focal cerebral damage, and Peterman (38) estimated 52% of febrile convulsions have an organic basis. Since Todd's pareses were included, it is impossible to enumerate correctly permanent disability in the 20% with neurological disorder reported by Millichap et al. (32).

Lower figures for continuing deficit are given where authors report unselected cases, or where clinical neurological signs have been associated with obvious disability (2,4,7). By restricting their remarks to permanent spasticity, Bamberger and Matthes (2) found only 1.3% of 314 cases were neurologically disabled. Degen and Goller (4) reported abnormality in 9.4% of 64 children reviewed when aged 8–13 years. An intermediate figure of 5.1% disabled amongst 522 children was found by Doose et al. (7). Even the lowest of these estimates (2) is a higher percentage disabled than would be expected in a normal population.

Once the existence of signs compatible with the minimal cerebral dysfunction syndrome is recognised, the total incidence of neurological disorders increases. Zellweger (54) makes repeated references to the frequency of *neurologischen mikrosymptomen* but does not give a precise percentage for their occurrence. In a follow-up study of the Edinburgh children (51),

103 (77%) of the original 134 cases were neurologically examined 8–10 years after their initial fit. They were between 8 years 9 months and 14 years of age. There were 63 males and 40 females. The sex ratio, age at first fit, family history, and perinatal details were entirely comparable with the 31 children who were not reviewed. A trend towards a complicated initial convulsive episode in those who were re-examined was not significant (χ^2 3.16, df 1, not significant). Fifty-eight (56%) of those reviewed had had more than one convulsion; 72 (70%) of the 103 children were considered to have some neurological abnormality. This was in no case severe, but moderate disability was found in 15 males and 1 female, representing 15.5% of the total sample and 24% of the males.

The type of neurological disorder suffered is rarely categorised. Bamberger and Matthes (2) mention permanent spasticity. Because of their selection of cases, hemiplegia was commonest in the series of Gastaut et al. (15). Horstmann and Schinnerling (18) do not give precise details of diagnoses, but case histories suggest that some children were severely damaged. It is not possible to distinguish chronic from acute neurological abnormalities in their report, but strabismus, hypotonia, hyperkinesia, and retarded motor development are reported by Millichap et al. (32). Zellweger (54) examined 47 of a group of 105 children more than 4 years after their initial fit. Minor central nervous system signs were common and included bi- and unilateral pyramidal tract disorders, unilateral dysdiadokinesis, and 1 case of Horner's syndrome. One-fourth of the children were hypotonic with brisk tendon reflexes. Of 36 whose heads were measured at follow-up, 17 were larger and 6 smaller than expected.

Developmental histories were taken for all 103 Edinburgh children at follow-up. Some evidence for an increase in manipulative or sequencing difficulties was obtained. At ages of 8 years 9 months or more, 9 children were still having difficulty in fastening buttons; 27 (43%) males and 9 (23%) females were unable to tie laces before age 7, and 13 (21%) males and 5 (12%) females were over 9 years before this was achieved. Parents were asked about hand dominance in the siblings, and this was compared with that in the patients reviewed. There was a significant excess of ambidexterity or left-handedness amongst the patients (χ^2 8.52, df 1, p 0.02). This supports the contention that within an unselected population of children who convulse with fever, there is an excess of brain-damaged individuals. Although delay or aberration of speech development were significantly increased in patients whose first fit occurred after the age of 2 years, when examined as a whole and corrected for sex, speech disorders had not been significantly commoner in the 103 children reviewed than in their siblings (χ^2 2.38, not significant). In particular, of the 4 children who acquired right hemiplegia only 1 who was moderately disabled had had any delay in speech development, and even she was speaking in sentences before age 3 years.

The findings on examination are shown in Table 2. Pyramidal tract ab-

TABLE 2. *Clinical neurological diagnoses 8–10 years after the initial convulsion*

Neurological findings[a]	Males (N = 63)	Females (N = 40)
Hemiplegia, right		
Moderate	0	1
Mild	4	2
Minimal	6	7
Hemiplegia, left		
Mild	3	2
Minimal	15	15
Diplegia (mild)	3	0
Cerebellar ataxia		
Right (mild)	1	0
Left (minimal)	1	1
Bilateral		
Moderate	3	0
Mild	4	1
Minimal	1	0
Choreoid syndrome		
Right (mild)	1	0
Left (mild)	1	0
Bilateral		
Moderate	3	0
Mild	1	2
Minimal	2	0
Dyspraxia		
Moderate	11	0
Mild	1	3
Minimal	6	2
UMN facial weakness (without hemiplegia)		
Right	6	2
Left	4	1
Incoordinated eye movements	1	0
Deafness	1	0
Brachial plexus injury	1	0
Normal	18	13

[a] More than one (up to three) abnormalities were present in 17 males and 10 females.

normalities were present in 71 but were associated with moderate disability in only 1 child. Cerebellar ataxia occurred bi- or unilaterally in 12 children (moderate in 3), choreoid movements in 10 (moderate in 3) and dyspraxia in 23 (moderate in 11). Incoordinated eye movements, deafness, and brachial plexus injury were each present in 1 child. Seventeen males and 10 females had more than one (up to three) types of disability. Dyspraxia or ataxia occurring with pyramidal tract lesions were the most common combinations. Although the percentage of children with abnormalities was comparable to that within 24 hr of the first fit and higher than that of the subsequent 6 months, no parent remarked on further acute alterations in motor or other abilities. It was possible to approach neurological examination with greater sophistication in children over 8 years old than in those younger than 3 years, and the increase in number and variation in type of disabilities found at follow-up is probably a reflection of the children's improved ability to cooperate with testing. Since neurological abnormality in these children was significantly correlated with their scores on the Wechsler Intelligence Scale for Children (WISC), full scale and performance, and on the Oseretsky Test of Motor Proficiency, their neurological findings cannot have been entirely spurious.

Five of the 6 children whose parents had originally commented on a change in ability were reviewed. (Since the sixth had emigrated to Australia at age 9 years, it can be presumed that he is not seriously neurologically disturbed.) All 5 showed residual signs of the abnormality originally noted: 4 with right hemiplegia and 1 with left hemiplegia. One of the 4 with right hemiplegia was moderately disabled, and only 1 used the right hand for writing. Even he, at 10 years old, still had difficulty in fastening buttons with this hand. Additional disabilities in these 5 children were dyspraxia (moderate in 1 and mild in 1).

Factors which might predispose to, or mitigate against later, neurological abnormality were examined. When family history of convulsive disorders was correlated with neurological abnormality, there appeared to be no relationship unless socioeconomic status was also taken into account. A clustering of females with central nervous system abnormalities was then found in the families of manual workers whose histories were otherwise negative for convulsive disorders. Males from the higher social classes who were family history-negative were most likely to be neurologically abnormal. In both cases, compared with other groups the trend is not significant. Perinatal abnormalities were likely to be associated with continuing deficits, but significance was not reached (χ^2 3.63). Unlike other studies, there was a trend towards girls with younger age of onset (14 months or less) having normal neurological findings at follow-up, and a higher likelihood of continuing deficit if the first fit occurred at 15 months or more (χ^2 3.72, not significant). All 3 girls who definitely acquired abnormality had their first fit with later age of onset. No association of neurological abnormality with younger or older age of onset could be determined for the males, even if those with moderate disability were considered separately. A complicated initial fit was not more likely to be associated with continuing neurological deficit, nor were initial fits with unilateral features significantly correlated with asymmetry on later neurological examination. It can only be surmised that regardless of whether neurological abnormality is found the final picture results from many apparently unrelated factors.

CONTINUING INTELLECTUAL DEFICITS

The overall incidence of global intellectual deficits are considered initially. Mental retardation is mentioned as a later complication in most series of children who have convulsed with fever, but exact measurements and details of tests used are rarely given.

As with the neurological findings, groups of cases selected by referral to specialist clinics are likely to be more severely affected. After episodes of status 48% of children were mentally retarded (1). Younger children appeared more vulnerable. In patients with temporal lobe epilepsy preceded by febrile status, performance and verbal quotients on the WISC were commonly reduced, especially if status had occurred during the first year (37); 22% of 240 children selected by attendance at an EEG department had IQs of less than 80 (22).

Where children had apparently not been selected for severity of sequelae, the incidence of mental retardation varied from 1.9% to 17% (2–4,9,11, 18,19,32,47,54), but in only three series (4,47,54) was the frequency more than 10%. The lowest figure (4 of 208 children) comes from the Danish study (11). Because of their policy of admitting all children with febrile convulsions to hospital, this incidence may give a truer overall picture than those of other studies, where because of selective hospitalisation there is an initial bias towards more severely ill children. However, the criteria for the diagnosis of mental retardation are not clear. The number of convulsions suffered by children in any sample may affect the incidence of mental retardation, as may the age range at the time of the first fit. Nelson et al. (35) reported on data from the Collaborative Perinatal Project NINDS in which 47,222 children who convulsed with fever during the first year of life were identified. When a simple febrile convulsion had occurred, the IQ at age 4 years was within normal limits and comparable with IQs of siblings; but when there had been several febrile convulsions, although the IQ at age 4 was within normal limits it was significantly reduced when compared with the siblings' IQs. The worst prognosis appeared to be associated with repeated convulsions on the first day of the initial illness. A tendency for reduced intelligence to be more likely where fits recurred has been noted by other authors (2,3,18).

After eliminating possible cases of brain damage, Schiottz-Christensen and Bruhn (42) investigated intelligence in 14 monozygous twin pairs who were discordant for febrile convulsions. They found that the twins who had not convulsed were better in tests of logical memory, Wechsler digit symbol test, block design, and part B of the trail-making test. Most difference between the twin pairs was found on the WISC performance scale (p 0.001). Having excluded children with birth injuries, they conclude that the convulsion must be the damaging factor.

The review of the 103 Edinburgh children included psychological testing in 102 (3). This was approached without the psychologist having prior knowledge of school placement or details of the medical history. The following tests were administered: Draw-a-person, WISC, Bender Gestalt,

Oseretsky Test of Motor Proficiency, and Neale Analysis of Reading Ability.

As a whole the children performed badly on the Draw-a-person test. Ten percent had above-average and 54% below-average scores, with 20% well below average. Poor drawing was significantly related to unilateral features in the initial fit (χ^2 10.84, df 4, p 0.03), but neither side seemed more likely to have been affected. Poor drawing was also significantly related to recurrence of febrile fits (χ^2 17.08, df 8, p 0.03), grand mal attacks without fever (χ^2 15.6, df 4, p 0.004), and continuing fits up to the time of review (χ^2 17.08, df 4, p 0.03).

WISC full scale IQs ranged from 60 to 139 (mean 100.5, SD 19.4). Eight children had IQs of less than 70; 6 of these had had evidence of suboptimal development prior to their first fit. Significant associations were obtained between reduced full-scale IQs and low socioeconomic status (χ^2 11.72, df 2, p 0.003), neurological abnormality (χ^2 11.46, df 2, p 0.003), complicated initial fits (χ^2 16.46, df 8, p 0.04), and convulsions other than grand mal occurring without fever (χ^2 17.4, df 4, p 0.002). The verbal scale ranged from 58 to 136 (mean 100.2, SD 18.7). Significant relationships were found between lower verbal IQ and socioeconomic status (χ^2 16.53, df 2, p 0.003), recurrence of fits with fever (χ^2 15.36, df 8, p 0.05), and afebrile fits other than grand mal (χ^2 12.6, df 4, p 0.01). The performance scores ranged from 53 to 140 (mean 101.6, SD 18.7). Significant reduction on this scale occurred with low socioeconomic status (χ^2 7.52, df 2, p 0.02), neurological abnormality (χ^2 6.33, df 2, p 0.04), grand mal when afebrile (χ^2 9.35, df 4, p 0.05), and the use of anticonvulsants other than barbiturates before the age of 7 (χ^2 9.88, df 4, p 0.04). At least 15 points difference between verbal and performance scores was obtained in 27 children. A significant excess of these children were neurologically abnormal (χ^2 6.44, df 1, p 0.02), but the expected correlation between laterality of the first fit, asymmetry of neurological findings, and reduction of either verbal or performance abilities was not found. The suggestion that children with repeated fits during the first day of illness have a high risk of subsequent retardation (35) was not confirmed with material from a wider age range. Thirty-three Edinburgh children had more than one fit during the initial illness. Their full-scale IQs ranged from 65 to 139 (mean 97.1, SD 19.72). Only 3 (9%) had full-scale scores of less than 70, and none of these had had initial fits during the first year of life. The mean of the verbal scores was 95.5 (SD 17.54) and of the performance scores 101.1 (SD 19.56). There was thus a tendency—which was more marked in the females than the males and observed in 22 of the 33 children—for there to be lower verbal than performance IQs in those children who had had repeated fits during the initial episode.

Error scores on the Bender Gestalt ranged from 0 to 17 (mean 4.1, SD

3.6). Most of the errors were distortions of form. High-error scores correlated significantly with grand mal while afebrile (χ^2 15.18, df 5, p 0.01) and current treatment with anticonvulsants other than barbiturates (χ^2 18.02, df 5, p 0.003).

On the Oseretsky Test of Motor Proficiency the score was within normal limits for age in 74% of children; 13% were slightly and 13% severely clumsy for age. The clumsier children had significant increases in neurological abnormality (χ^2 7.5, df 2, p 0.02), grand mal when afebrile (χ^2 11.14, df 2, p 0.004), convulsions continuing up to the time of review (χ^2 20.12, df 4, p 0.0005) and current receipt of anticonvulsants other than barbiturates (χ^2 6.61, df 2, p 0.04).

Six of the 102 children were unable to read. After assessment on the Neale Analysis of Reading Ability, and calculating reading retardation from the discrepancy between mental age and reading age, 19% of the children were found to be retarded in reading skill and 12% in reading comprehension. This could be compared with reading retardation in 7% of the control children used by Rutter et al. (41). Poor readers had poor Bender scores and low IQs significantly more often, with most correlation being present between scores on the WISC performance scale and reading ability. It was felt that the group as a whole showed average reading ability, but there was a subset of less-able children with poor visuomotor skills who had difficulty.

No significant correlation was found between any test used and sex, age at onset, family history, or barbiturates given either during early childhood or at the time of review.

In her assessment of the psychological aspects of these 102 Edinburgh children, Cull (3) felt that her findings did not support the view (42) that a child who has a convulsion with fever suffers, as a result of the fit, some cerebral damage which can be detected in general intellectual functioning or in specific developmental delay. She found that complicated initial fits were associated with lower intellect, but there was no evidence for a necessary relationship. Since seizures occurring early during the child's life and fits associated with persistent neurological abnormality also seemed to have a detrimental effect on cognitive capacity, the isolation of the severity of the initial convulsion seemed unjustified. Her final conclusions are that larger and more detailed studies are required and that clarification of the role of the febrile convulsion in producing psychological changes depend on the discovery of whether children who convulse when febrile can ever truly be said to have been normal.

CONCLUSIONS

Evidence is presented that children who convulse when febrile have an increased incidence of factors associated with suboptimal neurological development. Minor delays or deviations from normal in the acquisition of skills are commonly apparent before the first fit, and most reported series contain a greater number of seriously disabled children than would be expected in the general population. Long-term neurological findings in most cases probably reflect the preseizure state, but a small group of children, perhaps 5% of the total, appear definitely to acquire new abnormalities in association with the illness during which a fit occurs. The role of viral infection requires further investigation in this context. Mental retardation is generally commoner than would be expected in an unselected group of children. Many of the children whose IQs fall within the normal range score unevenly on subtests. There is little evidence that intellectual deficits are necessarily sequelae rather than precursors of the initial convulsion with fever. It is suggested that a convulsion in a febrile child is drawing attention to a developmental defect.

ACKNOWLEDGMENTS

All the paediatricians at the Royal Hospital for Sick Children, Edinburgh, kindly allowed their patients to be studied. Dr. T. T. S. Ingram, Professor J. O. Forfar, and Professor O. P. Gray have given much support and encouragement. Continuous help has been received from many members of the secretarial staffs of the Department of Child Life and Health, University of Edinburgh, and the Department of Child Health, Welsh National School of Medicine. Between 1964 and 1968 the author was in receipt of a grant from the fund given to the University of Edinburgh by the Distillers Company. In 1974 the follow-up study was made possible through the generosity of the Scottish Council for the Care of Spastics.

REFERENCES

1. Aicardi, J., and Chevrie, J. J. (1970): Convulsive status epilepticus in infants and children. *Epilepsia,* 11:187–197.
2. Bamberger, P., and Matthes, A. (1959): *Anfälle im Kindersalter,* pp. 376–380. Karger, Basel.
3. Cull, A. M. (1975): Some psychological aspects of the prognosis of febrile convulsions. M.Phil. thesis, University of Edinburgh.
4. Degen, R., and Goller, K. (1967): Die sogenannten Fieberkrämpfe des Kindesalters und ihre Beziehungen zur Epilepsie. *Nervenarzt,* 38:55–61.
5. Dignam, W. J. (1967): Fetal survival with premature delivery in complications of pregnancy. *Am. J. Obstet. Gynecol.,* 98:587–593.
6. Dobbing, J. (1974): The later development of the brain and its vulnerability. In: *Scientific Foundations of Paediatrics,* edited by J. A. Davis and J. Dobbing, pp. 565–577. Heineman, London.
7. Doose, H., Petersen, C. E., Volke, E., and Herzberger, E. (1966): Fieberkrämpfe und Epilepsie. I. Ätiologie, klinisches Bild und Verlauf der sogenannten Infekt-oder Fieberkrämpfe. *Arch. Psychiatr. Nervenkr.,* 208:400–412.
8. Drillien, C. M., Ingram, T. T. S., and Wilkinson, E. M. (1966): *The Causes and Natural History of Cleft Palate.* Livingstone, Edinburgh.

9. Ekholm, E., and Niemineva, K. (1950): On convulsions in early childhood and their prognosis. *Acta Paediatr. (Stockholm)*, 39:481–501.
10. Falconer, M. A. (1974): Mesial temporal (Ammon's horn) sclerosis as a common cause of epilepsy. *Lancet*, 2:767–770.
11. Frantzen, E., Lennox-Buchthal, M. A., and Nygaard, A. (1968): Longitudinal EEG and clinical study of children with febrile convulsions. *Electroencephalogr. Clin. Neurophysiol.*, 24:197–212.
12. French, F. S., and Van Wyk, J. J. (1964): Fetal hypothyroidism. *J. Pediatr.*, 64:589–600.
13. Friderichsen, C., and Melchior, J. (1954): Febrile convulsions in children: Frequency and prognosis. *Acta Paediatr. (Stockholm)* [*Suppl. 100*], 43:307–317.
14. Gardiner, P. A., and Griffiths, J. (1960): Association between maternal disease during pregnancy and myopia in the child. *Br. J. Ophthalmol.*, 44:172–178.
15. Gastaut, H., Poirier, F., Payan, H., Salamon, G., Toga, M., and Vigouroux, M. (1960): HHE syndrome: Hemiconvulsions, hemiplegia, epilepsy. *Epilepsia*, 1:418–447.
16. Gruneberg, R. N., Leigh, D. A., and Brumfitt, W. (1969): Relationship of bacteriuria during pregnancy to acute pyelonephritis, prematurity and fetal mortality. *Lancet*, 2:1–3.
17. Herlitz, G. (1941): Studien uber die sogenannten initialen Fieberkrämpfe bei Kindern. *Acta Paediatr. (Stockholm)* [*Suppl. 1*], 29:40–44.
18. Horstmann, W., and Schinnerling, W. (1963): Zur Prognose der sogenannten Fieber-krämpfe. *Monatsschr. Kinderheilk.*, 111:52–57.
19. Hrbek, A. (1957): Fieberkrämpfe im Kindersalter. *Ann. Paediatr.*, 188:162–182.
20. Ingram, T. T. S., and Russell, E. M. (1961): The reproductive histories of mothers of patients suffering from congenital diplegia. *Arch. Dis. Child.*, 36:34–41.
21. Kass, E. H. (1970): Pregnancy, pyelonephritis and prematurity. *Clin. Obstet. Gynecol.*, 13:239–254.
22. Lennox, M. A. (1949): Febrile convulsions in childhood: A clinical and electroencephalographic study. *Am. J. Dis. Child.*, 78:868–882.
23. Lennox, W. G. (1953): Significance of febrile seizures. *Pediatrics*, 11:341–357.
24. Lennox-Buchthal, M. A. (1973): *Febrile Convulsions. A Reappraisal.* Elsevier, Amsterdam.
25. Lilienfeld, A. M., and Pasamanick, B. (1954): Association of maternal and fetal factors with the development of epilepsy. I. Abnormalities in the prenatal and paranatal periods. *JAMA*, 155:719–724.
26. Livingston, S., Bridge, E. M., and Kajdi, L. (1947): Febrile convulsions: A clinical study with special reference to heredity and prognosis. *J. Pediatr.*, 31:509–512.
27. Man, E. B., Shaver, B. A., and Cooke, R. E. (1958): Studies of children born to women with thyroid disease. *Am. J. Obstet. Gynecol.*, 75:728–741.
28. McDonald, A. D. (1961): Maternal health in early pregnancy and congenital defect. *Br. J. Prev. Soc. Med.*, 15:154–166.
29. Meldrum, B. S., Horton, R. W., and Brierley, J. B. (1974): Epileptic brain damage in adolescent baboons following seizures induced by allylglycine. *Brain*, 97:407–418.
30. Melekian, R., Laplane, R., and Debray, P. (1962): Considérations cliniques et statistiques sur les convulsions au cours des deshydrations aigues. *Ann. Pediatr.*, 9:290–302.
31. Millichap, J. G. (1968): *Febrile Convulsions.* Macmillan, New York.
32. Millichap, J. G., Madsen, J. A., and Aledort, L. M. (1960): Studies in febrile seizures. V. Clinical and electroencephalographic study in unselected patients. *Neurology (Minneap.)*, 10:643–653.
33. Myant, N. B. (1963): Foetal effects of maternal thyrotoxicosis. *Dev. Med. Child. Neurol.*, 5:652–653.
34. Neligan, G., and Prudham, D. (1969): Norms for four standard developmental milestones by sex, social class, and place in family. *Dev. Med. Child. Neurol.*, 11:413–422.
35. Nelson, K., Rubenstein, D., and Beadle, E. L. (1972): Seizures with fever beginning in the first year of life. Presented at Child Neurology Society Meeting.
36. Ounsted, C. (1971): Some aspects of seizure disorders. In: *Recent Advances in Paediatrics*, edited by D. Gairdner and D. Hull, pp. 363–400. Churchill, London.
37. Ounsted, C., Lindsay, J., and Norman, R. (1966): *Biological Factors in Temporal Lobe Epilepsy.* Heineman, London.
38. Peterman, M. G. (1952): Febrile convulsions. *J. Pediatr.*, 2:536–540.

39. Pharaoh, P. O. D., Butterfield, I. H., and Hetzel, B. S. (1971): Neurological damage to the foetus resulting from severe iodine deficiency during pregnancy. *Lancet,* 1:308–310.
40. Roseman (1955): Personal communication to Schmidt and Ward, ref. 43.
41. Rutter, M., Tizard, J., and Whitmore, K. (1970): *Education, Health and Behaviour.* Longmans, London.
42. Schiottz-Christensen, E., and Bruhn, P. (1973): Intelligence, behaviour and scholastic achievement subsequent to febrile convulsions: An analysis of discordant twin pairs. *Dev. Med. Child Neurol.,* 15:565–575.
43. Schmidt, R. P., and Ward, A. A., Jr. (1955): Febrile convulsions. *Epilepsia,* 4:41–47.
44. Speidel, B. D., and Meadows, S. R. (1972): Maternal epilepsy and abnormalities of the foetus and newborn. *Lancet,* 2:839–843.
45. Talbert, L. M., Thomas, C. G., Holt, W. A., and Rankin, P. (1970): Hyperthyroidism in pregnancy. *Obstet. Gynecol.,* 36:779–785.
46. Taylor, D. C., and Ounsted, C. (1971): Biological mechanisms influencing the outcome of seizures in response to fever. *Epilepsia,* 12:33–45.
47. Thom, D. A. (1942): Convulsions in early life and their relation to chronic convulsive disorders and mental defect. *Am. J. Psychiatry,* 98:574–580.
48. Wallace, S. J. (1972): Aetiological aspects of febrile convulsions. *Arch. Dis. Child.,* 47:171–178.
49. Wallace, S. J. (1974): The reproductive efficiency of parents whose children convulse when febrile. *Dev. Med. Child Neurol.,* 16:465–474.
50. Wallace, S. J. (1975): Factors predisposing to a complicated initial febrile convulsion. *Arch. Dis. Child.,* 50:943–947.
51. Wallace, S. J. (1976): Developmental histories and neurological signs in children who convulse with fever (*in preparation*).
52. Wallace, S. J.: Unpublished data.
53. Wallace, S. J., and Zealley, H. (1970): Neurological, electroencephalographic and virological findings in febrile children. *Arch. Dis. Child.,* 45:611–623.
54. Zellweger, H. (1948): Krämpfe in Kindesalter. *Helv. Paediatr. Acta (Suppl. 5),* 3:1–195.

Brain Dysfunction in Infantile Febrile
Convulsions, edited by M. A. B. Brazier and
F. Coceani. Raven Press, New York © 1976.

Genetic Messages and Convulsive Behaviour in Pyrexia

Christopher Ounsted

Human Development Research Unit, The Park Hospital for Children, Old Road,
Headington, Oxford, England

To understand the relationship between genetic messages and convulsive behaviours, it is necessary to rethink both the ethological status of seizures and the kind of questions we may properly ask about genetic messages in relation to them. Some texts still persevere in asking of behaviour such as epilepsy: Is it genetic or acquired? Such questions are scientifically improper and so are their more sophisticated forms such as: how much of the variance is genetic? Sir Peter Medawar dismissed such false dichotomizing in his brilliant aphorism: "Hereditary proposes and development disposes."

In another context Taylor and I (13) outlined what we think are the seven useful groups of questions which may be properly asked about genotypic propositions and developmental dispositions:

1. What is the formal nature of the message? What kind of laws does it impose on development? What anatomical histological and biochemical systems are involved?

2. At what moment in development is the message delivered? Is it fundamental to the development of the organism? Can the organism survive without it? At what stage in development does its presence or absence become recognisable?

3. Over what period in development does the genetic message endure? What processes inhibit its expression? Is there a dose effect?

4. How is the message translated developmentally? What physiological steps lie between the gene and its final expression in the behaviour of the phenotype? How can we mimic the genetic message? What do they tell us about the nature of the natural phenomena?

5. Which contingencies limit and which promote the expression of a particular message? Do these contingencies themselves reside in the genome, or are they dependent on the vagaries of the idiosyncratic environment?

6. How frequently and with what consequences does the genetic order go wrong? In what situations is an instruction harmless and in what disastrous?

7. How does the genetic message relate to the evolution of the particular species? What advantages does it confer? What consequences has it for the ecology of each species? Is it disadvantageous to the individual but advantageous to the gene pool from which that individual arises?

In this chapter I try to give some tentative answers to some of these questions. First, however, let us reconsider what seizures really are.

Seizure disorders are usually treated as a group of diseases: some of known and some of unknown pathology and etiology. The attacks themselves traditionally have been regarded as something alien from the behavioural repertoire of the organism. Hippocrates himself wrote that "this disease is not like any other." Homer nodded here, for, viewed biologically, seizures belong to quite a large class of behaviours that have many aspects in common. I suggested that the mammalian ethogram contains a large number of behaviours which can usefully be grouped in a common class category as "the paroxysmal behaviours" (12).

Coughing, sneezing, yawning, startle with gasping, hiccupping, laughing, weeping, sobbing, raging, screaming, vomiting. labour, orgasm, defecation, and urination are the commonest of the paroxysmal behaviours, and all have much that is similar to the seizure behaviours themselves.

PAROXYSMAL BEHAVIOURS

Neuronal Circuitry Genomically Specified

The genome specifies the nature and the circumstances in which paroxysmal behaviours occur. Phylogenetically the genomic message is, for many of these, buried deeply. The sneeze of the cat and a baby do not differ greatly. The fits that can be induced in both are closely similar in behavioural morphology. All human beings show all the behaviours I listed, and all human beings can be induced to have seizures.

Ontogenetic Stability

Certain seizures characterize certain developmental epochs; but once a particular form (e.g., grand mal) has been established, its nature, given adequate provocation, remains stable over the ontogeny. For instance, every physician has smiled at the old man's yawn in the premature nursery.

Prodrome

Many epileptics have uncomfortable and restless periods before the seizure strikes them. They use this warning in some cases to seek an environment where they privately can induce the seizure they need by subjecting themselves to appropriate stimulation. Prodromes are common also in the other paroxysmal behaviours: Consider sneezing, weeping, sobbing, vomiting, and orgasm.

Aura

Most of the paroxysmal behaviours, including some types of seizures, have warnings that can be described. This warning period is a particularly interesting one because it is the time when intervention by external or self-administered stimuli may inhibit both the epileptic and the other paroxysms. Most epileptics believe that specific action by them enables them to "fight off" many fits. It has been demonstrated in our laboratory that a stimulus which in one brain in one particular state releases seizures in another brain or in another state inhibits them. Here again there is an analogy with other paroxysmal behaviours, all of which can be delayed or wholly inhibited by the organism's experience.

State

The state of the brain in Prechtl's sense influences the occurrence of all paroxysmal behaviours, including seizures. Fairweather and Hutt (4) quantified the effect of level of arousal on epileptic paroxysms and showed that it was sharp and quantitative.

The Absolute System

Once the paroxysmal behaviours have passed the aura phase, they all become "absolute" for a greater or lesser duration of time. The sequence of events marches forward now regardless of what is done to the organism. The similarity between labour and orgasm and seizure is here evident.

It is the inevitability in orgasm, labour, and seizure which renders them all to some persons both repugnant and frightening. Taylor (17) suggested that psychodynamically the fear is one of loss of control and the sense of being possessed by forces no longer subject to any kind of ego influence.

Mass Reflex of Voluntary Muscle

In the paroxysmal behaviours voluntary muscles of the limbs and trunk together with those surrounding the eyes and mouth enter into mass reflex tonic and clonic activity. Thus vomiting and fits of laughter are associated with jactitations as violent as those of epilepsy.

Exocrine Secretion

Lacrimation, salivation, and sweating are all integral parts of many of the paroxysmal behaviours, any one of which when attaining major force is associated with excess exocrine activity.

Vascular Alterations

Flushing and blanching are regular features of the limbic ictus and also occur in many of the other paroxysmal behaviours, as do elevation of the blood pressure and the pulse rate simultaneously.

Contraction of Smooth Muscle

The contraction of smooth muscle and the relaxation of sphincters occurs in most of the paroxysmal behaviours at their extremes of violence.

Primitive Respiratory Movements

Primitive respiratory gasping is a feature of nearly all paroxysmal behaviours including major seizures.

Afterglow

After any paroxysmal behaviour including seizures there is often a change of mood. The temperament of Ginsburg's mice (5) became milder after a fit. The induced seizure may lift mood from profound depression to euphoria. The afterglow is accompanied by a sense of lassitude and a physiologically refractory period.

Social Unacceptability

In most societies and on most occasions the paroxysmal behaviours at their extreme are contrary to the mores of society. It is here we come to the possible biological significance of seizures. The seizure is repellent, and in this, Chance (3) suggests, lies its biological value. *Peromyscus,* the deer mouse, is polyethic for seizures. Approximately 5% of the feral population are genetically disposed to convulsions from which they may die. The timing of this propensity in the ontogeny coincides with the period of habitat exploration and habitat imprinting. It has been proposed that the convulsions which occur when the mice are predated train predators to avoid *Peromyscus* and hence reduce predation on the total deer mouse population. Similarly, the seizures of the epileptic mouse are precisely those that would be aversive to a cat when tossing the mouse in the air or holding him in his mouth. When adequately shaken at the right age the epileptic mouse suddenly stiffens, saliva pours from his mouth, and urine and faeces are emitted. He next jactitates in the clonic phase and finally goes limp as though he were dead. He becomes a very unappetizing morsel. It is an interesting fact that man too, at least during childhood, has an approximately 5% propensity to convulse. No homology is intended, but one of the unsolved problems of the convulsive disorders is to find some biological explanation for their polyethism in man. Since these behaviours are potentially lethal, we require an explanation for why the genomically determined propensity should be so frequent in our species.

Specific Inhibition

Inhibition of the paroxysmal behaviours may occur at any level. Chance (3) showed that the adolescent deer mouse convulses to auditory shock. He put such mice in a free field, i.e., in a territory of some size but one from which they could not escape. In one corner of the field he placed a little hutch. If between the administration of the stimulus and the final onset of seizure the mouse reached the hutch, it did not convulse. It seemed that reaching sanctuary was sufficient to inhibit the seizure. After the mouse had been trained to escape in this way, the hutch was gradually taken apart until it was finally removed. It was now sufficient to reach that corner of the free field where a hutch had stood for the mouse to remain free and protected from fits. Inhibition of the paroxysm of vengeful aggression is similarly echoed in the games of children and in ecclesiastical history. Staveley (15) traced the development and decline of church sanctuary in England. At their height such sanctuaries were remarkably elaborate in the safety they conferred and in the penalties for their infringement. At the monastery of Hagulstad, for example, the penalties for the infringement of asylum were quantitatively related to the distance between the miscreant at the point of capture and the centre of the great church.

The reader may well ask what this long prodrome has to do with the down-to-earth problem of febrile infants having fits. I think it is relevant for both understanding and action. The instruction to convulse inheres in every mammalian genome: The critical path that leads to seizure is a stochastic sequence peculiar to each case. Many of the muddles about fits arise because these behaviours can themselves devastate the brain, and it is hard to accept that a natural behaviour can do that until we reflect that most paroxysmal behaviours can lead to death in a suitably weakened person.

Nearly 50% of children under 4 years with purulent meningitis have fits; over the age of 4 the risk rapidly falls. For these seizures no specific predisposition is needed (11). Other seizures with fever sometimes require a specific genetic predisposition. Lennox-Buchthal's trenchant review (8) suggests the trait is transmitted as a single autosomal gene manifest in the heterozygote (dominant). The frequency of the gene cannot be known since only a limited number of those who carry it show its effects. A parsimonious estimate would be 5%. If this is so, then 1 in 20 marriages will take the form shown in Fig. 1. It also follows that 1 in 400 marriages will be in the form shown in Fig. 2. In such families two out of four children will have a single gene for febrile convulsions, and 1 in 4 will have a double dose of the gene.

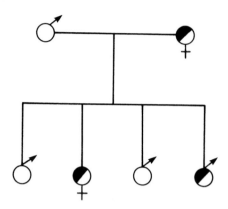

FIG. 1. A single gene promotes seizures in fever. One in 20 carries a tendency to convulse with fever. The expression is age- and sex-dependent. The heterozygotes are otherwise healthy.

Lindsay (9) drew attention to the strikingly analogous situation in the work of Kurokawa et al. (7) in the Japanese epileptic mouse. This inbred strain is homozygous for alleles whose formal instruction is to convulse to a specific stimulus, viz., shaking through an angle greater than 15°. The phenotypic expression of the gene is age-dependent and appears at approximately 7 weeks. This age dependence is dose-dependent. The epileptic mice were outbred with the nonconvulsive gpc strain: the F_1 offspring were seizure-prone but not until 30 weeks. Is there a similar dose dependence in man? The question can be answered. My own tentative figures suggest that where febrile convulsions run in a family and where one infant has protracted seizures leading to mesial temporal sclerosis with epilepsy his affected siblings with convulsions have milder fits at a later age.

All studies concur in showing that febrile convulsions are strictly age-dependent: Taylor and I (18) showed that this has the corollary that they are sex-dependent. Those who have febrile convulsions dependent on the specific gene show an age and gender dependency strikingly different in pattern from those not gene-dependent. Figure 3 shows a large sample of unselected children with febrile convulsions. The probands are assigned

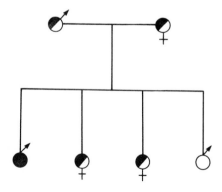

FIG. 2. A possible dose effect on timing and severity. One in 400 marriages could take the form shown. A dose effect could determine earlier susceptibility and greater risk of mesial temporal sclerosis.

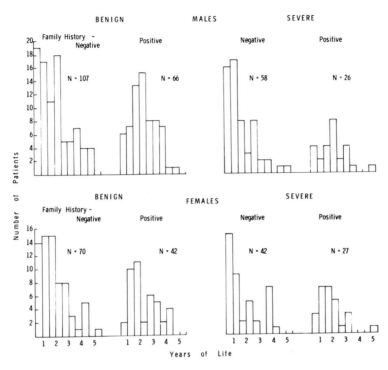

FIG. 3. Onset of febrile convulsions by age and sex and severity of outcome.

to eight histograms by gender, family history, and outcome. Each incorrect assignment would tend to blur differences — yet the results are quite clear-cut. All four family history-positive groups are alike, as are all four family history-negative groups. Furthermore, the sex of the proband can be used delicately to probe these data. In each of the four male histograms risk continues for 6 months longer than in the equivalent female group, reflecting precisely the half-year advantage in maturity which girls have over boys at this age.

In the epileptic mouse it seems that the physiological anomaly relates to the balanced overproduction of gamma-aminobutyric (GABA) acid and acetylcholine. Seizure depletes both the excess of excitatory and inhibitory transmitter.

Hertz et al. (6) clearly showed that febrile convulsions could be induced in DBA mice by pyrexia. This proclivity was strictly age-dependent. Underlying the susceptibility, four linked quantitative chemical differences were found. At the age of peak susceptibility, but not before or after, the brains of DBA mice had marked diminution in Na,K-activated ATPase, diminished concentration of K^+, diminished K^+-stimulated release of GABA, and diminished oxygen uptake. Thus it begins to seem very likely that human susceptibility to seizures during fever, when familial, rests on some homologous or analogous base.

Now turn to phenocopies. Some infections cause febrile convulsions without specific predisposition, but these infections do not arise at random. We must ask what specific settings allow the release of the general genetic predisposition to convulse during infections. Consider meningitis due to *Haemophilus influenzae* type b. This disease is a cause of severe convulsions with fever. Finding the organism in the cerebrospinal fluid (CSF) so focusses attention on eradicating the invader that seizure control is neglected. (The danger of seizures in this disease was not mentioned in four recent publications.) Yet it has been known for a quarter of a century that the prognosis for treated meningitis is directly related to the frequency and intensity of the seizures it promotes. Chronic epilepsy, often with hemiplegia, results. Here then is a phenocopy of the protracted familial febrile convulsions (Fig. 4). In the light of our proper questions, we must push matters further and ask in what particular environment did this meningitis arise? A specific microenvironment seems necessary, i.e., that the infant affected shall be living in close contact with siblings in the age range in which immunity to *H. influenzae* is rising but incomplete (10). This setting generates that dose of the capsulated type b strain which can reach the infant brain.

An even more precisely defined environment seems needed for the infective phenocopy of exanthema subitum. Lennox-Buchthal's cogent analyses (8) suggest that it is the youngest of an all-male single-sex sibship

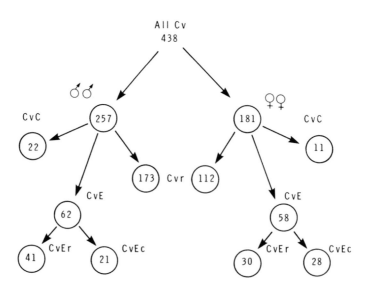

FIG. 4. Febrile convulsions (FC) by sex and outcome. CvC, death during FC. CvR, benign FC. CvEr, FC and remittent epilepsy. CvEc, FC and drug-resistant epilepsy.

who convulses to this otherwise harmless and omnipresent microorganism. Figure 5 illustrates the pattern.

Thus we see that the universal and genetic propensity of infants to convulse is not randomly released but always the endpoint of a stochastic process. Both the bacterium and the virus need these unexpected settings to undergo a presumably genetic change from which their pathogenicity derives.

How often does the instruction to convulse go wrong? I think the answer varies widely and depends critically on the duration of the seizure, which in turn varies from population to population. In recent papers Aicardi and Chevrie (1) described large series of children who have hemiplegic epilepsy after convulsions lasting many hours or even days. In my own studies between 1948 and 1954 (Fig. 4) approximately 8% of convulsing children died and a similar proportion lived with chronic drug-resistant epilepsy.

The instruction to convulse usually carries the corollary to inhibit the convulsion as soon as possible; but, as in any paroxysmal behaviour, runaway may occur. When this happens and the child goes into febrile status epilepticus, a specific subsystem of one hemisphere is at risk for destruction: This system involves parts of Ammon's horn, within which the Sommer sector is selected but the h_2 sector is preserved. The cerebellar cortex shows a patchy loss of Purkinje cells. The cerebral cortex may have

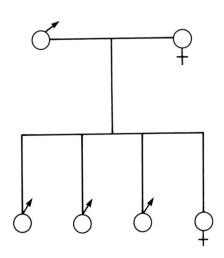

FIG. 5. A bacterial phenocopy. Convulsions often occur in infants with *Haemophilus influenzae* type b meningitis. These infants' families contain partially immune siblings.

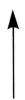

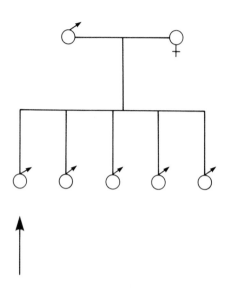

FIG. 6. A viral phenocopy. The setting of an all-male single-sex sibship promotes a seizure-evoking infection with the virus exanthema subitum.

laminar atrophy. The thalamus, corpus striatum, and inferior olive may be involved to a lesser degree. This is the pattern of lesions designated by the term mesial temporal sclerosis (14). Such lesions have been known since the classic papers of Bouchet and Cazauvieilh in 1825 (2). The provenance of the lesions was much debated. At one time a curious notion was considered that these scars were mechanically produced. The mesial temporal brain was imagined to have herniated over the sharp free edge of the tentorium cerebelli either during birth or during an episode of raised intracranial pressure. Within the prolapsed brain the anterior choroidal artery was nipped. Occlusion followed; an infarct formed; and "incisural sclerosis" followed. There was no evidence to support this strange idea, and it has no place in modern epileptology.

The concept of the convulsive destruction of particular brain areas immediately raises the question of laterality. How can a generalised insult produce a lesion in one hemisphere and leave the other unharmed? The answer seems to lie in the exquisitely timed pattern of brain maturation, which differs between the sexes and between the hemispheres (Fig. 7). Taylor's clear analyses show that the age-dependent pattern of risk differs between the sexes and between the hemispheres (16). Female and left-sided vulnerability are packed during the early months of life; male and right-sided vulnerability are delayed to a later epoch.

Thus in the production of mesial temporal sclerosis we see an aetiology which can be understood only in terms of a genomically controlled pattern of maturation. The convulsive insult hits very selectively at a system whose susceptibility is itself genomically determined.

In Copenhagen now it seems likely that postconvulsive brain damage

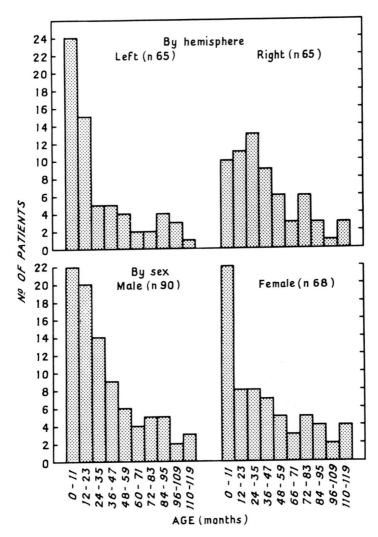

FIG. 7. Age-of-onset histograms of patients with temporal lobe epilepsy showing differences between hemispheres and between sexes.

is much reduced by careful prophylaxis and rapid treatment of seizures accompanied by fever. The human tendency to seizure is innate, however: "Man is built to convulse" wrote William Gordon Lennox. The specific gene to febrile convulsions is too widespread ever to be eliminated. The tendency seriously to convulse with fever can, however, be overcome by means already available, and the prevention of prolonged seizures is likely to have a major impact on the frequency of chronic drug-resistant epilepsy.

REFERENCES

1. Aicardi, J., Amsili, J., and Chevrie, J. (1969): Acute hemiplegia in infancy and childhood. *Dev. Med. Child Neurol.,* 11:162–173.
2. Bouchet and Cazauvieilh (1825): De l'épilepsie considerée dans ses rapports avec aliéna-tion mentale. *Arch. Gen. Med.,* 9:510–542.
3. Chance, M. R. A. (1957): The role of convulsions in behaviour. *Behav. Sci.,* 2:30–37.
4. Fairweather, H., and Hutt, S. J. (1969): Inter-relationships of EEG activity and informa-tion processing on paced and unpaced tasks in epileptic children. *Electroencephalogr. Clin. Neurophysiol.,* 27:7–701 (abstract).
5. Ginsberg, B. E. (1967): Genetic parameters in behavioural research. In: *Behaviour-Genetic Analysis,* edited by J. Hirsch, pp. 135–154. McGraw-Hill, New York.
6. Hertz, L., Schousboe, A., Formby, B., and Lennox-Buchthal, M. (1974): Some age-dependent biochemical changes in mice susceptible to seizures. *Epilepsia,* 15:619–632.
7. Kurokawa, M., Naruse, H., and Kato, M. (1966): Metabolic studies on ep mouse, a special strain with convulsive predisposition. In: *Correlative Neurosciences: Part A. Fundamental Mechanisms,* edited by T. Tokizane and J. P. Schadé, pp. 112–130. Elsevier, Amsterdam.
8. Lennox-Buchthal, M. (1973): Febrile convulsions: A reappraisal. *Electroencephalogr. Clin. Neurophysiol. (Suppl.),* 32:1–135.
9. Lindsay, J. M. M. (1971): Genetics and epilepsy: A model from critical path analysis. *Epilepsia,* 12:47–54.
10. Ounsted, C. (1949): Haemophilus influenzae meningitis treated with streptomycin. *Lancet,* 2:639–643.
11. Ounsted, C. (1951): Significance of convulsions in children with purulent meningitis. *Lancet,* 1:1245–1248.
12. Ounsted, C. (1971): Some aspects of seizure disorders. In: *Recent Advances in Paediatrics* 4th ed., edited by D. Gairdner and D. Hull, pp. 371–374. Churchill, London.
13. Ounsted, C., and Taylor, D. C. (1972): The Y chromosome message: a point of view. In: *Gender Differences: Their Ontogeny and Significance,* edited by C. Ounsted and D. C. Taylor, pp. 241–262. Churchill Livingstone, London.
14. Ounsted, C., Lindsay, J., and Norman, R. (1966): *Biological Factors in Temporal Lobe Epilepsy.* Clinics in Developmental Medicine No. 22. Heinemann, London.
15. Staveley, T. (1712): *The History of the Churches of England: Wherein Is Shown, The Time, Means, and Manner of Founding, Building, and Endowing of Churches Both Cathedral and Rural with Their Furniture and Appendages,* edited by T. Davies. Covent Garden, London.
16. Taylor, D. C. (1969): Differential rates of cerebral maturation between sexes and between hemispheres. *Lancet,* 2:140–142.
17. Taylor, D. C. (1973): Aspects of seizure disorders: On prejudice. *Dev. Med. Child Neurol.,* 15:91–94.
18. Taylor, D. C., and Ounsted, C. (1971): Biological mechanisms influencing the outcome of seizures in response to fever. *Epilepsia,* 12:33–45.

Brain Dysfunction in Infantile Febrile Convulsions, edited by M. A. B. Brazier and F. Coceani. Raven Press, New York © 1976.

Treatment and Prevention of Infantile Febrile Convulsions: The Clinical Problem

Joseph H. French

Department of Pediatrics, Albert Einstein College of Medicine, 1300 Morris Park Avenue, Bronx, New York 10461

The propensity for a convulsive episode to occur when a young child experiences a febrile illness was probably known during prehistory. A recent encyclopedic review documents that in ancient times an occidental physician wrote about this unique seizural susceptibility of the developing nervous system (16). By the dawn of the Age of Reason, it was suggested that a genetic factor contributed to this temporal relationship of youthfulness, fever, and convulsions (16). Contemporary investigations and reviews suggest that "febrile convulsions" have potentially lethal (16,17) and disabling connotations (7,15,23,25) even though the folk wisdom of some developing cultures anticipates them as a natural event (18).

This disorder or group of disorders occurs in a significant proportion of the population. Lennox-Buchthal (16) reviewed incidence studies performed prior to 1970 and found an average rate of 29/1,000 children (range 19–33). Subsequent studies utilizing retrospective survey of birth date cohorts (22,24) and retrospective medical record survey methodology (11) are shown in Table 1. A recent prevalence study of febrile convulsions and epilepsy utilized a household survey instrument technology in an American metropolis. The epilepsy estimate was based on a random sample of 760 persons surveyed via personal interview, telephone, and mail modes of inquiry: 16/1,000 cases of epilepsy were found in all ages and 19/1,000 in children less than 10 years (10). The febrile convulsion estimate of 46/1,000 was based on a random sample of 562 persons containing 131 children less than 10 years of age. The febrile convulsion sample was surveyed by personal interview and telephone modes of inquiry only (10). "Nontarget," previously diagnosed cases and their surrounding households were blindly assigned to interviewers and questions designed to detect diseases with a well-known prevalence were included in the survey instrument. These controls establish the efficacy of this epidemiologic technique for studying seizure disorders in large, potentially mobile urban populations (10).

Many studies support the presence of a genetic determinant for febrile convulsions (16,26). Two recent reports (8,20) conclude that the pattern of transmission is consistent with autosomal dominant inheritance. Auto-

TABLE 1. *Recent prevalence studies of febrile convulsions*

Author	Population	Ascertainment method	Rate (per 1,000)
Stanhope et al. (24)	Chamorro, Mariana Islands	Retrospective birth cohorts survey	114
Ross (22)	England, Scotland, Wales	Retrospective birth cohorts survey	21
Hauser and Kurland (11)	Midwestern United States	Retrospective medical records survey	33

somal dominant transmission with penetrance modification by other genes has been found in audiogenic seizure-susceptible mice (12). Audiogenic seizures, like febrile seizures, are an age-dependent, transient behavior. Seizures provoked by body temperature elevation have been reported recently in a mouse strain known to be susceptible to audiogenic seizures (13). Unfortunately, a biochemically quantifiable gene product(s) has not been found in either human febrile convulsions or in susceptible mutant mice.

Single seizures transiently disrupt the acquisition of new memory traces. Prolonged seizures of any etiology, including febrile convulsions, may result in death or subsequent fixed neurologic deficit (Table 2). The poor prognosis of prolonged convulsions may be the consequence of the apnea that often accompanies the forceful muscular contractions of severe convulsions. The associated anoxic anoxia in human and experimental status epilepticus is objectively documented by a lowered arterial oxygen concentration and pH, as well as increased arterial carbon dioxide and lactic acid concentrations (21). Even in well-oxygenated experimental animals that experience seizures, brain metabolism is altered (Table 3). It is hypothesized that these findings are a result of an increased neuronal utilization of chemical energy stores, adenosine triphosphate (ATP), for monovalent

TABLE 2. *Prognosis in pediatric status epilepticus*

No. of cases	% Associated with febrile convulsions	Total mortality (%)	Total CNS morbidity rate (%)	0.5–3 year age range CNS morbidity rate (%)
239[a]	28[b]	11	45	58

Modified from Aicardi and Chevrie, ref. 1.
[a] There were 79% of cases in 0.5–3 year age range.
[b] Maximum incidence age range for febrile convulsions etiology was 0.5–3 years.

TABLE 3. *Physiological chemistry of feline flurothyl-induced seizures*

Chemistry	During seizure	30 sec post seizure	5 min post seizure	15 min post seizure
A-V O$_2$ Δ[a]	Decreases	Diminished decrement	Near control value	Control value
A-V CO$_2$ Δ[b]	Decreases	Increased decrement	Near control value	Control value
Lactate content cerebral cortex	Increases	Near control value	Control value	Control value
Lactate/pyruvate cerebral cortex[c]	Increases	Near control value	Control value	Control value
Phosphocreatine content cerebral cortex	Decreases	Control value	Control value	Control value
ATP content cerebral cortex[d]	Decreases	Control value	Control value	Control value

Modified from Plum et al., ref. 21.

[a] Cerebral arteriovenous oxygen concentration difference.
[b] Cerebral arteriovenous carbon dioxide difference.
[c] Ratio of cerebral cortex lactate and pyruvate contents.
[d] ATP (adenosine triphosphate).

ion pumping during paroxysmal discharges (21). A transient, age-dependent diminution of sodium-potassium adenosine triphosphatase activity has been reported in mice susceptible to audiogenic seizures as well as febrile convulsions (13).

Figure 1 lists potential biochemical changes secondary to augmented adenosine diphosphate (ADP) production associated with an increased neuronal utilization of ATP (a, Fig. 1). Increased cellular ADP produced

a) ATP + Creatine $\xrightarrow[\text{Creatine Kinase}]{}$ ADP↑ + Creatine Phosphate

b) ADP↑ + Substrate↑ $\xrightarrow[\text{Respiratory Chain}]{O_2}$ ATP + H_2O (mitochondria)

c) Isocitrate $\xrightarrow[\text{Mg, ADP↑}]{NAD^+, H^+}$ ∝-ketoglutarate + NADH + CO_2 (mitochondria)
Mitochondrial Isocitrate Dehydrogenase

d) 1, 3-Diphosphoglycerate $\xrightarrow[\text{Mg}]{ADP↑}$ 3-Phosphoglycerate + ATP
Phosphoglycerate Kinase

e) 2 ADP↑ $\xrightarrow[\text{Adenylate Kinase}]{}$ ATP + AMP

f) Fructose-6-Phosphate $\xrightarrow[\text{Mg, AMP↑, Pi↑}]{ATP}$ Fructose-1, 6-diphosphate + ADP
Phosphofructokinase

g) Glyceraldehyde-3-Phosphate $\xrightarrow[\text{Glyceraldehyde-3-Phosphate}]{NAD^+, Pi}$ Glyceraldehyde-1, 3-Diphosphate + NADH +H^+
Dehydrogenase

h) Pyruvate $\xrightarrow[\text{Lactate Dehydrogenase}]{NADH↑, H^+↑}$ Lactate + NAD^+

i) Dihydroxyacetone-Phosphate $\xrightarrow[\text{Glycerol-3-Phosphate}]{NADH, H^+}$ Glycerol-3-Phosphate + NAD^+ (cytosol)
Dehydrogenase

j) Glycerol-3-Phosphate $\xrightarrow[\text{∝-Glycerol-Phosphate}]{}$ Dihydroxyacetone-Phosphate + Reduced flavin adenine dinucleotide (mitochondria)
Dehydrogenase

FIG. 1. Potential biochemical changes associated with increased neural activity of seizures. Pi, inorganic phosphate.

by ATP hydrolysis may increase oxidative metabolism via positive modulation of isocitric dehydrogenase (c, Fig. 1), the rate-limiting activity of the tricarboxylic acid cycle, and mitochondrial respiration (b, Fig. 1), as well as anaerobic glycolysis via the 3-phosphoglycerate kinase reaction (d, Fig. 1) and adenylate kinase-produced adenosine monophosphate (AMP) (e, Fig. 1). AMP is a positive modulator for phosphofructokinase (f, Fig. 1), the rate-limiting activity for anaerobic glycolysis. The anaerobic glycolysis pathway-produced reduced diphosphopyridine nucleotide (NADH) in the glyceraldehyde-3-phosphate dehydrogenase reaction (g, Fig. 1) increases in the presence of an adequate supply of oxidized diphosphopyridine nucleotide (NAD$^+$). Increased cytosol NADH favors augmented anaerobic glycolysis-produced pyruvate transformation to lactate via the lactate dehydrogenase reaction (h, Fig. 1). The cytosol [NAD$^+$]/[NADH] is, in part, also regulated by glycerol-3-phosphate dehydrogenase activity (i, Fig. 1). This reaction may also serve as a mitochondrial entry shuttle for cytosol NADH-reducing equivalents when coupled with its mitochondrial, flavin cofactor counterpart (j, Fig. 1).

Mitochondrial metabolism is altered in a medium containing the convulsant agent 1,5-pentamethylene tetrazole (Metrazol®). Figures 2 and 3 demonstrate that increasing concentrations of 1,5-pentamethylene tetrazole are associated with a progressive inhibition of the state 4–3 transition when added prior to ADP. Higher concentrations ($\geqslant$ 140 μg/ml) are required to inhibit the succinate-linked state 4–3 transition and calcium transport (19).

Therefore in febrile convulsion status epilepticus, as with status epilepticus secondary to other causes, it is imperative to ventilate the convulsing patient promptly and adequately, safely terminate the convulsion, reestablish euthermia, and eradicate the febrile precipitant (4). Only symptomatic treatment is currently available to assist in the acute suppression of seizures; diazepam administration by slow, intravenous push (1.5 mg/min) is preferred by the author. Appropriate ventilation-support equipment should be available for the rare patient who experiences brief apnea during administration of this drug.

Specific therapies are required for some causes of status epilepticus which may mimic febrile convulsions. Thus all appropriate clinical and laboratory examinations must be performed to exclude central nervous system (CNS) infections, disturbances of electrolyte homeostasis, intoxications, occasional genetic diseases other than febrile convulsions, and rare nutritional disorders. The following list includes some conditions seen by the author which were misdiagnosed as febrile convulsions by physician trainees:

Lead encephalopathy
Atropine intoxication
Parathion poisoning
Cerebral infarction 2° to hemoglobinopathy S
Vitamin D deficiency rickets

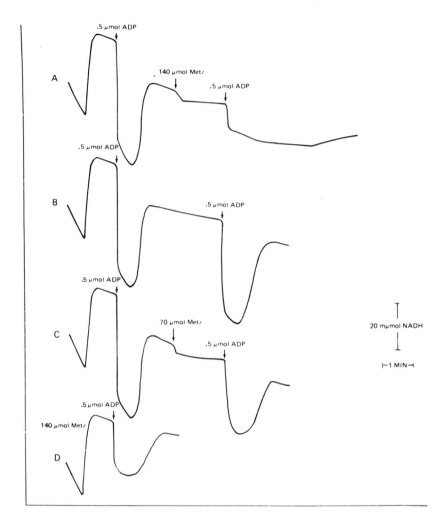

FIG. 2. 1,5-Pentamethylene tetrazole (Metz) inhibition of rat brain mitochondrial state 4–3 transition. Abscissa is time; ordinate is [NADH]. Arrows indicate points at which the indicated substances were added. Glutamate and malate were used as substrates. Downward deflection indicates NADH oxidation. Trace A: ADP (0.5 μmoles) initiated NADH oxidation in absence and presence of Metz (140 μmoles). ADP initiated NADH oxidation, state 4–3 transition, is inhibited by prior addition of Metz. Trace B: Equivalent state 4–3 transitions initiated by repeated ADP additions (0.5 μmoles) in absence of Metz. Trace C: [Metz] dependence of state 4–3 transition inhibition. Lower Metz concentration (70 μmoles) is associated with less inhibition of NADH oxidation than in trace A. Trace D: Diminished state 4–3 transition inhibition, compared to trace A, of Metz (140 μmoles) added prior to initial ADP-stimulated NADH oxidation. Modified from Moore and Gamble, ref. 19.

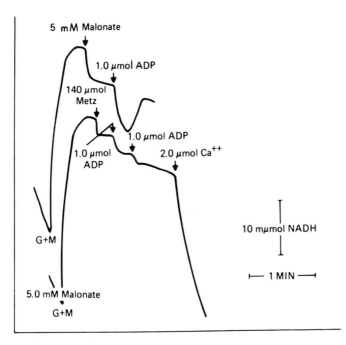

FIG. 3. Effect of malonate on succinate oxidation in 1,5-pentamethylene tetrazole (Metz) state 3 respiration-inhibited rat brain mitochondria. Abscissa is time; ordinate is [NADH]. Arrows indicate points at which the indicated substances were added. G + M, glutamate and malate (10 μmoles each). Downward deflection indicates NADH oxidation. Upper trace: Malonate inhibition of succinate oxidation with glutamate + malate supported NAD$^+$ reduction in the absence of Metz. Lower trace: Metz inhibition of state 4–3 transition with glutamate + malate-supported respiration in the presence of malonate. Metz diminishes state 4–3 transition as in Fig. 2, indicating negligible succinate oxidation in any residual state 4–3 transition. Calcium-induced oxidation persists as indicated. Modified from Moore and Gamble, ref. 19.

Since both febrile convulsions and pyogenic meningitis are relatively common in infants and young children, a prior diagnosis of febrile convulsions should not lull a physician into complacency and delay diagnosis of a treatable bacterial infection in the patient with both conditions.

A nonrandomized, prospective study of compliant febrile convulsion patients demonstrates effective prophylaxis with chronic oral phenobarbital administration if the serum phenobarbital concentration is maintained in excess of 15 μg/10^{-3} ml (6). Thus there is no literature disagreement that all patients who have experienced febrile convulsion status epilepticus should be given long-term treatment with this medication.

Children who chronically receive anticonvulsant medications, including phenobarbital, frequently demonstrate elevations of serum gamma-glutamyl transferase and less frequently alkaline phosphatase activities (2). Augmentation of the gamma-glutamyl transferase activity is attributed to induction of bile duct epithelium microsomal enzymes. Serum alkaline phosphatase elevations and diminished serum calcium concentrations coexist in some children chronically given anticonvulsant medications (3,14). Radiographically documented rickets with serum alkaline phosphatase elevation is described in two older infants with normal nutrition receiving phenobarbital and diphenylhydantoin (5). Moderate elevations of coagulation factor V are also known to occur in some children receiving anticonvulsant drugs (2). The incidence of these findings and their impact on growth and development in febrile convulsion patients who receive phenobarbital prophylaxis is not known.

Phenobarbital administration is occasionally associated with akathisia. Unaffected siblings of febrile convulsion patients receiving phenobarbital have potential access to an intoxicant and possible drug-abuse agent. The incidence of these potential complications of phenobarbital prophylaxis and their impact on the personal-social development of febrile convulsion patients is unknown.

In the absence of an easily demonstrated gene-product abnormality, specific at-risk febrile convulsion patients cannot be detected prior to experiencing their first febrile convulsion. Thus total prevention of febrile convulsions in a specific patient is not feasible at present.

Currently the diagnosis of febrile convulsion is made when a child 6 months to 5 years of age convulses during the temperature elevation associated with a non-CNS infection. Clinical and laboratory assessment must fail to reveal any other known cause. However, the diagnosis is not proved with certainty until the patient, if unscathed by the febrile convulsion, continues to develop, experiences no afebrile seizures, and does not convulse during febrile illnesses beyond 5–7 years of age. The difficulty posed by this operational definition is in documenting "unscathed." To date there appears to be no objective, precise marker which quantitates acute neural tissue loss in young children. Thus it is difficult to state categorically that phenobarbital prophylaxis is indicated in all febrile convulsion patients who have experienced a single, brief attack. There is currently no precise comparative at-risk data on minimal nervous system injury due to a future, brief convulsion which might be suppressed by phenobarbital prophylaxis versus the incidence and impact of the discussed potential iatrogenic risks. Hopefully they will become available from prospective studies which include randomized untreated controls as well as compliance assessment (27).

In summary, febrile convulsions are a significant health problem. If current prevalence estimates of febrile convulsions are applied to a developing nation where 60% of the population is composed of mothers and children, such as West Africa with an estimated population base of 160 million (9), the enormity and potential impact of this problem is obvious. Prolonged febrile convulsions may be lethal or cause CNS sequelae. Thus febrile convulsion status epilepticus is a medical emergency. Phenobarbital prophylaxis is indicated in febrile convulsion patients who have had prolonged or multiple attacks. Prospective clinical research, randomly assigning phenobarbital prophylaxis, as well as a placebo control treatment strategy in febrile convulsion patients who have experienced only a single brief convulsion appears to be justified. Basic science investigations designed to elicit the gene product abnormality in febrile convulsions have the potential of achieving case identification before clinical expression occurs.

REFERENCES

1. Aicardi, J., and Chevrie, J. J. (1970): Convulsive status epilepticus in infants and children: A study of 239 cases. *Epilepsia*, 11:187–197.
2. Bartels, H., Evert, W., Hauck, W., Petersen, C., Putzki, H., and Schulze, W. (1975): Significance of increased serum gamma-glutamyltransferase activity during long-term anticonvulsive treatment: Clinical and experimental studies. *Neuropaediatrie*, 6:77–89.
3. Borgstedt, A. D., Bryson, M. F., Young, L. W., and Forbes, G. B. (1972): Long-term administration of antiepileptic drugs and the development of rickets. *J. Pediatr.*, 81:9–15.
4. Carter, S., and Gold, A. P. (1969): The critically ill child: Management of status epilepticus. *Pediatrics*, 44:732–733.
5. Crosley, C. J., Chee, C., and Berman, P. H. (1975): Rickets associated with long-term anticonvulsant therapy. *Pediatrics*, 56:52–57.
6. Faerø, O., Kastrup, K. W., Lykkegaard, N. E., Melchior, J. C., and Thorn, I. (1972): Successful prophylaxis of febrile convulsions with phenobarbital. *Epilepsia*, 13:279–285.
7. Falconer, M. A. (1971): Genetic and related aetiological factors in temporal lobe epilepsy: A review. *Epilepsia*, 12:13–31.
8. Frantzen, E., Lennox-Buchthal, M., Nygaard, A., and Stene, J. A. (1970): A genetic study of febrile convulsions. *Neurology (Minneap.)*, 20:909–917.
9. French, D. M., and Latham, M. (1975): World hunger, health and refugee problems. VI. Special study mission to Africa, Asia and the Middle East. Hearings Before the U.S. Senate Subcommittees on Health and Refugees, 94th Congress, 1st Session, June 10 and 13.
10. French, J. H., Rowan, A. J., and Hyman, H. (1975): Unpublished data.
11. Hauser, W. A., and Kurland, L. T. (1975): The epidemiology of epilepsy in Rochester, Minnesota, 1935 through 1967. *Epilepsia*, 16:1–66.
12. Henry, K. R., and Haythorn, M. M. (1975): Albinism and auditory function in the laboratory mouse. I. Effects of single-gene substitutions on auditory physiology, audiogenic seizures, and developmental processes. *Behav. Genet.*, 5:137–149.
13. Hertz, L., Schousboe, A., and Lennox-Buchthal, M. (1974): Some age-dependent biochemical changes in mice susceptible to seizures. *Epilepsia*, 15:619–631.
14. Hunter, J., Maxwell, J. D., Stewart, D. A., Parsons, V., and Williams, R. (1971): Altered calcium metabolism in epileptic children on anticonvulsants. *Br. Med. J.*, 4:202–204.
15. Ingram, T. T. (1973): The treatment of febrile convulsions in childhood. *Dev. Med. Child Neurol.*, 15:531–533.
16. Lennox-Buchthal, M. (1973): Febrile convulsions: A reappraisal. *Electroencephalogr. Clin. Neurophysiol. (Suppl.)*, 32:1–138.
17. Lennox-Buchthal, M. A. (1974): Febrile convulsions. In: *Handbook of Clinical Neurology*, Vol. 15, edited by O. Magnus and A. M. Lorentz de Haas, pp. 246–263. Elsevier, Amsterdam.
18. Lessell, S., Torres, J. M., and Kurland, L. T. (1962): Seizure disorders in a Guamanian village. *Arch. Neurol.*, 7:37–44.
19. Moore, C. L., and Gamble, R. (1972): The effect of Metrazol® on mitochondrial oxidative phosphorylation. In: *Proceedings: Biophysical Society Annual Meeting, Toronto*, Vol. 16, p. 129a (abstract).

20. Ounsted, C. (1971): Some aspects of seizure disorders. In: *Recent Advances in Pediatrics,* 4th ed., edited by D. Hull and D. Gairdner, pp. 371–374. Churchill, London.
21. Plum, F., Howse, D. C., and Duffy, T. E. (1974): Metabolic effects of seizures. *Assoc. Res. Nerv. Ment. Dis. Res. Publ.* 53:141–156.
22. Ross, E. M. (1974): Proceedings: Convulsive problems in the national child development study. *Arch. Dis. Child.,* 49:820.
23. Schiøttz-Christensen, E., and Bruhn, P. (1973): Intelligence, behavior and scholastic achievement subsequent to febrile convulsions: An analysis of disconcordant twin-pairs. *Dev. Med. Child Neurol.,* 15:565–575.
24. Stanhope, J. M., Brody, J. A., Brink, E., and Morris, C. E. (1972): Convulsions among the Chamorro people of Guam, Mariana Islands. II. Febrile convulsions. *Am. J. Epidemiol.,* 95:299–304.
25. Taylor, D. C., and Ounsted, C. (1971): Biologic mechanisms influencing the outcome of seizures in response to fever. *Epilepsia,* 12:33–45.
26. van den Berg, B. J. (1974): Studies on convulsive disorders in young children. IV. Incidence of convulsions among siblings. *Dev. Med. Child Neurol.,* 16:457–464.
27. Wolf, S. M., Carr, A. C., Hanson, R. A., Dale, E. P., Davis, D. C., Goldenberg, E. D., Lulejian, G. A., Sharpe, K. S., Treitman, P., and Weinstein, A. W. (1973): Parental compliance in the continuous administration of phenobarbital for the prevention of febrile seizures. *J. Pediatr.,* 83:1085–1086.

Brain Dysfunction in Infantile Febrile Convulsions, edited by M. A. B. Brazier and F. Coceani. Raven Press, New York © 1976.

Treatment of Convulsions with Fever

Sheila J. Wallace

Department of Child Health, University Hospital of Wales, Heath Park, Cardiff CF4 4XW, Wales

When a convulsion with fever has been prolonged, unilateral, or repeated within the same illness, there is an increased risk of recurrence of febrile convulsions, later grand mal or temporal lobe epilepsy, neurological abnormalities, and mental retardation (1,4,7,8,11,20,21,26). Children with repeated seizures with fever are more likely to develop spontaneous attacks (12,16), be at greater risk of having a severe attack (11), and have a significant reduction in the verbal score on the Wechsler Intelligence Scale for Children (WISC) (3).

Two points seem important: No convulsion should be allowed to persist longer than 30 min, and recurrence of attacks with fever should be avoided if possible. The most effective method for terminating an acute episode of status is to give an intravenous injection of diazepam. Alternatively, sodium amytal or paraldehyde may be given intramuscularly. These have a less immediate but more prolonged action.

The use of continuous anticonvulsant therapy in the prevention of febrile convulsions has been discussed for many years (2,12,13,17,24). Because of the ill-substantiated view that such seizures are associated with a benign prognosis, it is probable that many of the early studies were half-hearted or relied partially on intermittent therapy. It is also possible that those anticonvulsants given were not prescribed in a dosage high enough to achieve effective blood levels.

A controlled trial has shown that phenobarbitone 30 mg given with salicylates at the onset of fever did not prevent a febrile convulsion (13). During this study it also became obvious that parents had difficulty in deciding when their children were ill enough to be given medication. Failure of phenobarbitone given at the onset of fever to prevent convulsions is not surprising since it is impossible to achieve a therapeutic level in the serum until 48 hr after treatment has been started, even if double the usual dosage is given (6). However, if continuous daily phenobarbitone is received and the serum barbiturate level is maintained above 15 mg/liter, children are unlikely to convulse when febrile (6). In contrast, it has been suggested that febrile seizures are not prevented in children under 3 years by phenytoin, even if the serum level is within the range usually regarded as therapeutic (15). Nevertheless, phenytoin appears to reduce the likelihood of the occurrence

301

of a prolonged convulsion, although the numbers have been too small to make this finding significant.

A study comparing recurrence of febrile convulsions in treated and untreated children who had factors associated with a high incidence of repeated attacks has been conducted (27). A total of 199 children who convulsed when febrile were examined at the Royal Hospital for Sick Children, Edinburgh, and Cardiff Royal Infirmary; 117 had had either an initial fit lasting more than 30 min, repeated attacks during the same illness, or both a history of fits in siblings or parents or both, and a neurological disorder persisting longer than the acute illness. An untreated group of 68 children did not receive anticonvulsants after their first fit; and the other 49 were treated after the initial seizure. Phenobarbitone 2–4 mg/kg body weight/day was prescribed for 27 and primidone 10–15 mg/kg/day for 22. Allocation of patients to treatment with phenobarbitone or primidone was largely on a random basis, but there was a bias towards the use of primidone when neurological signs persisted. Therapy was discontinued almost immediately by the parents in 6 of the children on phenobarbitone and 3 of those on primidone. In 3 on phenobarbitone and 1 on primidone, overactivity and irritability were intolerable. In the other 5 cases, parents were unwilling for their children to have long-term drugs, which they feared might be addictive in nature or lead to delay in development. The treated group, used for comparison with the 68 untreated, finally consisted of 40 children. No significant difference between those treated and those untreated was present for sex, age at first fit, family history, or severity of first fit. The treated children were significantly more likely to have persisting neurological abnormality (p 0.01). All 108 children were followed for a minimum of 18 months.

The effects of anticonvulsant therapy were dramatic. Those children treated were very significantly less likely to have another fit if they became febrile again. Seven of the 40 who were treated and 40 of the 68 untreated had a fit with a subsequent febrile illness (χ^2 13.24, df 1, $p < 0.005$). Recurrence of convulsions was equally uncommon whichever anticonvulsant had been used; 3 of the 19 on primidone and 4 of the 21 treated with phenobarbitone had another fit when febrile. Blood levels of the anticonvulsants were not measured, but subsequent experience of the dosage per body weight used in this study suggests serum values usually considered as therapeutic would not have been achieved. Nevertheless, the incidence of recurrence of febrile convulsions in treated children was very significantly reduced. Therefore it is possible that the barbiturate level of over 15 mg/liter suggested by Faerø et al. (6) may be higher than is entirely necessary. Further investigation of this is in progress (28).

Although convulsions can be prevented by continuous treatment with barbiturates, there are disadvantages in their use. Ataxia and drowsiness may occur. A clinical impression that these are comparatively uncommon with the dosage normally given for febrile convulsions tends to be confirmed by the finding that impairment of motor tasks occurs only if a high plasma level is present (10). Specific psychological changes have been observed after giving barbiturates to adults. Alterations in short-term memory and more specifically in those links of the psychological chain of memory involved with visual perception, attention, organisation, and rehearsal have been noted (5,9,14,18,19,22,25). It has been concluded that barbiturates impair both learning and retention, and that these impairments are most noticeable in adults with poorer learning ability. The effects of barbiturates on psychological functioning in children under age 7 have not been adequately examined. However, a study of 102 children between 8 and 10 years after their initial convulsion showed no significant difference in psychological functioning between the 50 who had received barbiturates for at least 1 year before the age of 7 years and those 52 who had not been so treated (3). The tests used were Draw-a-person; WISC full scale, verbal, and performance; Bender Gestalt; and the Oseretsky Test of Motor Proficiency. On the Rutter Behavior Scale, children who had previously received barbiturates were not more likely to be disturbed at ages 8–14 years.

The most dramatic side effects of barbiturates are those associated with gross behaviour disorders. At least 20% of all young children treated with phenobarbitone are so intolerant that discontinuance is necessary (23,28). A small series of children are currently under investigation for the effects of phenobarbitone on their behaviour (28). An attempt is being made to qualify and, if possible, quantify behavioural changes. So far it has been necessary to discontinue phenobarbitone in 9 of 27 treated. All 9 were excessively irritable; and overactivity, temper tantrums, and poor concentration were each noted in at least 5 of the 9. Where serum barbiturate levels were available, there appeared to be no relationship to the severity of the disturbance. There was an impression from the previous investigation of anticonvulsants in the prevention of febrile convulsions that primidone was better tolerated than phenobarbitone (27). Therefore a trial of primidone was given to the first 7 in the series of 9 children who were disturbed by phenobarbitone; 4 were equally intolerant of primidone, and this policy has now been discontinued. There thus remains a group of perhaps 20–30% of children in whom it would be desirable to prevent subsequent convulsions but who are intolerant of barbiturates.

Phenytoin has been shown to reduce the likelihood of a severe convulsion, even if complete prevention is not achieved (15). Its effect on cognitive functioning in small children has not been adequately studied. Of those tested by Cull (3), the children who had received anticonvulsants other than barbiturates for at least a year before the age of 7 had a significant reduction in their WISC performance scores at ages 8–14 years (χ^2 9.88, df 4, p 0.04). Although ethosuximide and sulthiame had also been given to some of these children, most had received phenytoin. Those children still receiving phenytoin at the time of follow-up had significantly increased error scores on the

Bender Gestalt test (χ^2 18.02, df 5, *p* 0.003) and a significant excess of clumsiness on the Oseretsky Test of Motor Proficiency (χ^2 6.61, df 2, *p* 0.04). It is impossible, however, to be certain that these observations are due to the phenytoin rather than the underlying cerebral condition necessitating its use. Further investigation of this problem is obviously required.

In conclusion, it is possible to control most convulsions which occur with fever by the use of continuous prophylactic phenobarbitone or primidone. In children whose behaviour is not seriously disturbed, it appears that long-term psychological damage is not sustained, whereas recurrence of convulsions has been associated with significant reduction on the WISC verbal scale. Between a fifth and a third of children are intolerant of barbiturates. Phenytoin reduces the severity of convulsions, although it may not completely avert them. Its use can be associated with alterations in cognitive functioning. It is suggested that only in the children where there is a high risk of subsequent attacks should continuous anticonvulsant therapy be given after the first seizure, but that all who have a second episode should be treated thereafter. Those whose initial fits are prolonged, repeated during the same illness, or unilateral; who have their first seizure before the age of 18 months; whose family history is positive for convulsive disorders; and who have persisting neurological disorders have a high risk of recurrence. It is proposed that they receive either phenobarbitone or primidone as a first choice of treatment, and that phenytoin be reserved for those intolerant of barbiturates. It is further suggested that continuous therapy be given for 2 years provided no subsequent attack occurs; that if a seizure does occur during therapy, 3 clear years should elapse before medication is discontinued; and that it is necessary in any child to continue with anticonvulsants until the age of approximately 5 years.

ACKNOWLEDGMENTS

Paediatricians at the Royal Hospital for Sick Children in Edinburgh, the Cardiff Royal Infirmary, and the University Hospital of Wales in Cardiff kindly allowed their patients to be studied. The secretarial staffs of all three institutions have given invaluable aid.

REFERENCES

1. Aicardi, J., and Chevrie, J. J. (1970): Convulsive status epilepticus in infants and children. *Epilepsia*, 2:187–197.
2. Carter, S. (1964): Diagnosis and treatment: Management of the child who has had one convulsion. *Pediatrics*, 33:431–434.
3. Cull, A. M. (1975): Some psychological aspects of the prognosis of febrile convulsions. M.Phil. thesis, University of Edinburgh.
4. Degen, R., and Goller, K. (1967): Die sogennanten Fieberkrampfe des Kindersalters und ihre Beziehungen zur Epilepsie. *Nervenarzt*, 38:55–61.
5. Evans, W. O., and Davies, K. E. (1969): Dose-response effects of secobarbital on human memory. *Psychopharmacologia*, 14:46–61.

6. Faerø, O., Kastrup, K. W., Lykkegard Nielson, E., Melchior, J. C., and Thorn, I. (1972): Successful prophylaxis of febrile convulsions with phenobarbital. *Epilepsia,* 13:279–285.
7. Falconer, M. A., Serafetinides, E. A., and Corsellis, J. A. N. (1964): Etiology and pathogenesis of temporal lobe epilepsy. *Arch. Neurol.,* 10:232–248.
8. Gastaut, H., Poirier, F., Payan, H., Salamon, G., Toga, M., and Vigouroux, M. (1960): H.H.E. syndrome: Hemiconvulsions, hemiplegia, epilepsy. *Epilepsia,* 1:418–447.
9. Grove-White, I. G., and Kelman, G. R. (1971): Effect of methohexitone, diazepam, and sodium-4-hydroxybutyrate on short term memory. *Br. J. Anaesth.,* 43:113–116.
10. Hutt, S. J., Jackson, P. M., Belsham, A., and Higgins, G. (1968): Perceptual motor behaviour in relation to blood phenobarbitone level: A preliminary report. *Dev. Med. Child Neurol.,* 10:626–632.
11. Lennox-Buchthal, M. A. (1973): *Febrile Convulsions. A Reappraisal.* Elsevier, Amsterdam.
12. Livingston, S., Bridge, E. M., and Kajdi, L. (1947): Febrile convulsions; A clinical study with special reference to heredity and prognosis. *J. Pediatr.,* 31:509–512.
13. Mackintosh, T. F. (1970): Studies on prophylactic treatment of febrile convulsions in children. *Clin. Pediatr.,* 9:283–286.
14. Malpas, A., and Joyce, C. R. B. (1969): Effects of nitrazepam, amylobarbitone and placebo on some perceptual, motor and cognitive tasks in normal subjects. *Psychopharmacologia,* 14:167–177.
15. Melchior, J. C., Buchthal, F., and Lennox-Buchthal, M. A. (1971): The ineffectiveness of diphenylhydantoin in preventing febrile convulsions in the age of greatest risk, under 3 years. *Epilepsia,* 12:55–62.
16. Millichap, J. G. (1968): *Febrile Convulsions.* Macmillan, New York.
17. Millichap, J. G., Aledort, L. M., and Madsen, J. A. (1960): Critical evaluation of therapy of febrile convulsions. *J. Pediatr.,* 56:364–368.
18. Mirsky, A. F., and Kornetsky, C. (1964): On the dissimilar effects of drugs on the digit symbol substitution and continuous performance tests. *Psychopharmacologia,* 5:161–177.
19. Osborn, A. G., Bunker, J. P., Cooper, L. M., Frank, G. S., and Hilgard, E. R. (1967): Effects of thiopental sedation on learning and memory. *Science,* 157:574–576.
20. Ounsted, C., Lindsay, J., and Norman, R. (1966): *Biological Factors in Temporal Lobe Epilepsy.* Clinics in Developmental Medicine No. 22. Heineman, London.
21. Schmidt, R. P. (1958): Sequelae of febrile convulsions. *Med. Clin. North Am.,* 42:389–397.
22. Talland, G. A., and Quarton, G. C. (1965): The effects of methamphetamine and pentobarbital on running memory span. *Psychopharmacologia,* 7:379–382.
23. Thorn, I. (1975): A controlled study of prophylactic long-term treatment in febrile convulsions. *Acta Neurol. Scand. [Suppl.],* 60:67–73.
24. Van den Berg, B. J., and Yerushalmy, J. (1971): Studies on convulsive disorders in young children. II. Intermittent phenobarbital prophylaxis and recurrence of febrile convulsions. *J. Pediatr.,* 78:1004–1012.
25. Van Felsinger, J. M., Lasagna, L., and Beecher, H. K. (1953): The persistence of mental impairment following a hypnotic dose of a barbiturate. *J. Pharmacol. Exp. Ther.,* 109:284–291.
26. Wallace, S. J. (1974): Recurrence of febrile convulsions. *Arch. Dis. Child.,* 49:763–765.
27. Wallace, S. J. (1975): Continuous prophylactic anticonvulsants in selected children with febrile convulsions. *Acta Neurol. Scand. [Suppl.],* 60:62–66.
28. Wallace, S. J. (1976): Anticonvulsants in the prophylaxis of convulsions with fever. First European Regional Conference on Epilepsy.

Brain Dysfunction in Infantile Febrile Convulsions, edited by M. A. B. Brazier and F. Coceani. Raven Press, New York © 1976.

Surgical Treatment of Sequelae of Severe Febrile Convulsions

Murray A. Falconer

Neurosurgical Unit of Guy's, Maudsley, and King's College Hospitals, London SE5 8AZ, England

Although it has been known for several generations that a febrile illness in childhood may be accompanied by convulsions and coma, and be followed by epilepsy (21,22,44,49,52,57), it has only become accepted in recent years that a severe febrile convulsion during infancy or a series of convulsions in close succession may of themselves produce severe focal damage in the brain that after healing can become an epileptogenic lesion. The most important of these lesions appears to be the one long known as Ammon's horn sclerosis but which, as it often involves other structures in the mesial part of the temporal lobe such as the amygdala and the uncus, we prefer to term mesial temporal sclerosis (11,16,20). In yet other cases the febrile convulsive process may be followed by an acute infantile hemiplegia and then be known by such rubrics as *lobar sclerosis* (22), the *HHE syndrome* of Gastaut et al. (23), and *cerebral hemiatrophy* (39). As the epilepsy which results from these lesions can often be improved by judicious surgical treatment, the salient points of the pathology and pathogenesis of these lesions is first reviewed followed by a consideration of findings noted in their surgical treatment. Even now the precise pathogenesis of these lesions is still a matter of speculation, and this of course is reflected in the conclusions which can be drawn from their surgical treatment.

RATIONALE OF SURGICAL TREATMENT

At the present time the surgical treatment of epilepsy is diverging in two separate directions: first, the excision of abnormal epileptogenic tissue; and second, the stereotactic destruction of intracranial neuronal masses or of their fiber connections so as to interfere with the generation and propagation of seizure discharges. The whole field of stereotactic surgery in epilepsy was recently reviewed by Ojemann and Ward (42), who concluded that the results of this form of surgical therapy are not as dramatic as those following lobectomy and other excision procedures but may have a place where the site of origin of the seizure discharges is indefinite or bilateral, or where a unilateral lobectomy has failed and there is evidence of a contralateral epileptogenic focus. From the viewpoint of etiology, a defect of the stereotactic procedures is that they usually fail to disclose the pathological substrate.

My philosophy of "the rationale of surgical treatment of epilepsy, whether in the temporal lobe or elsewhere, is that the surgeon maps out by clinical, neuroradiological, EEG, or other means a zone of tissue which he can then excise in one block suitable for detailed histological examination without adding appreciably to the patient's handicaps" (14). This is a concept similar to that offered previously by Green (24) and Rasmussen (46), except that both stressed that the surgeon should remove the area of maximum epileptogenicity as determined by electrocorticography. Neither evidently practised *en bloc* resections but did their removals by a piecemeal technique, which was probably as effective therapeutically as the *en bloc* resection practised by myself (12); it did not, however, provide them with a specimen so suitable for histological demonstration of the lesion. By following the principle of *en bloc* resections both in temporal lobe epilepsy and in hemispherectomy, we have been able to make clinicopathological correlations which would not have been possible if we had not demonstrated the pathological substrate (13).

PATHOLOGICAL SUBSTRATES

Mesial Temporal (Ammon's Horn) Sclerosis

The most important of the pathological substrates is the one long known as Ammon's horn sclerosis but which we prefer to term mesial temporal sclerosis (Figs. 1 and 2). I have twice traced its long circuitous history (11,

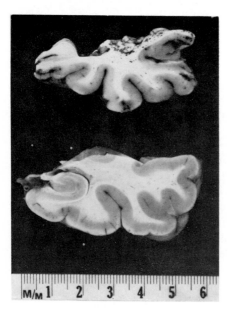

FIG. 1. Top: Cross section of resected temporal lobe from epileptic male with antecedent history of a febrile infantile convulsion showing a scarred Ammon's horn. **Bottom:** Normal control.

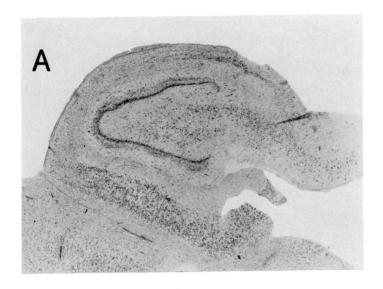

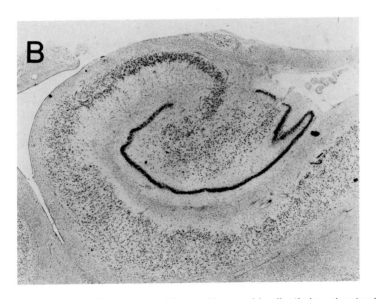

FIG. 2. A: Ammon's horn (hippocampus) from a 12-year-old epileptic boy showing loss of the Sommer sector (h_1) above and to the left, and of the end-folium ($h_{3,4,5}$) in the center. Some cells of the resistant sector (h_2) remain above and slightly to the right. **B:** Normal Ammon's horn at the same magnification. Cresyl violet. ×11.

16). It is a process which essentially involves usually one but sometimes both temporal lobes. During the past century and a half many postmortem studies of the brain of chronic epileptics who died a natural death have demonstrated its presence in more than half of them (27,32,47). The lesion is thus frequent and also is clearly of anoxic origin with its main brunt falling on the Ammon's horn (hippocampus) where there is a selective loss in the Sommer sector (h_1) and in the end-folium (h_3, h_4, and h_5) with preservation of cells in the "resistant" sector (h_2). However, it also often involves the amygdala as well (11,16,20). Sometimes it is the only lesion present in the brain in epilepsy, and postmortem studies suggest that whenever it is present it is unilateral in 80% of instances (32). No one has yet explained fully why it is so often unilateral. However, using case material drawn from my surgical patients as well as medically treated patients of their own, Taylor and Ounsted (51) argue that males tend to be involved more than females, in the ratio 1.4:1. In their view girls mature faster than boys, while the right hemisphere with its visuospatial functions tends to mature before the left hemisphere with its language functions. The tendency to incept febrile convulsions thus falls more rapidly in girls than in boys. They think this explains why girls and the right hemisphere are involved more frequently during the first 18 months of life, while boys and the left hemisphere are involved more frequently after that than are girls. Paradoxically, those females who do convulse are more prone to serious sequelae, as they convulse more frequently at a younger age.

Ammon's horn sclerosis is also a lesion which Meldrum and Brierley (34) showed can often be produced experimentally in immature baboons by the induction of many serial grand mal attacks following intravenous injection of allyl glycine in an appropriate amount, and it may often develop only on one side and as the sole abnormality. Moreover, it is often associated with a patchy loss of Purkinje cells of the cerebellum together with patchy laminar cell loss in the cerebral cortex and patchy cell loss in the thalamus and corpus striatum but usually sparing the putamen and the calcarine cortex, thereby indicating that the pattern of damage was in no way caused by a tentorial pressure cone provoked either by cerebral oedema or by birth trauma that would have compressed the anterior choroidal or posterior cerebral arteries (20,39). The concept of "incisural sclerosis" due to birth injury cannot, we think, be upheld (11,20,39,44). It is our belief that a severe febrile convulsion during infancy is frequently an important factor in the production of mesial temporal or Ammon's horn sclerosis, as evidenced by the frequency with which it occurs in our epilepsy case material (*vide infra*), but just how it acts or whether it always acts in the same way we do not know.

Others have shown that Ammon's horn sclerosis similar to that found in epilepsy can occur after other anoxic states such as carbon monoxide poisoning, hypoglycemia, strangulation, or administration of some anesthetic gases (4,36). Still others say it can result from severe asphyxia at birth (31), although Norman held that asphyxia neonatorum damaged the h_2 sector rather than the Sommer sector (44). Zimmerman (57) reported it as occurring in a child following prolonged asphyxial episodes caused by pertussis without a convulsion. It can occur also in mental defectives who have not had clinical epilepsy (7). Norman as well as Zimmerman reported that occasionally a child may die of a severe status without showing changes in the Ammon's horn, although usually in children following status the Ammon's horn shows marked damage (40,44,57). Again Meldrum and his colleagues (35) showed in their baboons that if, once the convulsions appear, they are then controlled by muscle relaxants and artificial ventilation while systemic hyperpyrexia, hypoglycemia, and hypoxia are also controlled, the animal still goes on to develop Ammon's horn sclerosis provided electro-encephalographic (EEG) evidence of continuing seizure disturbances continue in the brain. This led us to postulate, as do Meldrum and his colleagues, that it is a local consumptive anoxia of the discharging hippocampal cells that in a sense leads to their own selective destruction (16). The only facts that various authorities are agreed on is that, whatever its precise etiology, Ammon's horn sclerosis usually arises during infancy or early childhood and that severe febrile convulsions play an important part in its etiology (20,44). As supportive evidence for this it is not uncommon in an elder child or adult to see in X-ray films of the skull that the middle cranial fossa on the affected side is slightly smaller than the other, indicating an underlying atrophic process dating from early life, while the air encephalogram may show slight signs suggesting atrophy of the mesial temporal structures (18,24,38).

Margerison and Corsellis (32) pointed to the difficulties incurred when comparing the cell changes observed in the mature lesion of Ammon's horn sclerosis in chronic epilepsy with the acute changes noted in the hippocampal cells after asphyxial illnesses in infants and children. The survival period in the latter was usually short, and often the degree of damage in other parts of the brain besides the hippocampus was extensive and not compatible with their clinical recovery except as severely demented patients. Epilepsy has not been a necessary sequel in such circumstances. Margerison and Corsellis then go on to say: "It may therefore be misleading to equate unreservedly the pathology of hypoxia in general with that of chronic epilepsy. The development of temporal lobe attacks is not merely a function of the scarred hippocampus in isolation but is probably also dependent upon the relative integrity of other parts of the brain" (32). Norman and his colleagues (41) recently published a similar caution.

Cerebral Hemiatrophy

The pathogenesis of a second entity, cerebral hemiatrophy, which affects primarily one whole cerebral hemisphere, is even more speculative than that of mesial temporal sclerosis, which affects one or sometimes both temporal lobes. William Osler in 1889 from Philadelphia (43), Sigmund Freud in 1897 from Vienna (22), Ford and Schaffer from The Johns Hopkins Hospital (21), and Lyon, Dodge, and Adams from the Massachusetts General Hospital (30) have all written extensively on these illnesses which quickly supervene on various acute infections like pertussis, diphtheria, pneumonia, and otitis media, or may suddenly attack apparently healthy infants or young children; James Taylor in 1905 from the National Hospital in London gave a long clinical description without committing himself to etiology or providing a bibliography (52). Coma and convulsions with or without fever are usually prominent at the outset, and when the convulsions subside the child is left with a severe and permanent hemiplegia. Freud in particular surveyed the previous literature and concluded that since the hemiplegia was sudden in onset the initial lesion was likely to be vascular (22). He pointed out, however, that the lobar sclerosis found at autopsy was a mature endproduct and went on to say: "The nature of the original vascular lesion is still questionable – whether it is a mechanical one (plugging of a vessel by an embolus?) or, as Pierre Marie indicated, whether organisms causing inflammation or products of inflammation had reached a specific arterial region, radiating a chronic, damaging effect. Both theories present certain problems." Osler reported 120 cases, in 89 of which he could give no explanation (43), while Ford and Schaffer analyzed 43 cases (21). They concluded that, in the ones with antecedent fever at the onset, vascular lesions in the cerebral hemispheres were largely responsible; but for the cases that began without fever they had no explanation and pointed to the paucity of postmortem evidence. Lyon et al. described 16 cases of acute encephalopathy in infants and young children in most of whom the illness began rapidly with fever, convulsions, and coma (30). Only two survived; and of the 14 cases who came to autopsy, a swelling of the brain was found in all but three. These authors felt that they could distinguish the illness they were reporting from a primary systemic electrolyte or fluid abnormality, arterial or venous thrombosis, meningitis, and encephalitis. They wrote "that in all probability [the illness] is closely related to febrile convulsions and febrile delirium." All the authors quoted above, from Osler and Freud onwards, have been mystified by the etiology of acute infantile hemiplegia and some by its relationship to cerebral diplegia. Furthermore, a theory by Strümpell that the condition was due to poliomyelitis has long been disproved (22,27, 43).

Whatever the causal factors or how they interplay, they lead to gross atrophy of more or less the whole of one cerebral hemisphere together with relative smallness of the opposite cerebellar hemisphere (Figs. 3 and 4). In 1963 Norman wrote that, although it is often the result of vascular thrombosis (both arterial and venous) precipitated by sepsis or dehydration and possibly by birth trauma, there is the additional and highly important factor

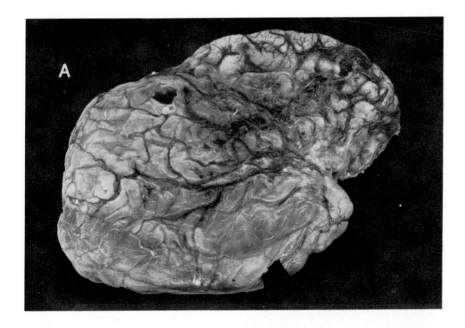

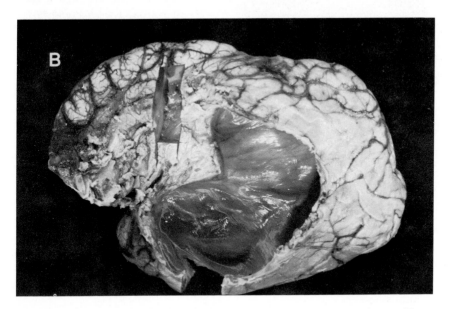

FIG. 3. Convexity **(A)** and mesial aspect **(B)** of resected right hemisphere from a 17-year-old male whose birth was somewhat traumatic and whose left infantile hemiplegia and epilepsy followed a severe convulsion at 1 year. Portions of the hemisphere have been removed for histology; the epilepsy was relieved following the operation. The preoperative IQ was 90 (F.S. WISC).

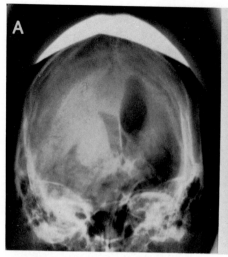
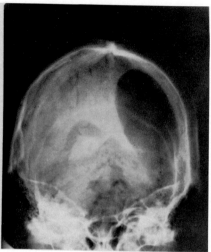

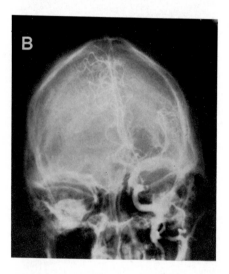

FIG. 4. Radiological studies of an 18-year-old girl who had a normal birth and normal milestones. At 18 months she had an unexplained high fever followed by convulsions for 2 weeks and then by an infantile hemiplegia and epilepsy. Speech was retarded until 5 years, but her IQ at 18 years was 74 (F.S. WISC). **A:** Pneumoencephalogram (left A.P., right P.A.) shows a small left cerebral hemisphere with a uniformly dilated ventricle and thickened cranial vault on that side. **B:** Left carotid arteriogram shows patency of major intracranial arteries with preferential filling of both anterior cerebral arteries from the carotid artery of the diseased side, a not-uncommon finding. The epilepsy was completely relieved following a left hemispherectomy.

of the severe epilepsy itself, which so often ushers in the illness (39). It is this idea—that the severe convulsion during infancy may of itself play a crucial role—which is the chief problem posed in this volume. Lobar sclerosis in this respect has many similarities to the pathogenesis of mesial temporal sclerosis.

It seems that an occasional case is the sequel of patchy thrombosis of the superior longitudinal venous sinus and others the result of thrombosis of the middle cerebral artery either at birth or later during infancy (19,39,56). This typically leads to a cicatrix or porencephaly in the territory of the middle cerebral artery, and there is a hemiplegia, usually without an associated hemianopia. However, even though the hemiplegia dates from birth, it does not become apparent until the child is several months old. Post-mortem examinations during the early stages of this type of hemiplegia may show no changes in the Ammon's horn but only infarcts of the hemisphere (39,44).

The most important cause appears to be a severe hemiconvulsion, and the process is now often known as the HHE syndrome of Gastaut (23). The usual story is that of an infant or child between the ages of 6 months and 2 years (but sometimes older) who suddenly develops a severe and pro-longed hemiconvulsion which may become generalised and sometimes lasts longer than 24 hr. When the child recovers, it exhibits an infantile hemi-plegia and sometimes also an homonymous hemanopia, which may remain permanently (1,23). Almost all children who convulse recover with some mental deterioration, which may be severe (1,3). Aicardi and Baraton (2) showed that, in children with hemiplegia, if a pneumoencephalogram is performed immediately after the status is over the affected hemisphere is often found to be swollen with the ipsilateral ventricle showing generalised compression and the midline structures displaced towards the opposite hemisphere. Then if the pneumoencephalogram is repeated a few weeks later, the ipsilateral ventricle is found to be enlarging fast and the cortical mantle is thinned, indicating gross atrophy of the affected hemisphere. Furthermore, there is usually no arteriographic evidence of obstruction of the cerebral arteries or cortical veins in this type of case (1). Patchy throm-bosis of the superior longitudinal sinus has been evoked to explain part of the syndrome (23), but it has not yet been satisfactorily demonstrated either radiologically or at postmortem examination, possibly because the throm-bosis may affect the lower levels of the superior longitudinal sinus or may resolve and recanalize quickly (39). The whole pathological basis of this syndrome is thus still a mixture of fact and speculation, but Aicardi et al. (1) strongly argue that whenever there is a prolonged convulsion anoxic changes occur widely among the neurons throughout the affected hemi-sphere, leading presumably to their death from consumptive anoxia and subsequent replacement by gliosis (1–3). A marked Ammon's horn sclerosis is always a feature of these cases (39).

Occasionally the hemiplegia appears abruptly in the somewhat older child (up to approximately 13 years of age), without a convulsion. Aicardi et al. (1) report that such children do not deteriorate mentally to the same degree as those who have had a convulsion, while carotid arteriography may show evidence of porencephaly and thrombotic lesions of the middle cerebral artery. Presumably such cases may not show hemianopia. Ammon's horn sclerosis may not be present (39).

However, in whatever way the infantile hemiplegia is produced, as the child grows older it shows spasticity and defective development of the affected limbs, which become relatively shorter. Whereas the child with a fully developed case is able to move the shoulder and elbow weakly, he cannot extend the wrist and individual finger movements are absent. In the lower limb he retains weak movements of the hip and knee but usually shows a spastic talipes equinus with no voluntary movements of the ankle and toes. Crude sensations to pinprick are preserved, and there is only moderate impairment of two-point discrimination and postural sense on the affected limb. The child can usually walk and run, but because the affected leg is shorter than its fellow he does not need to circumduct it. Hemianopia may be detected only if someone stands behind the child and brings his hands in from behind. The child himself is usually not aware of the defect in his vision and may bump into objects on the affected side as he walks.

Needless to say, both pathological substrates — mesial temporal sclerosis and lobar sclerosis — are sometimes bilateral. As a bilateral temporal lobectomy is impracticable because of the gross defect of recent memory it provokes (53), and bilateral cerebral hemispherectomies are equally impracticable, it is in such cases that stereotactic surgery offers the best hope of amelioration (42).

PERSONAL OBSERVATIONS OF SURGICAL THERAPY OF THE SEQUELAE OF SEVERE CONVULSIONS

Temporal Lobe Epilepsy

I have personally performed anterior temporal lobectomy for epilepsy in more than 300 patients, and my colleagues and I have reported the results of three separate series, the first two comprising 100 patients each (18,20), and the third 40 consecutive children under the age of 16 years (8). These three reports form the basis of the present discussion. Some observations in the first two series have already been summarised in a fourth report (13).

In general the basis of selection of these cases for operation has always been fourfold (8,18,20). Firstly, they have had frequent attacks of drug-resistant epilepsy; secondly, neuroradiological studies have apparently ruled out a sizeable space-occupying lesion; thirdly, many EEG studies employing particularly sphenoidal electrodes under intravenous thiopentone (Pentothal®) narcosis have disclosed a spike discharging which, if bilateral, was predominant on the side that was subsequently resected; and finally, apart from mental deficiency (IQ below 70), which we took to indicate bilateral pathology, we accepted patients with various psychiatric and personality disorders. As time went by we sometimes found that the data obtained were conflicting. However, we learned that there are sometimes small points about the neuroradiological and EEG findings which may be pathognomonic (10,38). In all patients *en bloc* resection of the temporal lobe was undertaken in order to determine the precise detailed histological examination.

Throughout, the pathological lesions disclosed in the resection specimens can be categorized into four subgroups:

1. Mesial temporal (Ammon's horn) sclerosis was uncovered in approximately half of my patients.

2. Hamartomas and other discrete developmental anomalies, usually of glial origin, were found in a fifth to a fourth of the cases.

3. Miscellaneous lesions such as scars and infarcts were found in a tenth of adults, but there were none in children.

4. Nonspecific lesions in which there might be gliosis but not neuronal abnormalities were found in the remaining fifth to fourth of patients.

In all three published series we clearly showed that, in the group with mesial temporal sclerosis as the substrate, there was a highly significant incidence of severe antecedent febrile convulsions or status epilepticus which was not found with the other pathological substrates (8,10,18). In our first two series the patients were mainly adults, and we noted that most of the patients with this particular substrate had their onset of habitual seizures during the first decade of life, whereas patients with other pathologies tended to have a later onset of seizure (18,20). Moreover, of the remaining patients with mesial temporal sclerosis, nearly all had developed habitual epilepsy by the time they had reached their teens. Furthermore, a family history of epilepsy was obtained in a fifth to a sixth of them, suggesting a genetic factor (13).

Table 1 gives the actual incidence of antecedent febrile convulsions in the three different series. In all three series we ignored cases in which the convulsions had lasted but a few minutes, as we had been impressed by the then prevailing and possibly misleading concept of "benign febrile convulsions" (29,37). In the first series we merely recorded the "severe and prolonged" febrile seizures, which had an incidence of 40%. In the second and third series, however, influenced by Ounsted et al. (44), we described a seizure that lasted longer than half an hour as a "status." In the second series the incidence of "status" was 30%, but in the third series in children

TABLE 1. *Onset of epilepsy with prolonged febrile convulsions in three series*

Series	No. in series	Patients with mesial temporal sclerosis	
		No.	Febrile convulsions or status
1. Mostly adults[a]	100	47	19 (40%)
2. Mostly adults[b]	100	47	14 (30%)
3. Children under 16 years[c]	40	24	19 (79%)

[a] Falconer et al. (18).
[b] Falconer and Taylor (19).
[c] Davidson and Falconer (8).

it became 79%. There are two principal explanations for the apparent rise in the incidence of febrile convulsions in our third series. Firstly, as Lennox-Buchthal (28) pointed out, the memory of witnesses for these events grows shorter for the older patients, and secondly my group for years had been telling our pediatric colleagues who referred their patients to us that a potent cause of mesial temporal sclerosis and so of habitual epilepsy was a severe febrile convulsion (14). This undoubtedly influenced their selection of patients for reference to us. At this stage I must point out that our published indices for febrile convulsions are probably an underestimate, as we excluded the less severe cases. Moreover, many of our patients had had several recurrent febrile convulsions. The published incidence in the community of febrile convulsions in children averages 40–50 infants per 1,000; in Newcastle-upon-Tyne it was recorded to be as high as 72/1,000, of whom 20% died; in Boston an incidence of 67/1,000 was reported, of whom 19% died; and in different series 1–20% of the surviving infants subsequently developed continuing epilepsy (28). Recent reliable statistics for Rochester, Minnesota, compiled by Hauser and Kurland (26) give an incidence of past febrile convulsions in the general community of approximately 32/1,000; of these, 2.3% of the individuals subsequently developed habitual epilepsy (i.e., 1–2/1,000). I must also point out how difficult it often is to tell whether an infant has had a convulsion, and then to determine its duration. Quite often a mother has told me that she did not realise that anything was amiss until she had gone upstairs and opened the bedroom door to find her child in a convulsion. Again, many of our patients had had more than one febrile convulsion before the habitual epilepsy began, the initial convulsions often being mild. We can testify, as Lennox-Buchthal (28) pointed out, that there is a strong tendency for febrile infantile convulsions to be recurrent.

Thus the frequency with which febrile convulsions have occurred in our patients with mesial temporal sclerosis is clearly significantly high to indicate it must have some special importance. Others such as Haberland (25) from Budapest, Green (24) from Phoenix, Mathieson (33) from Montreal, and Van Buren and his colleagues (54) from Bethesda recorded an appreciable incidence of antecedent febrile convulsions in their surgically treated cases of temporal lobe epilepsy but without specifying the substrate. There is also in our material an antecedent positive family history of epilepsy in first-degree relatives in approximately 13–20%, suggesting an important genetic factor (13). In an earlier paper I mentioned that I had performed a temporal lobectomy on a 14-year-old girl whose two siblings were epileptic as were her mother and some uncles, indicating a strong family history of epilepsy (20). Her epilepsy and that of one sibling began with a severe febrile convulsion, the sibling developing an infantile hemiplegia with epilepsy. Both girls benefited from surgery, the first now completely fit-free and off drugs for more than 12 years, and the hemispherectomized one now almost fit-free. These two cases reinforce our view that the epileptogenic lesions were mesial temporal sclerosis and lobar sclerosis, respectively.

The third point about mesial temporal sclerosis is that our best results of surgery, not only in regard to the relief of epilepsy but also in the improvement in social adaptation has occurred whenever this substrate was encountered at operation, suggesting that it was responsible for the habitual drug-resistant epilepsy. The results regarding relief of epilepsy are summarized in Table 2. In the first series, following the criteria of Penfield and Paine (45) we grouped together those patients who subsequently became fit-free and those who had only two or three seizures a year, calling them our "success group." Later we became aware that there is a great difference between becoming fit-free and having only an occasional seizure, for among other things those in the former group can qualify for a driving licence. In general the cases listed as fit-free have usually given up medication. Table 2 clearly shows that slightly more than half our patients with mesial temporal sclerosis have become fit-free, and most of the others benefited.

It was not until we were collecting our second series that we attempted to quantify the degree of social improvement that had occurred in our patients. The most marked social improvement occurred particularly when the substrate was mesial temporal sclerosis (8,18,50). We have had at least one patient gain a Ph.D.; several have done well in professions, music, and business; and several have become successful parents. There have of course been some disappointments, but no patient has become seriously involved with the law. Aggression in particular has often been relieved (15). For some reason, inexplicable to us, whenever psychosis has become associated with temporal lobe epilepsy the substrate is more likely to be a hamartoma than mesial temporal sclerosis, and a common experience has been that temporal lobectomy has relieved the epilepsy but not the psychosis (15).

TABLE 2. *Epilepsy relief following anterior temporal lobectomy correlated with pathological findings in three series*

Series no. and pathological substrates	No. in series	Fit-free	Almost fit-free	50% improved	Others
1. Mostly adults[a]	100				
Mesial temporal sclerosis	47	28 (60%)		15 (32%)	4 (9%)
Other pathologies	53	25 (47%)		15 (28%)	13 (25%)
2. Mostly adults[b]	100				
Mesial temporal sclerosis	47	24 (51%)	8 (17%)	13 (28%)	2 (4%)
Other pathologies	53	18 (34%)	12 (23%)	9 (17%)	14 (27%)
3. Children under 16 years[c]	40				
Mesial temporal sclerosis	24	14 (58%)	6 (25%)	4 (17%)	0
Other pathologies	16	9 (56%)	1 (6%)	1 (6%)	5 (31%)

[a] Falconer et al. (18).
[b] Falconer and Taylor (19).
[c] Davidson and Falconer (8).

Thus in our experience an antecedent febrile convulsion appears often to have played a significant part in the subsequent development of mesial temporal sclerosis. Others who described Ammon's horn sclerosis in neurosurgical case material with a frequency similar to ours include Haberland (25), Green (24), and Brown (5). How it does this is still a matter of conjecture, but its effect seems roughly proportional to the severity and duration of the febrile seizures. Corsellis (6) told me that in our case material the lesion of mesial temporal sclerosis is mostly mature as shown by paraffin and celloidin preparations, but recently Scheibel et al. (48) presented evidence from a study of Golgi preparations that the effects of recent nonfebrile habitual convulsions may have an additional cumulative effect on the development of the lesion. We have not performed such histological studies.

Infantile Hemiplegia

In the past I have written only sketchily about my experiences of hemispherectomy for infantile hemiplegia. In 1969 Wilson and I related our experiences in 18 consecutive cases operated on between 1952 and 1967; we reported these cases in order to report particularly four cases of delayed hemorrhage into the cranial cavity and how to recognize and treat this complication surgically (19). Since then I have been called on to perform the operation two or three times a year (8), with a total of over 40 cases now, but I do not have the same details in my records postoperatively as I have on the epilepsy cases. However, my conclusions are in general agreement with those of my collaborator Wilson (56), who also conducted a long-term follow-up of 50 cases operated by McKissock, and with the views of Aicardi and his colleagues on etiology (1,3).

When accepting patients for hemispherectomy we like to see the full-blown signs of an infantile hemiparesis down one side and no evidence of a hemiplegia on the other side. An associated hemianopia is not mandatory but is desirable. Similarly radiological evidence of an intact hemisphere on the sound side contralateral to the one with a lobar sclerosis is essential. Often one finds EEG abnormalities over both hemispheres with a tendency to flattening of the record over the sclerosed side. Epileptic activity in the form of spike discharges and sharp waves may be even more marked than over the sclerosed hemisphere; but other things being equal this should not deter the surgeon, for after removal of the sclerosed hemisphere the chances are that the EEG activity over the sound hemisphere will return to normal.

In general the type of infantile hemiplegia that apparently dates from birth occurs without a convulsion and usually takes the form of a large cicatrix or more often of a porencephaly in the territory of the middle cerebral artery. It is the more common type of case which usually commences with a convulsion during infancy or early childhood that takes the form of a lobar sclerosis with or without associated hemianopia and with marked Ammon's horn sclerosis. I think it important therefore that when excising the affected lobe the hippocampal structures be deliberately included in the resected lobe. I have had at least one striking success, over a 12-year follow-up, with a patient who had an infantile hemiplegia that followed a febrile convulsion at the age of 3 years and who developed severe habitual seizures at the age of 4½ years. The child was submitted to an anterior temporal lobectomy at age 13 years, leaving the rest of the hemisphere *in situ,* and has been fit-free and readily manageable for the 12 years since. The resected temporal lobe had a gross Ammon's horn sclerosis. I therefore regret that I have not tried this procedure as a first procedure more often, although I also had an early failure; it is also difficult always to make the wisest choice before the event. Wilson reported that in one of McKissock's cases there had been a previous unsuccessful corpus callosum section and in two others an unsuccessful temporal lobectomy.

My results of hemispherectomy (9,19) in general are similar to those reported by Wilson (56). These patients usually suffer from intractable epilepsy of psychomotor or convulsive type, with a high proportion of lateralized convulsions and frequently also a severe aggressive behavioral disorder. Both features are usually strikingly benefitted by hemispherectomy, and I think that approximately three-fourths of my cases are rendered fit-free regardless of whether their illness began with a severe febrile convulsion. In the long term, however, complications like stricture of the aqueduct or delayed hemorrhage into the cerebral cavity occur which mar the ultimate prognosis (19). A striking finding in cases that come to autopsy is the smallness of the contralateral cerebellar hemisphere. This presumably is the result of transneuronal influences from the atrophic cerebral hemisphere whatever the factor that triggers off the febrile convulsion.

Typically it is the fever that initiates the convulsion, which in turn leads to the anoxic factor responsible for the brain damage whether limited to the temporal lobe or involving the whole hemisphere; the problem of pathogenesis is not always as simple, however. Firstly, although fever is apparently often a factor in the onset of the convulsion, the initial fever is not always high. Aicardi and Chevrie (3) place it at 38.5°C. In most of our patients the onset of the convulsion was associated with some such illness as an upper respiratory infection, teething, measles, pertussis, immunizations, etc., and we cannot determine the level of fever at the onset of the convulsion. Anyway, an infant in a convulsion develops additional hyperpyrexia from the excessive muscular contractions. Moreover, we know from experimental work in baboons that the lesion of Ammon's horn sclerosis develops even if the convulsion, temperature, and systemic blood sugar levels are controlled, provided evidence of the seizure discharges in the brain continues to be recorded on the EEG (35). Again Ammon's horn sclerosis and possibly also lobar sclerosis causing infantile hemiplegia can develop after purely anoxic lesions without an antecedent convulsion (4,36).

Aicardi and Chevrie (3), while agreeing that antecedent fever prior to the onset of convulsions is important, say it is not essential, a view which conflicts with that of many pediatricians but which also appears to have been the opinion of both Osler (43) and Freud (22). They state: "We would like to suggest that febrile, cryptogenic status epilepticus is only the most severe expression of idiopathic convulsions and differs from the common, brief benign seizures in severity, not in nature" (3). From our experience I think this view is correct.

THE FACTOR THAT TRIGGERS THE CONVULSION

It is generally accepted that a study of what happens in identical twins affords some sort of control of etiological factors. We have one pair of identical twins in our hemispherectomy material, and a second pair has been reported in the literature.

Case 1 (17): An 8-year-old girl, proved by blood grouping and dermatoglyphics to be an identical twin, was born second by a breech delivery, the first twin having had a normal vertex delivery. She experienced some anoxia at birth and was slightly smaller (birth weight 1.5 kg) than her twin (birth weight 2.0 kg) but otherwise seemed well. After a few minor convulsions during early infancy, which her twin did not have, she developed normally until the age of 2 years 4 months, at which time she had a status epilepticus and recovered with a dense left hemiplegia, a left homonymous hemianopia, and some mental retardation. The ability to walk and talk was slowly regained, and presumably her speech functions were transferred to the right hemisphere. At age 8 years, because of drug-resistant epilepsy as well as hyperkinesis and uncontrolled aggression, she underwent a right hemispherectomy. The resected specimen showed gross hemispheral atrophy with marked Ammon's horn sclerosis. The hemiplegia and hemianopia were not increased by the operation. She was reported by us initially because of marked coarsening of her features produced by prolonged anticonvulsant drug therapy, but her convulsions occurred before her habitual epilepsy started and drug therapy was commenced.

Case 2 (55): This child was also a second twin, born after a difficult breech delivery (birth weight 1.9 kg). The first twin had had a normal vertex delivery and was slightly lighter (birth weight 2.4 kg). Both were males, and evidence of identical twinning was afforded by blood grouping, dermatoglyphics, and a common placenta. During the first 3 days the second-born twin looked poorly, breathed irregularly, and at times had a temperature up to as high as 41°C. Both twins regained their birth weights by the 14th day. From birth, however, the second twin was slower than his brother with his milestones. Then at 16 months he had a febrile status, the duration of which was not stated. He deteriorated after this and had many hospital admissions for epilepsy. He died at 3 years 4 months, while his brother continued to thrive and had a normal EEG. At postmortem examination his brain showed numerous areas of cortical atrophy, particularly in the right cerebral hemisphere, and well-marked Ammon's horn sclerosis on the right side.

I cite these two sets of identical twins because in both sets one twin had a difficult breech delivery. Neither set had a family history of epilepsy. In both the evidence was strong that it was the birth injury which was the factor leading to subsequent events. Norman (40,44) reported some other children who came to postmortem examination following status epilepticus; he found evidence in these of previous brain damage due to birth injury, including one patient with a lesion on the resistant (h_2) sector of Ammon's horn which he regarded as pathognomonic of severe asphyxia neonatorum. Yet in our three reported series we felt we could discount birth injury as a cause of subsequent epilepsy because the incidence of difficult birth in each of the four pathological subgroups was the same and no higher than in the community at large (13). It may well be, however, that the degree of birth injury which acts as the trigger may be apparently mild and not appreciated before the actual convulsion.

CONCLUSIONS

The work outlined in this chapter was done in a neurosurgical unit, but it involved close collaboration of people from many disciplines: clinicians, neurophysiologists, neuroradiologists, neuropathologists, and psychologists who helped work up the various cases and assisted in their long follow-up. As time has gone by our knowledge and experience have increased steadily. We showed that in temporal lobe epilepsy, mesial temporal or Ammon's horn sclerosis is the pathological substrate in approximately half the cases, and that whenever this lesion is encountered at operation we can expect good results not only in regard to the relief of the epilepsy but also with the patient's subsequent rehabilitation into society. Clearly mesial temporal sclerosis, which is the most common single lesion found at autopsy in patients who die a natural death, is an important epileptogenic lesion in its own right. Its causation is still a matter for discussion, but our finding of a strikingly high antecedent incidence of a severe febrile convulsion with this particular substrate suggests that such convulsions are an important cause of the lesion, which then matures into an epileptogenic one. There is also often a genetic factor.

Likewise our findings with hemispherectomy in infantile hemiplegia epilepsy show that lobar sclerosis has many causes. Some are clearly due to birth trauma, but in many patients a severe convulsion during infancy is a potent causal factor. There may likewise be a genetic factor both in the production of Ammon's horn sclerosis in temporal lobe epilepsy and of lobar sclerosis in infantile hemiplegia. The early literature for both conditions was reviewed to show how our elders were mystified by the factors which provoked these lesions. It is only since a severe generalised convulsion causing widespread neuronal damage during early life was accepted as an important factor that the etiology and pathogenesis of these lesions has begun to make sense (20,44).

Our surgical studies were limited by our choice of operated material. We did not resect brain tissue in cases of mental deficiency or cerebral diplegia, for in such cases both cerebral hemispheres are presumably damaged and operation by cortical resection would not benefit the patient. Hence we have no observations to make in such types of cases, but by analogy we believe that antecedent convulsions often play an important part in their causation also, a view expressed long ago by Freud (22).

Two cases of these lesions occurring in one each of a pair of identical twins are reported to remind us that other factors such as birth trauma may also play an important causal role. We do not understand fully the interplay of the various factors we have been considering, or whether there are missing factors not yet mentioned.

However, it is clear from our surgical experience that a severe febrile convulsion sometimes plays a decisive role in producing temporal lobe epilepsy and/or acute infantile hemiplegia in many patients. The degree of damage it causes seems roughly proportional to the duration and severity of the seizure (1,3,39,44). Although their full significance has not yet been unravelled, on the evidence available we agree that a febrile convulsion should be regarded as an emergency and prompt steps taken to cut the cerebral discharges short, as by the injection of diazepam, clonazepam, or sodium amytal (28,44). Supporting therapy alone (e.g., administration of oxygen or measures designed to cool the child) is not sufficient (35). It will be interesting to learn ultimately whether such measures and also prophylactic therapy to prevent a recurrent seizure cut down the incidence of habitual epilepsy during childhood (28).

ACKNOWLEDGMENTS

I wish to thank my various colleagues who helped me throughout these studies, and in particular Drs. J. A. N. Corsellis and D. C. Taylor who helped me in the compilation of this chapter.

REFERENCES

1. Aicardi, J., Amsili, J., and Chevrie, J. J. (1969): Acute hemiplegia in infancy and childhood. *Dev. Med. Child Neurol.*, 11:162–173.
2. Aicardi, J., and Baraton, J. (1971): A pneumographic demonstration of brain atrophy following status epilepticus. *Dev. Med. Child Neurol.*, 13:660–667.
3. Aicardi, J., and Chevrie, J. J. (1970): Convulsive status epilepticus in infants and children: A study of 239 cases. *Epilepsia*, 11:187–197.
4. Brierley, J. B., Meldrum, B. S., and Brown, A. W. (1973): The threshold and neuropathology of cerebral "anoxic-ischemic" cell change. *Arch. Neurol.*, 29:367–375.

5. Brown, W. J. (1973): Structural substrates of seizure foci in the human temporal lobe. In: *Epilepsy: Its Phenomena in Man,* edited by M. A. B. Brazier, pp. 329–374. Academic Press, New York.
6. Corsellis, J. A. N. (1975): Personal communication.
7. Crome, L. (1955): A morphological critique of temporal lobectomy. *Lancet,* 2:882–884.
8. Davidson, S., and Falconer, M. A. (1975): Outcome of surgery in 40 children with temporal-lobe epilepsy. *Lancet,* 1:1260–1263.
9. Davidson, S., Falconer, M. A., and Stroud, E. C. (1972): The place of surgery in the treatment of epilepsy in childhood and adolescence: A preliminary report in 13 cases. *Dev. Med. Child Neurol.,* 14:796–803.
10. Engel, J., Driver, M. V., and Falconer, M. A. (1975): Electrophysiological correlates of pathology and surgical results in temporal lobe epilepsy. *Brain,* 98:129–156.
11. Falconer, M. A. (1968): The significance of mesial temporal (Ammon's horn) sclerosis in epilepsy. *Guys Hosp. Rep.,* 117:1–12.
12. Falconer, M. A. (1971): Anterior temporal lobectomy for epilepsy. In: *Operative Surgery, Vol. 14: Neurosurgery,* edited by V. Logue, pp. 142–149. Butterworths, London.
13. Falconer, M. A. (1971): Genetic and related aetiological factors in temporal lobe epilepsy: A review. *Epilepsia,* 12:13–21.
14. Falconer, M. A. (1972): Temporal lobe epilepsy in children and its surgical treatment. *Med. J. Aust.,* 1:1117–1121.
15. Falconer, M. A. (1973): Reversibility by temporal-lobe resection of the behavioral abnormalities of temporal lobe epilepsy. *N. Engl. J. Med.,* 289:451–455.
16. Falconer, M. A. (1974): Mesial temporal (Ammon's horn) sclerosis as a common cause of epilepsy: Aetiology, treatment, and prevention. *Lancet,* 2:767–770.
17. Falconer, M. A., and Davidson, S. (1973): Coarse features in epilepsy as a consequence of anticonvulsant therapy: Report of cases in two pairs of identical twins. *Lancet,* 2:1112–1114.
18. Falconer, M. A., and Taylor, D. C. (1968): Surgical treatment of drug-resistant epilepsy due to mesial temporal sclerosis. *Arch. Neurol.,* 18:253–261.
19. Falconer, M. A., and Wilson, P. J. E. (1969): Complications related to delayed hemorrhage after hemispherectomy. *J. Neurosurg.,* 30:413–426.
20. Falconer, M. A., Serafetinides, E. A., and Corsellis, J. A. N. (1964): Etiology and pathogenesis of temporal lobe epilepsy. *Arch. Neurol.,* 10:233–248.
21. Ford, F., and Schaffer, A. (1927): The etiology of infantile (acquired) hemiplegia. *Arch. Neurol. Psychiatry,* 18:323–347.
22. Freud, S. (1897): *Die infantile Centrallähmung.* Translated by L. A. Russin and reprinted (1968) as *Infantile Cerebral Paralysis.* University of Miami Press, Coral Gables, Florida.
23. Gastaut, H., Poirier, F., Payan, H., Salamon, G., Toga, M., and Vigoroux, M. (1960): H.H.E. syndrome: Hemiconvulsions, hemiplegia, epilepsy. *Epilepsia,* 1:418–467.
24. Green, J. R. (1967): Temporal lobectomy, with special reference to selection of epileptic patients. *J. Neurosurg.,* 26:584–597.
25. Haberland, C. (1958): Histological studies in temporal lobe epilepsy based on biopsy materials. *Psychiatr. Neurol. (Basel),* 135:12–29.
26. Hauser, W. A., and Kurland, L. T. (1975): The epidemiology of epilepsy in Rochester, Minnesota, 1953 through 1967. *Epilepsia,* 16:1–66.
27. Kinnear Wilson, S. A. (1940): In: *Neurology,* Vol. 2, edited by A. N. Bruce, pp. 770–778 and 1513–1514. Arnold, London.
28. Lennox-Buchthal, M. A. (1973): Febrile convulsions: A reappraisal. *Electroencephalogr. Clin. Neurophysiol. (Suppl. 32).*
29. Livingstone, G. (1968): Infantile febrile convulsions. *Dev. Med. Child Neurol.,* 10:374–376.
30. Lyon, G. Dodge, P. R., and Adams, R. D. (1961): The acute encephalopathies of obscure origin in infants and children. *Brain,* 84:680–708.
31. Malamud, N. (1958): Some observations on the pathology of epilepsy following birth trauma and post-natal infection in the light of temporal lobe epilepsy. In: *Temporal Lobe Epilepsy,* edited by M. Baldwin and P. Bailey, pp. 149–165. Charles C Thomas, Springfield, Ill.
32. Margerison, J. H., and Corsellis, J. A. N. (1966): Epilepsy and the temporal lobes: A

clinical, electroencephalographic and neuropathological study of the brain with particular reference to the temporal lobes. *Brain*, 89:499–530.

33. Mathieson, G. (1975): Pathologic aspects of epilepsy with special reference to the surgical pathology of focal cerebral seizures. *Adv. Neurol.*, 8:107–138.

34. Meldrum, B. S., and Brierley, J. B. (1972): Neuronal loss and gliosis in the hippocampus following repetitive epileptic seizures induced in adolescent baboons by allyl glycine. *Brain Res.*, 48:361–365.

35. Meldrum, B. S., Vigoroux, R. A., and Brierley, J. B. (1973): Systemic factors and epileptic brain damage: Prolonged seizures in paralyzed, artificially ventilated baboons. *Arch. Neurol.*, 29:82–87.

36. Meyer, A. (1963): Intoxications. In: *Greenfield's Neuropathology*, 2nd ed., edited by W. Blackwood, W. H. McMenemey, A. Meyer, R. M. Norman, and D. S. Russell, pp. 235–287. Arnold, London.

37. Millichap, J. G. (1968): *Febrile Convulsions*. Macmillan, New York.

38. Newcombe, R. L., Shah, S. H., Hoare, R. D., and Falconer, M. A. (1975): Radiological abnormalities in temporal lobe epilepsy and clinicopathological correlations. *J. Neurol. Neurosurg. Psychiatry*, 38:279–287.

39. Norman, R. M. (1963): Acute encephalopathies of vascular origin originating in early life and post-encephalitic encephalopathy. In: *Greenfield's Neuropathology*, 2nd ed., edited by W. Blackwood, W. H. McMenemey, A. Meyer, R. M. Norman, and D. S. Russell, pp. 401–405. Arnold, London.

40. Norman, R. M. (1964): The neuropathology of status epilepticus. *Med. Sci. Law*, 4:46–51.

41. Norman, R. M., Sandry, S. A., and Corsellis, J. A. N. (1974): The nature and origin of pathoanatomical change in the epileptic brain. In: *Handbook of Clinical Neurology, Vol. 15: The Epilepsies*, edited by O. Magnus and A. M. Lorento de Haas, pp. 611–620. North-Holland Publishing Co., Amsterdam.

42. Ojemann, G. A., and Ward, A. A. (1975): Stereotactic and other procedures for epilepsy. *Adv. Neurol.*, 8:241–263.

43. Osler, W. (1889): *The Cerebral Palsies of Childhood*. Lewis, London.

44. Ounsted, C., Lindsay, J., and Norman, R. (1966): *Biological Factors in Temporal Lobe Epilepsy*, Heinemann, London.

45. Penfield, W., and Paine, K. W. (1955): Results of surgical therapy for focal epileptic seizures. *Can. Med. Assoc. J.*, 73:515–531.

46. Rasmussen, T. (1968): The role of surgery in the treatment of focal epilepsy. *Clin. Neurosurg.*, 16:288–314.

47. Sano, K., and Malamud, N. (1953): Clinical significance of sclerosis of the cornu ammonis. *Arch. Neurol. Psychiatry*, 70:40–53.

48. Scheibel, M. E., Crandall, P. H., and Scheibel, A. B. (1974): The hippocampal-dentate complex in temporal lobe epilepsy. *Epilepsia*, 15:55–80.

49. Shanks, R. A. (1948): The historial background of convulsions in childhood. *Arch. Dis. Child.*, 24:257–267.

50. Taylor, D. C., and Falconer, M. A. (1968): Clinical, socio-economic, and psychological changes after temporal lobectomy for epilepsy. *Br. J. Psychiatry*, 114:1247–1261.

51. Taylor, D. C., and Ounsted, C. (1971): Biological mechanisms influencing the outcome of seizures in response to fevers. *Epilepsia*, 12:39–43.

52. Taylor, J. (1905): *Paralysis and Other Diseases of the Nervous System in Childhood and Early Life*. Churchill, London.

53. Terzian, H. (1958): Observations on the clinical symptomatology of bilateral, partial or total removal of the temporal lobes. In: *Temporal Lobe Epilepsy*, edited by M. Baldwin and P. Bailey, pp. 501–529. Charles C Thomas, Springfield, Ill.

54. Van Buren, J. M., Ajmone Marsan, C., Mutsaga, N., and Sadowsky, D. (1975): Surgery of temporal lobe epilepsy. *Adv. Neurol.*, 8:155–181.

55. Weller, S. D. V., and Norman, R. M. (1955): Epilepsy due to birth injury in one of identical twins. *Arch. Dis. Child.*, 30:453–456.

56. Wilson, P. J. E. (1970): Cerebral hemispherectomy for infantile hemiplegia: A report of 50 cases. *Brain*, 93:147–179.

57. Zimmerman, H. M. (1938): The histopathology of convulsive disorders in children. *J. Pediatr.*, 13:859–890.

Brain Dysfunction in Infantile Febrile Convulsions, edited by M. A. B. Brazier and F. Coceani. Raven Press, New York © 1976.

A Summing Up: Clinical Session

Margaret A. Lennox-Buchthal

Institute of Neurophysiology, University of Copenhagen, Juliane Mariesvej 36, 2100 Copenhagen, Denmark

A volume on convulsions with fever shows how much interest there is for this rather common illness of childhood. The authors in this section have presented evidence on the clinical aspects that is new or not generally recognized; some of it has been incomplete and some conflicting. I shall try to supplement it, reconcile divergent views when possible, or point out which view has the best evidence in its favor. We could not hope to cover all aspects and so chose to concentrate on genetics, mechanisms, sequelae, and treatment.

DEFINITION

Let us first define convulsions with fever, commonly called febrile convulsions (FCs). The definition used by authors in this volume is that any child who has had a convulsion with a (rectal) temperature of 38°C or more has the specific genetic trait(s) "susceptibility to convulsions with fever" and should be classified as such, whether he has had previous afebrile (e.g., neonatal) convulsions; subsequent afebrile convulsions, few or many; a relative who has had febrile or afebrile seizures; or whether his own convulsion was short or long, generalized or unilateral. This definition is different from the one advocated by Livingston (45), who believes that there are two clinical entities—simple FCs and fever-triggered epilepsy—and that the two entities are distinct. According to him, simple FCs are brief, single, generalized convulsions that occur soon after the onset of fever, when the age is 9–18 months, a relative has had FCs, and the electroencephalogram (EEG) is normal after the temperature has been normal for a week. Subsequent epilepsy occurs in 3%. He distinguishes fever-triggered epilepsy when the convulsion is long or focal at any time during fever, when the child is over 5 years old, and when the EEG is paroxysmal. Only 3% have a relative with convulsions. The prognosis is the same as for afebrile convulsions at the same age. Although many other workers have used his classification, those who have not categorized children *a priori* according to his scheme have not *post hoc* been able to confirm his delineation (3,24,32,58). Therefore the concept that there are two distinct entities—

simple FCs and fever-triggered epilepsy — is useless for diagnosis when the child is seen for his first convulsion.

The group defined as having FCs can be subdivided. Most workers exclude from the group those children whose febrile illness was due to infection of the central nervous system (CNS), arguing that the damage caused by the infection makes it impossible to determine whatever features one is interested in. Only Ounsted and his colleagues (58) contend that convulsions with meningitis, encephalitis, and brain abscess are FCs like any other, especially since fits are much more frequent under than over the age of 4 years ($p < 0.05$) (53). He points out, however, that the incidence of convulsions in the siblings of probands who have a convulsion with fever due to CNS infection makes it likely that the fits of the probands are due to gross organic brain damage with little evidence of a specific genetic trait: The sibs are no more at risk for FCs than the population at large (3%), whereas the sibs of probands whose convulsions are associated with fever that does *not* involve the CNS have a 20% risk for FCs (Fig. 1).

Subgroups under the main classification "FCs" can be dealt with for the purpose of comparison, but subgroups should not be excluded unless the reason is compelling. For example, when factors related with the kind and incidence of neurological sequelae are to be studied, it is defensible to exclude those children who had gross neurological deficits before the FC,

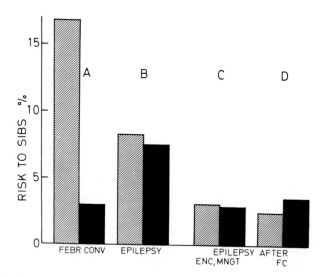

FIG. 1. Risk to sibs (ordinate) of probands with FCs or epilepsy (43). **A:** Probands with simple FCs (570 sibs) and with febrile and transient afebrile seizures (116 sibs). **B:** Probands with epilepsy, i.e., with recurrent afebrile seizures (274 sibs). **C:** Probands with FCs followed by epilepsy (75 sibs). **D:** Probands with epilepsy subsequent to massive insult to the brain (meningitis, encephalitis, and other causes; 182 sibs). Hatched columns: simple FCs and transient afebrile convulsions (groups CVR, CVER, and ER) (58). Solid columns: epilepsy (group EC) (58). (Redrawn from 58, Lennox-Buchthal, ref. 43.)

as Aicardi and Chevrie have done (3,4,14). Whether the children with antecedent neurological deficit have inherited a susceptibility to FCs in a different way is not known but should be studied (see under *Genetics,* below).

When a prospective study is planned, it is reasonable to accept into the group consecutive children seen with their first convulsion if it was accompanied by fever, i.e., the first convulsion (after the neonatal period) solely with fever. The general statement that "febrile convulsions apply to convulsions occurring solely with fever" (43) is blatantly false. In fact the child with FCs (an estimated 5–10%) may have an occasional afebrile convulsion, usually one or two, and often under certain conditions such as after a slight blow on the head or during violent struggling and crying (both examples are from ref. 49). These convulsions under certain conditions are presumably what Hochsinger (35) meant when he described *Gelegenheitskrämpfe.* After first FCs a few children may even have repeated afebrile convulsions to a degree that the child is considered to have developed epilepsy; but these convulsions may then cease, and after a 2-year seizure-free interval without medication the diagnosis of epilepsy, in the sense of chronic afebrile convulsions, must be withdrawn (25). Ounsted called the condition "epilepsy which remits" (55) and Lennox (41) spoke of it as "transient" as opposed to "chronic" epilepsy, including as transient both the transitory susceptibility to convulsions during childhood and the rare convulsions in adult life that some of these individuals may have. When rare convulsions occur in adults under certain circumstances, often in those with a history of FCs, they have been called "stress" convulsions (26).

The purpose of discussing the definition of FCs at such length is to underline that any study should make clear precisely which definition is being used. Differences may explain some of the points of disagreement in the literature and may reconcile some of the divergent findings reported in this volume.

PREVALENCE

How frequent is this fairly common illness of childhood? Four studies have been reported in which all mothers attending a well-baby clinic or in a certain area were asked in detail and in words they would understand whether the child had ever had a convulsion, stiffening or jerks with unconsciousness, a fit with a febrile illness, teething fits, etc. The mother was asked when the baby was at least 3 years old and under school age (15,59), or in primary school (37) or under 20 years of age (69), when she would not have forgotten. Agreement was rather close (respectively, 31,32,23, and 36/1,000); an epidemiological study with detailed follow-up found 33/1,000 (32). Thus a mean of 31/1,000 normal children have had FCs, accounting for approximately half the convulsions under 5 years. Two studies were prospective ones; consecutively born children were followed for 3–5 years.

In the series with the most detailed information on illnesses during the first 5 years of life (49), the prevalence of FCs was 33/1,000, as in the surveys described above. In a large series of 18,500 consecutively born babies, only 2% had an FC (80), the same as the 20/1,000 in the epidemiological study during the years when follow-up was not so detailed (32). Other American studies have found a higher prevalence, from 4% to 4.8%, whether ascertained by study of boys 8–9.5 years old in a school (88), ambulatory clinics (90), a prospective study (the Collaborative Perinatal Project, ref. 30), or questionnaire (63). Gates thought the high rate in her prospective study was due to more complete ascertainment. It is conceivable that differences in definition play some role, since some rates in North America are the same as the European ones and some are 50% higher.

GENETICS

Usual Mode of Inheritance

There seems little doubt — although doubt has been expressed (50) — that the child who has a convulsion with fever has the specific genetic trait for susceptibility to FCs, a trait distinct from that predisposing to chronic afebrile daytime convulsions. Since FCs occur in 10% of the parents (25,41), 10% of the siblings of probands (25,41,54,60), i.e., approximately twice the incidence in aunts and uncles, and four times that in cousins (25), the conclusion is that the trait is an autosomal dominant one with incomplete penetrance. It was not possible to find subgroups of 208 probands where inheritance might be different according to the family history (25), clinical features, or EEGs of the probands (43), but the subgroups and the sibships were small. The incidence in siblings was close to 20% in one study (79), and in one it was 17% in parents and 15% in siblings (21).

Although the trait is thought to be rather frequent, it is often asked why only 10% of parents and sibs have manifest FCs. One view is that most FCs are extremely brief and many occur during sleep (42,43); and they may go unnoticed for both these reasons. Another view has it that the high degree of age dependence (Fig. 2) and the fact that fever is the necessary trigger (Fig. 3) are the explanation (13). Unless the child has a febrile illness at the age of peak susceptibility (9–20 months), he may never have a febrile convulsion. This view is as difficult to prove as it is to disprove. If true, age dependence must be exquisite in some children, since a higher fever a day or a few weeks after the first episode may fail to elicit a convulsion and the child may never have another one (Fig. 4). The mean period of highest susceptibility is probably 6–12 months, since 60–75% of recurrences occur within that time (25,31,43,78,85).

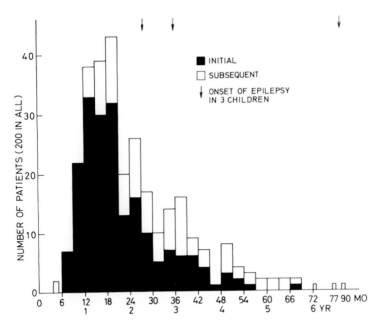

FIG. 2. Age incidence of initial and subsequent FCs of 200 consecutive children (patients reported by Frantzen et al., refs. 24, 25). The arrows show the age at onset of recurrent afebrile convulsions that have persisted, i.e., epilepsy. (From Lennox-Buchthal, ref. 43.)

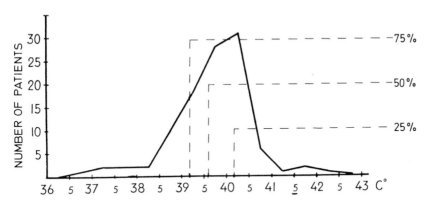

FIG. 3. Distribution of rectal temperatures at the time of an FC or within 0.5 hr in 104 babies. (From Herlitz, ref. 33.)

Dose Factor

There are a few facts about FCs that are difficult to explain unless a genetic dose factor is operating.

1. Boys are more susceptible to FCs than girls by a mean ratio of 1.4:1

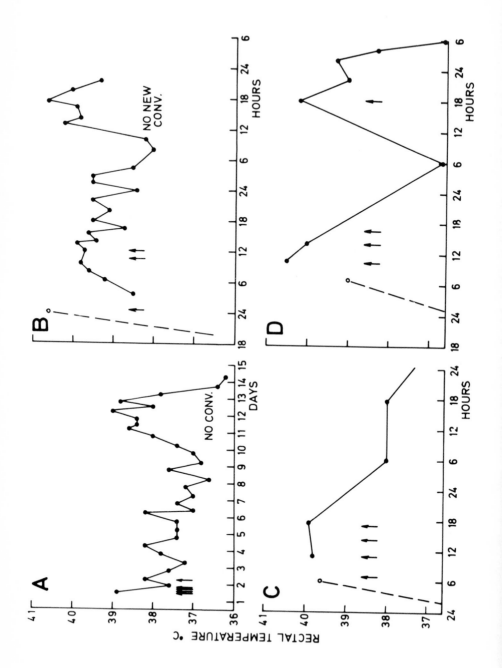

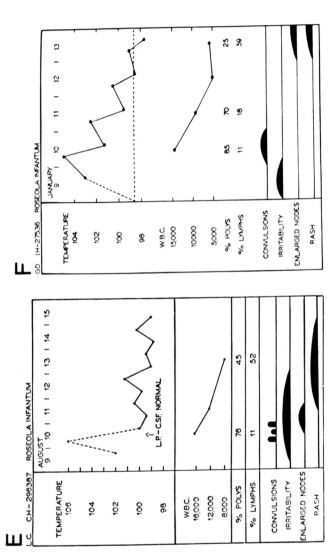

FIG. 4. Exceptions to the rule that the convulsion occurs as the temperature is increasingly rapidly to its peak. The rectal temperature (7°C) is shown on the ordinate, and the time is on the abscissa. The convulsions are indicated by arrows. **A:** The only convulsions of a girl at age 8 months. There were no more convulsions in spite of a higher fever 2 weeks and 2 and 4 months later; she was last seen at age 7. The EEG at 3 years 9 months showed 3/sec spike-wave paroxysms. Her mother has epilepsy. **B:** The only convulsions of a 3-year-old boy, first at a temperature of 40.6°C and repeated at 39.8°C. There were no further convulsions in spite of a new elevation to 40.6°C. The family history was negative. He later developed 3/sec spike-wave paroxysms in the EEG. He was last seen at age 7. **C** and **D:** Two FC episodes of a boy at 16 and 17 months of age. The family history was negative, and the eeg was normal. He was last seen at age 4 years. (The above patients are in the Gentofte series.) **E** and **F:** Convulsions and fever in two children with exanthem subitum (patients of Berenberg et al., 1949). (From Lennox-Buchthal, ref. 43.)

(50), yet girls have more severe convulsions and more recurrences than boys. The less susceptible sex needs a higher dose of the genetic factor to manifest FCs, and the higher dose accounts for more severe and repeated convulsions, the argument runs.

Girls have more "severe" (long or unilateral) convulsions than boys, especially under the age of 18 months (33,43). Unilateral convulsions were more frequent in girls, whether those during fever of nonspecific cause (4) or those due to exanthem subitum, common infectious diseases of childhood, or vaccination (4; for references see ref. 43). Infant girls were especially apt to have a high rate of recurrence (43,85). Girls were more apt to have a severe outcome, which could have been a recurrence since "severe outcome" was "any eventuality other than a single brief febrile convulsion" (74).

Although severe convulsions are much more frequent in infants, girls do not have more than boys because they are younger at the onset. In three large series totalling 1,464 patients (24,32,33)—all "selected" only in the sense that those patients were excluded whose fever was due to infection of the CNS—the proportion of boys and of girls with onset in the first year of life was the same (Table 1). Nor could Aicardi and Chevrie (4) confirm the supposition (74) that girls have more severe convulsions than boys because they are younger at the onset. CNS infections were included in that series (74), and (probably for that reason) there were many more infants with an onset under 6 months than in any other series.

2. Spike-and-wave paroxysms appear in the EEG of children with FCs (20,24), in about one-third of them (40,43,44), and usually at the age of 2.5 years old or more, i.e., some months to years after the first FC. They are twice as frequent (47%) in those children who have a relative with convulsions, regardless of whether they were febrile, than when the family history is negative for convulsions (24%) (25,43). This relation is baffling unless one assumes that children who develop spike-and-wave patterns have a higher genetic dose, as exemplified by more relatives with manifest convulsions.

3. The younger the infant the more frequent are severe convulsions, a

TABLE 1. *Age at onset of FC in boys and girls[a]*

Age (months)	Onset in boys (%)	Onset in girls (%)
0–11	26	22
12–23	43	44
24–35	18	20
36–47	7	8
48–59	2	3
60+	4	4
Total	100	101

[a] Series of refs. 32, 33, and 43.

finding that has not been satisfactorily explained. It can hardly be due to a dose factor since girls are not younger at the onset. No clues implicating some factor other than a genetic one were given by the description of normal neonatal cerebral development described in previous chapters.

4. Ounsted's (58) information on FCs in siblings suggests that children who develop temporal lobe epilepsy after a febrile status either have a higher dose (30% of their siblings had FCs) or they inherit the trait in a different way (children who developed temporal lobe epilepsy but who had no history of status had the usual 10% of siblings with FCs).

The Trait Inherited?

There is good evidence, from the incidence of seizure disorders in relatives (reviewed in ref. 43), that the specific trait susceptibility to FCs is inherited, not a general convulsive diathesis. There is also evidence—the kind of convulsive disorder in co-twins of monozygotic pairs, that FCs tend to occur in relation with sleep (42), and that some individuals with FCs themselves have nocturnal convulsions (43,55)—that the specific genetic trait may be related with a tendency to nocturnal convulsions. Finally, spike-and-wave discharges in the EEGs of children with FCs suggest that FCs may be genetically related with petit mal epilepsy (see above). There is one report of spike-and-wave discharges and of FCs in three generations of the same family (48). The 3/sec discharges in children with FCs have no clinical connotations, since these children are not apt to have more recurrences or to develop epilepsy more often than children whose EEGs never exhibit spike-and-wave patterns.

Is Inheritance Uniform?

One gets the impression that inheritance may be different when the child with FCs also has some antecedent brain damage, but it has not been possible to pin the difference down.

1. Of 208 consecutive children with FCs whose parents gave reliable information about convulsions in the family, there were 25 who had no relative with FCs but they did have a relative with epilepsy, i.e., recurrent afebrile seizures. Some abnormality in the pre-, peri-, or postnatal period of the probands was frequent (60%) whereas it was uncommon (23%) when a relative had FCs or when no relative had convulsions (25,43). The probands were not grossly different from those in the other groups, nor did their siblings have a different incidence of FCs (43); however, the sibships were generally small, and it is conceivable that a difference could have been hidden.

2. Of 19 pairs of monozygotic twins with FCs (42), concordance for convulsions was very high—100% when the intelligence quotient (IQ) was

alike or differed by no more than 12 IQ points. The sibships of these twins were larger than in the series of consecutive children (25), and there was a significant difference in the incidence of FCs in the siblings. When a parent had FCs 45% of the sibs had FCs, in contrast to the 13% when no parent had them ($p < 0.001$, 43). These two features—the very high degree of concordance in monozygotic twins and the higher incidence of FCs in sibs when a parent had FCs—suggest that inheritance was multifactorial (83) in the twins. Moreover, the ratio of FCs or occasional convulsions in first-, second-, and third-degree relatives was not 8:4:2, but 14:5:2, i.e., more reduction with degree of removal from the proband than with simple dominant inheritance (43,83). The feature that distinguished the twins (42) from the larger group of consecutive children (43) was the high incidence of an abnormal birth history: one twin or both of 10 pairs had a very abnormal birth, one of three pairs had a slightly abnormal birth, and only in two instances were both twins born normally (and both twins in both pairs had congenital idiocy). Concordance in monozygotic twins found through the Registry of Persons (i.e., not referred for a seizure disorder to a physician as in refs. 41–43) was reported to be lower (65) and fewer birth histories to be traumatic (66).

Is the Child With the FC Trait More or Less Apt To Be Damaged by Gross Lesions of the Brain Than the Child Without?

Evidence concerning gross brain lesions is conflicting. Ounsted (55,58) reported the risk to sibs of different groups of probands for FCs. It was 20% when the probands had simple FCs; it was much lower and approximately the same (3%) in two other groups: when the child developed epilepsy after a long FC or after gross insult to the brain (Fig. 1). This finding suggests that the child with the FC trait is no more susceptible to brain damage after gross insult than children without the genetic trait. On the other hand, children who developed temporal lobe epilepsy after a long FC had siblings with a 30% incidence of (brief) FCs, a very high figure indeed. Either the probands had a high genetic dose, or inheritance of the trait susceptibility to FCs was by some other mode (see above under *Dose Factor*, item 2). Probands with temporal lobe epilepsy who had neither gross insult to the brain nor febrile status had siblings with a 10% incidence of FCs—the "normal" incidence in the sibs of probands with FCs. Did the probands themselves have FCs? If so, they must have been more susceptible to brain damage than children without the FC trait.

MECHANISMS

Although study of the mechanisms responsible for this age-dependent transient convulsive disorder is one of the most important tasks in the field today—second only to the study of sequelae and their prevention—there is remarkably little information.

Twenty years ago Abood and Gerard (1) showed a transient enzymatic deficit in the brains of young mice during the period when they were susceptible to audiogenic seizures. We (34) found that during the same limited period around 30 days of age these mice also had a convulsion when their body temperature was raised, and Formby (34) confirmed the deficit in cerebral ATPase and showed that it was the form of ATPase implicated in neural activity: Na,K-activated ATPase. We did not take the next logical step to determine if the same deficit was present in the blood; if it were, the next step would have been to see if human infants had the same deficit at the time of susceptibility to FCs.

To the best of my knowledge, the single observation (9) has not been confirmed that the children have, at least at the time of the FC, a borderline deficit of vitamin B_6 as shown by an abnormal tryptophan loading test that returned to normal a week or so later. Whatever the mechanisms may be, they cannot be sought in normal processes of cerebral maturation "for as much as Children, who fall into Fevers about the time of breeding of Teeth, are not all tormented with Convulsions" (89).

SEQUELAE

Study of sequelae and related factors (the means of preventing them and treating them once they occur) is the largest practical problem in the field, and the one to which the last part of this volume is addressed. You have already read the evidence and views of leaders in the field, and there is little for me to add.

Incidence of Sequelae

When it is the custom to hospitalize infants with FCs, and feasible to arrest within minutes any convulsion lasting 10–20 min, the incidence of death, gross neurological sequelae, or epilepsy (defined as recurrent spontaneous afebrile seizures) is approximately 2–5% (reviewed in ref. 43). This is the population of children with FCs the practicing physician presumably sees. Since it may take him some years to accumulate 100 cases, it is natural that the two to five cases of death or severe sequelae disappear from his memory and he is left with the impression that FCs are benign, with treatment or prevention uncalled for.

When hospitalization is reserved for babies who are very sick, either by reason of the febrile illness or the convulsion, the incidence of sequelae is much higher—hence the death in 0.5–10% (for references see ref. 43) and the gross neurological deficit and epilepsy as defined above in 16–17% (5,40). The physicians who see these babies can tell us about the factors producing sequelae and means of preventing them.

The serious sequelae are: (a) gross neurological deficit, e.g., hemiparesis, regression in mental development, focal motor seizures (3,4,14,27); and

(b) temporal lobe epilepsy (58), often with severe behavioral difficulties such as hyperactivity (38,56), aggressiveness, and outbursts of rage (57).

Gross Neurological Deficit After FCs

There is little to add to the fine analysis presented in this volume (3,14). What you have read that is new is separate evaluations of long and unilateral seizures; usually they are classed together as "severe." We read that those features which favour severe sequelae include a long FC, young age, female sex, and some kind of abnormality during the pre-, peri-, or postnatal period. The only factor amenable to control is the duration of the FC. The health services must be arranged so that FCs longer than 30 min can be prevented — whether by teaching the mother or other lay persons, or by arranging emergency services; how this can best be accomplished is the task of each community. It is worth noting again how important definitions are. In the series in question (3), serious sequelae (hemiplegia, mental deficiency, focal seizures) and mild sequelae (a single afebrile seizure) are given equal weight and analyzed together.

Sequelae were less frequent when a relative had convulsions (3), whereas in Wallace's series (boys, 85) and ours (Fig. 5) children with a family history of convulsive disorders in parents or sibs were *more* apt to have recurrences. We all have a tendency to think that what we have found in our series applies to FCs in general. It does not. We should always specify "in our series."

This admonition applies to the contribution of Wallace (87) to this volume: can "children who convulse when febrile ever truly be said to have been normal?" (17) and "the child who convulses when febrile is drawing attention to a developmental defect" (87). Nonetheless Wallace admits that perhaps 5% of all her patients "appear to definitely acquire new abnormalities in association with the illness in which a fit occurs."

Now, let it be admitted at the outset that children with known brain damage — cerebral palsy (77) or spina bifida (87) — do have a higher than normal incidence of FCs. Let it also be admitted that in some hospital series these patients are probably overrepresented, but to generalize these findings to all children who convulse when febrile seems unjustified.

Space does not permit me to criticize the studies in detail, but I would like to draw attention to a few observations. One of Wallace's main arguments is her own study (84) of the birth histories of children with FCs compared with those in their siblings. Yet of six antenatal and six natal factors studied, only three (bleeding during the first and second trimesters, drugs other than iron given to the mothers, and fetal distress) were significantly different; viewed in the light of the large study of consecutive births (80), which showed no difference between probands and the whole cohort, her finding could as well be interpreted to mean there is no real difference between children with FCs and their sibs. The same criticism applies to the studies of

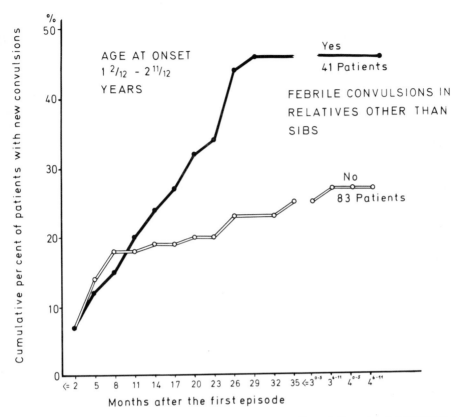

FIG. 5. Family history of FCs and the rate of recurrence. Cumulative rate of recurrence (ordinate) at quarterly intervals after the first FC (abscissa). The age at onset was 14–35 months. The rate is significantly higher in children with a relative with FCs ($\chi^2 = 6.84$, $p <$ 0.01). (From Frantzen et al., ref. 25.)

discordant monozygotic twins that Wallace cites (67,68): Of those items tested, too few were different to justify the conclusion that the child with FCs was different from his co-twin.

Another major support of Wallace's evaluation is the finding that children with FCs had an increased incidence of poor performance on psychological testing. Both she (87) and the psychologist (17) came to the conclusion that it seemed unjustified to isolate the severity of the FCs as an etiological factor, although that was the relation they found. She quotes, but does not consider in her final evaluation, the data (51) on the children (among a total group of 47,222) who had a convulsion within the first year of life. When one simple FC had occurred, the IQ at age 4 years was within normal limits and comparable with the IQ of siblings. After several FCs the IQ at age 4 was within normal limits but was significantly reduced when compared with the IQs of siblings.

To sum up, the balance of evidence points to the conclusion that, in general, FCs occur in normal children, and that any damage found is due to a long convulsion. Those children (and such a group undoubtedly exists) who have an increased susceptibility to FCs because of minimal or overt brain damage should be studied genetically and in other respects.

Temporal Lobe Epilepsy After Febrile Convulsions

It is to the credit of the English that they studied in detail what Bouchet and Cazauvieilh (6) originally described — sclerosis of mesial temporal structures in patients with epilepsy — and to add clinical, EEG, and pathological evidence (46). That a prolonged (>30 min) FC could be one of the causes was established incontrovertibly by the work of Ounsted (58) and Falconer (23) and their colleagues, and was demonstrated experimentally by Meldrum (47). Since Falconer (23) and Meldrum (47) contributed to this volume, there is no need for me to do other than to add a few key words. Questions about the genetic background of children with temporal lobe epilepsy have been discussed. In addition to epilepsy, hyperactivity (38,56) and episodes of rage (57) may accompany the syndrome. Even when epilepsy is not cured by resection of the affected anterior temporal lobe, these behavioural disorders often disappear; but epilepsy is cured or nearly so in 83% of the operated patients (23). Had Falconer not resected *en bloc*, there would have been no proof that the lesion which gives reversible symptoms is sclerosis of mesial temporal structures, nor that a history of long FCs during childhood is found in 79% of those operated early but not in patients with other types of temporal lobe pathology.

The contribution of Meldrum and his associates (47) has been to analyze the factors responsible for mesial temporal sclerosis and the often accompanying cerebellar and cortical neuronal loss. The key words here are the enormous increased cerebral demand for oxygen and for glucose caused in part by the seizure and in part by the fever. As a result, cerebral tissue is more than normally vulnerable if the blood pressure or glucose level falls, or if cerebral circulation is impaired, as it is during a convulsion, by increased intrathoracic pressure and by cerebral edema.

It must be admitted that the duration of the convulsions which produced lesions in adolescent baboons (47) was far longer than the 30-min limit tolerated with safety by the infant with FCs. The question whether the human infant's vulnerability is due to young age or a genetic factor might be answered experimentally.

TREATMENT AND PROPHYLAXIS

Treatment of Acute Attack

Treatment of the acute attack is obviously urgent and, fortunately, feasible. Since phenobarbital acts within hours (not minutes) and makes subsequent use of diazepam risky, it is contraindicated for the acute attack. At present diazepam is the drug of choice (28,29,50a). It is best given slowly intravenously; it can be stopped when the convulsion ceases and then given again if the convulsion recurs. The usual effective dose is 0.5–1 mg/kg (71). The rare complication of respiratory arrest has been reported mainly after phenobarbital had been given first. Diazepam acts nearly as fast when given intramuscularly, or when the *solution* is given several centimeters up into the rectum (2). *The suppository form available commercially is not effective* (2). In addition, the temperature can be lowered by removing blankets and heavy clothes, possibly by giving aspirin.

Prophylactic Treatment

If the mother or a health nurse or lay "visitor" can be instructed precisely how to give diazepam, or if the child can be taken to a physician at once, there is no need for prophylaxis. Furthermore, there is no need if the child has passed his third birthday and is seen during his first convulsion. However, if he is seen during his first convulsion and is not yet 3 years old, then 1 of 2 to 1 of 4 children will have another convulsion, and prophylaxis is advisable to the age of 3 years. If the child is having frequent convulsions, treatment is indicated at any age. In Wallace's series (85) children with long first convulsions were more liable to have a recurrence than children with brief first convulsions; in our series (43) there was no such tendency. The rate of recurrence in our series depended on the age (Fig. 6), sex (Fig. 7), and family history (Fig. 5). Recurrence in the same illness indicated a poor prognosis (51). As the number of episodes increased, the risk of severe convulsions (43) and of afebrile convulsions (11,78) increased. The differences between reports mean simply that different populations are being studied, and each hospital or clinic should try to establish the rate of recurrence and the prognostic features in the population it sees. In spite of the differences, the opinion is becoming more popular that it is wise to protect the child from further convulsions after the first convulsion (Table 2), at least to the age of 3 years. The aim of prophylaxis is that there be *no* new FCs to the age of 3 years, not simply fewer. Some physicians prefer to continue treatment to the age of 6, a practice that can be defended but is probably not necessary. Remember that it is the child and his convulsions that are being treated, not the EEG: Paroxysmal abnormalities in the EEGs are rather frequent although the child receives no treatment and never has another convulsion. Direct damage can be done by too-long and too-intensive treatment of a child who no longer has convulsions (16). *For clinical purposes the EEG is more often misleading than helpful,* and it would be wise not to obtain an EEG except for research purposes. The advice that paroxysmal abnormalities in the EEG constitute an indication for therapy is deplorable.

Drugs effective for prophylaxis are phenobarbital (22) (Table 2), primidone (12,86), and dipropylacetate (Depakine®) (12).

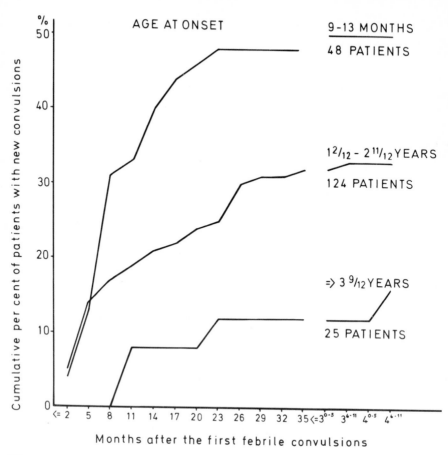

FIG. 6. Age at onset and the rate of recurrence. The cumulative rate of recurrence (ordinate) at quarterly intervals after the first FC (abscissa). The rate is significantly higher in the youngest patients ($p < 0.02$ and 0.01). (From Frantzen et al., ref. 25.)

Phenobarbital

Since the child metabolizes phenobarbital faster than adults (72,73), he needs a higher dose, 3–4 mg/kg (Fig. 8); a more level concentration is maintained if the drug is given twice a day. The symptoms most often reported in the children are hyperactivity and reversal of the sleep cycle. Both symptoms should be less if the drug is given in a single dose an hour before bedtime; when given this way, the dose should be 5 mg/kg in order to compensate for the usual 25% daily excretion by children. Since tolerance to the sedative effect of the drug is acquired within 1–2 weeks, a gradual increase should produce no sedative effect: 1 mg/kg/day for 1 week, increased by 1 mg/kg/day each week. In the hospital (22) children were given twice the usual dose for 2 days to bring their serum concentration to an effective level within

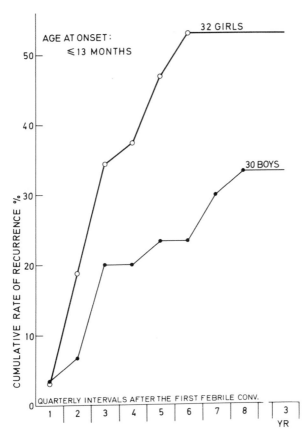

FIG. 7. Sex and the rate of recurrence. The cumulative rate of recurrence (ordinate) at quarterly intervals after the first febrile convulsion (abscissa) for 62 children $\leq$ 13 months old at onset. The rate is significantly higher in girls ($\chi^2 = 5.8$, $p < 0.02$). (Patients were in the Gentofte series.) (From Lennox-Buchthal, ref. 43.)

1–2 days; they then slept most of the time for up to a week, an effect which probably would not be tolerated at home.

The effective serum concentration is at the upper range of the effective concentration in adults—in the Copenhagen area >15 mg/liter (22). Since laboratories differ somewhat, it would be reasonable to measure the serum concentration when a child on treatment has an FC, thereby determining the effective concentration by the method used.

Finally, while medication is being given, the dose must be given every day. If the mother finds she has forgotten a day, she should give twice the dose the next day. If she has forgotten 2 days, she should give a double dose for 2 days. It is not advisable to give medication so irregularly, but it is better than omitting a day's dose entirely. Regular administration is easier for her if she puts the dose for a week into a container so she can see when she has

TABLE 2. Opinions[a] on prophylactic treatment for FCs

| Investigator | Treatment | | | | Recurrence (%) | | Toxic effects (%) | |
	Drug[b]	Dose (mg/kg/day)	Duration[c]	Indication	Control	Treated	Total	Requiring withdrawal
Denmark								
Faerø et al. (22)	Pb	3–5	6 mo trial	1st sz	20	4	10	7
Thorn (75)	Pb	3	2 yr	1st sz	26	13	58	21
Vestermark (82)	Pb			1st sz				
Yssing (91)	Pb	3–4	2 yr or to 4 yr	1st sz		Much less	<10	
France								
Graveleau (31)	Pb	5	"For years"	<1 yr, status, 2nd sz, EEG paroxysm				
Praud (61)	Pb			1st sz				
Roger (62)	Pb		To 6 yr	1st sz		Much less	Few	
Great Britain								
Brett (7)	Pb	3–4						
Ingram (39)	Pb		Long term	1st sz				
Scott and Swash (70)	Pb		2 yr or to 5 yr					
Tibbles (76)	Pb		To 5 yr					
Wallace (86)	Pb	2–4		"Atypical"			Some	
	Prim	10–15		High risk of recurrence	59	17	None	
Italy								
Cavazzuti (12)	Pb	5	1 yr	1st sz	55	0		
	Prim	25	1 yr	1st sz	55	6		
Scanabissi (64)	Dpk	20	Cont	1st sz	55	4		
Portugal								
De Freitas (19)			2 yr	2nd sz or abnormal EEG				

Study[a]	Drug[b]	Age (yr)	Duration	Criteria		
Spain						
Burlo and Vazquez (8)				For infants		
United States						
Carter (10)	Pb		Cont	1st sz		
David (18)	Pb		Int to 6 yr	First sign of illness		
Hauser and Kurland (32)	Pb		Int 13%	First sign of illness		
	Pb		Cont 13%			
Holowach et al. (36)			4 yr	Three episodes		
Livingston (45)	O			"Simple"		
	Pb		Cont	"Atypical"		
Ouellette (52)	Pb	3–6	3 yr sz-free	All except single brief		
Van den Berg and Yerushalmy (81)	Pb		Int	1st sz	30	20

[a] Most are found in *Epilepsy Abstracts*, 1972–1975.
[b] Pb, phenobarbital. Prim, primidone. Dpk, Depakine®.
[c] Sz, seizure. Cont, continuous. Int, intermittent.

Phenobarbital

Daily dose in mg

Body weight in kg	15	30	50	75	100	150	200	250	300	400	500
10	5	**15**	**25**								
15	5	**10**	**15**	25							
20	5	**10**	**10**	**20**	25						
25	5	5	**10**	**15**	**20**						
30		5	**10**	**15**	**20**						
35		5	**10**	**15**	**20**						
40		5	**10**	**15**	**20**						
50		5	**10**	**15**	**20**	30	40	50			
60		5	**10**	**15**	**20**	25	35	40	50		
70		5	5	**10**	**15**	**20**	30	35	45		
80			5	**10**	**15**	**20**	25	30	40	50	
90			5	**10**	**10**	**15**	**20**	30	35	45	
100			5	**10**	**10**	**15**	**20**	25	30	40	50
120				5	**10**	**10**	**15**	**20**	25	35	40

Serum level in μg/ml

FIG. 8. At the center are the serum concentrations of phenobarbital (milligrams per liter) to be expected when children with a given body weight (left) take a given daily dose (top). The effective anticonvulsant levels in adults are in bold type (72). The effective anticonvulsant concentration in children with FCs is over 15 mg/liter (22).

forgotten a dose. She can then lock the main supply out of reach lest the child or his siblings ingest a toxic dose.

Dipropylacetate

Cavazzuti (12) reported that dipropylacetate is just as effective as phenobarbital or primidone for prophylaxis. He gave 20 mg/kg/day in two daily doses and reported no side effects.

Recommendations for Prophylaxis

We had hoped to have more chapters in this volume on experience with prophylaxis; in their absence I tallied data from *Epilepsy Abstracts 1972–1975* (Table 2), supplemented by material from other sources when available.

Pediatricians in Holland prefer to rely on prompt treatment of the acute attack (*personal communication*). All other European reports favour continuous prophylactic treatment, most from the first seizure, and most for several years or to age 4, 5, or 6 years. Those who report the effect of prophylactic treatment found a much lower rate of recurrence in treated than untreated patients. The incidence of toxic effects is given as from under 10% to nearly 60%, a variation that must depend to some extent on the physician and the way he instructs the mothers since the populations were virtually the same.

In the United States, on the other hand, a minority of physicians advocate continuous medication from the first seizure. Although there is no pharmacological rationale for giving phenobarbital and aspirin at the first sign of illness, it is still advocated, if only to "give the parents something to do" (45).

Phenobarbital has been used for prophylaxis by nearly all physicians. Two recent reports offer dipropylacetate (12) and primidone (12,86) as effective substitutes in case phenobarbital causes intolerable side effects.

SUMMARY

The mean prevalence of FCs has been found to be 31/1,000, although recent studies in the United States found it to be 4–4.8%. The peak incidence is during the second year of life, with few occurring before 6 months and after 5 years. The temperature is usually high: >39.2°C in 75%. Most seizures are brief and half occur during sleep, so many are probably not noticed.

In the main, susceptibility to convulsions with fever is transmitted as a specific trait by a single dominant gene with low penetrance (10% in parents and sibs). Children with some brain damage are more liable to FCs than normal children, and inheritance may be multifactorial in them.

The likely mechanism is an age-dependent enzymatic deficit. Just such a genetically determined deficit of Na,K-activated ATPase was found in the brains of mice at the age when they had a convulsion with elevated body temperature. Clinical studies are notably few.

The incidence of severe sequelae (gross neurological deficit such as hemiparesis, focal motor seizures, temporal lobe epilepsy often with behavioural disorders) is variously estimated as 2–5% and even up to 20%. In the main, the incidence of sequelae is related to that of long or unilateral convulsions (contributions of Aicardi and Chevrie, and Falconer). In Wallace's series "suboptimal neurological development" was postulated. That a long seizure can cause the characteristic lesion — mesial temporal sclerosis — was demonstrated experimentally by Meldrum.

The lesion is amenable to surgical treatment, according to Falconer, although most European reports now favour prevention by continuous prophylactic treatment with phenobarbital, primidone, or dipropylacetate (Table 2) after the first seizure to age 3–4 and some to 6 years. Since the introduction of diazepam 10 years ago by the Marseille school, it has been the drug of choice for arresting seizures.

REFERENCES

1. Abood, L. G., and Gerard, R. W. (1954): A phosphorylation defect in the brains of mice susceptible to audiogenic seizure. In: *Biochemistry of the Developing System*, edited by H. Waelsch, pp. 467–472. Academic Press, New York.

2. Agurell, S., Berlin, A., Ferngren, H., and Hellström, B. (1975): Plasma levels of diazepam after parenteral and rectal administration in children. *Epilepisa,* 16:277–283.
3. Aicardi, J., and Chevrie, J. J. (1970): Convulsive status epilepticus in infants and children: A study of 239 cases. *Epilepsia,* 11:187–197.
4. Aicardi, J., and Chevrie, J. J. (1976): Febrile convulsions: neurological sequelae and mental retardation. *This volume.*
5. Bamberger, P., and Matthes, A. (1959): *Anfälle im Kindesalter.* Karger, Basel.
6. Bouchet and Cazauvieilh (1825, 1826): De l'épilepsie considérée dans ses rapports avec l'aliénation mentale. *Arch. Gen. Med.,* 9:510–542; 10:5–50.
7. Brett, E. M. (1973): Epilepsy in childhood. *Br. J. Hosp. Med.,* 9:177–190.
8. Burlo, J. M., and Vazquez, H. J. (1970): Electroencephalography in childhood febrile convulsions. *Arch. Fund. Roux Ocefa,* 4:59 (Spanish).
9. Careddu, P., Apollonio, T., and Giovannini, M. (1962): Troubles du métabolisme du tryptophane dans le mécanisme pathogénique des convulsions hyperpyrétiques. *Pediatrie,* 17:359–372.
10. Carter, S. (1964): Diagnosis and treatment management of child who has had one convulsion. *Pediatrics,* 33:431–434.
11. Cavazzuti, G. B. (1974): The fate of the child with febrile convulsions. *Clin. Pediatr. (Bologna),* 56:388–395 (Italian).
12. Cavazzuti, G. B. (1975): Prevention of febrile convulsions with dipropylacetate (Depakine®). *Epilepsia,* 16(4):647–648.
13. Chan, K. Y. (1974): Febrile convulsions in Singapore children. M.D. thesis, University of Singapore.
14. Chevrie, J. J., and Aicardi, J. (1975): Duration and lateralization of febrile convulsions: Etiological factors. *Epilepsia,* 16(5):781–790.
15. Costeff, H. (1965): Convulsions in childhood: Their natural history and indications for treatment. *N. Engl. J. Med.,* 273:1410–1413.
16. Covello-Harrison, A., and Lairy, G. C. (1974): Problèmes d'interprétation de l'E.E.G. en neuropsychiatrie infantile: Conséquences sur la conduite thérapeutique. *Rev. Electroencephalogr. Neurophysiol.,* 4:141–162.
17. Cull, A. M. (1975): Some psychological aspects of the prognosis of febrile convulsions. M.Phil. thesis, University of Edinburgh.
18. David, R. B. (1972): Febrile convulsions. *Va. Med. Mon.,* 99:955–959.
19. De Freitas, N. L. (1971): Febrile convulsions. *Rev. Med. Estado Guanabara,* 38:76–81 (Portuguese).
20. Doose, H., Völzke, E., Petersen, C. E., and Herzberger, E. (1966): Fieberkrämpfe und Epilepsia. II. Elektroencephalographische Verlaufsuntersuchungen bei sogenannten Fieber- oder Infektkrämpfen. *Arch. Psychiatr. Nervenkr.,* 208:413–432.
21. Escala, P.: Cited by Metrakos and Metrakos (1972): In: *The Epidemiology of Epilepsy. A Workshop,* pp. 97–102. NINDS Monograph No. 14.
22. Faero, O., Kastrup, K. W., Lykkegaard Nielsen, E., Melchior, J. C., and Thorn, I. (1972): Successful prophylaxis of febrile convulsions with phenobarbital. *Epilepsia,* 13:279–285.
23. Falconer, M. A. (1976): Surgical treatment of sequelae of severe febrile convulsions. *This volume.*
24. Frantzen, E., Lennox-Buchthal, M., and Nygaard, A. (1968): Longitudinal EEG and clinical study of children with febrile convulsions. *Electroencephalogr. Clin. Neurophysiol.,* 24:197–212.
25. Frantzen, E., Lennox-Buchthal, M., Nygaard, A., and Stene, J. (1970): A genetic study of febrile convulsions. *Neurology (Minneap.),* 20:909–917.
26. Friis, M. L., and Lund, M. (1974): Stress convulsions. *Arch. Neurol.,* 31:155–159.
27. Gastaut, H., Poirier, F., Payan, H., Salamon, G., Toga, M., and Vigouroux, M. (1960): H.H.E. syndrome: Hemiconvulsions, hemiplegia, epilepsy. *Epilepsia,* 1:418–447.
28. Gastaut, H., Naquet, R., Poiré, R., and Tassinari, C. A. (1965): Treatment of status epilepticus with diazepam (Valium®). *Epilepsia,* 6:167–182.
29. Gastaut, H., Roger, J., Soulayrol, R., Lob, H., and Tassinari, C. A. (1965): L'action du diazepam (Valium®) dans le traitement des formes non convulsives de l'épilepsie genéralisée. *Rev. Neurol. (Paris),* 112:99–118.

30. Gates, M. J. (1972): Age: risk of seizures in infants. In: *The Epidemiology of Epilepsy. A Workshop*, pp. 75–81. NINDS Monograph No. 14.
31. Graveleau, D. (1974): Les convulsions fébriles. *Concours Med.*, 96:5773–5785.
32. Hauser, W. A., and Kurland, L. T. (1975): The epidemiology of epilepsy in Rochester, Minnesota, 1935 through 1967. *Epilepsia*, 16:1–66.
33. Herlitz, G. (1941): Studien über die sogenannten initialen Fieberkrämpfe bei Kindern. *Acta Paediatr. Scand. (Suppl. 1)*, 29.
34. Hertz, L., Schousboe, A., Formby, B., and Lennox-Buchthal, M. (1974): Some age-dependent biochemical changes in mice susceptible to seizures. *Epilepsia*, 15:619–631.
35. Hochsinger, K. (1904): Krämpfe bei Kindern. *Dtsch. Klin.*, 7:479 (cited in ref. 5).
36. Holowach, J., Thurston, D. L., and O'Leary, J. (1972): Prognosis in childhood epilepsy. *N. Engl. J. Med.*, 286:169–174.
37. Hrbek, A. (1957): Fieberkrämpfe im Kindesalter. *Ann Paediatr. (Basel)*, 188:162–182.
38. Ingram, T. T. S. (1956): A characteristic form of over-active behaviour in brain-damaged children. *J. Ment. Sci.*, 102:550–558.
39. Ingram, T. T. S. (1973): The febrile convulsions in childhood. *Dev. Med. Child. Neurol.*, 15:531–533.
40. Laplane, R., and Salbreux, R. (1963): Les convulsions hyperpyrétiques. *Rev. Prat. (Paris)*, 13:753–761.
41. Lennox, W. G. (1960): *Epilepsy and Related Disorders*. Little, Brown, Boston.
42. Lennox-Buchthal, M. (1971): Febrile and nocturnal convulsions in monozygotic twins. *Epilepsia*, 12:147–156.
43. Lennox-Buchthal, M. (1973): Febrile convulsions: A reappraisal. *Electroencephalogr. Clin. Neurophysiol. (Suppl. 32)*.
44. Linda-Grossi-Bianchi, M. (1974): Reperti elettroencefalografici nelle convulsioni febbrili. *Clin. Pediatr.*, 56:411–449.
45. Livingston, S. (1972): *Comprehensive Management of Epilepsy in Infancy, Childhood and Adolescence*. Charles C Thomas, Springfield, Ill.
46. Margerison, J. H., and Corsellis, J. A. N. (1966): Epilepsy and the temporal lobes: A clinical, electroencephalographic and neuropathological study of the brain in epilepsy, with particular reference to the temporal lobes. *Brain*, 89:499–529.
47. Meldrum, B. (1976): Secondary pathology of febrile and experimental convulsions. *This volume*.
48. Meyer, J. G. (1973): Über die Vererbung von Spike-Wave-Komplexen und Fieberkrämpfen in drei Generationen. *Dtsch. Med. Wochenschr.*, 98:1717–1722.
49. Miller, F. J. W., Court, S. D. M., Walton, W. S., and Knox, E. J. (1960): *Growing up in Newcastle upon Tyne: A Continuing Study of Health and Illness in Young Children Within Their Families*. Oxford University Press, London.
50. Millichap, J. G. (1968): *Febrile convulsions*. Macmillan, New York.
50a. Naquet, R., Soulayrol, R., Dolce, G., Tassinari, C. A., Broughton, R., and Loeb, H. (1965): First attempt at treatment of experimental status epilepticus in animals and spontaneous status epilepticus in man with diazepam (Valium). *Electroencephalogr. Clin. Neurophysiol.*, 18:427 (abstract).
51. Nelson, K., Rubenstein, D., and Beadle, E. L. (1972): Seizures with fever beginning in the first year of life. *Child Neurology Society Meetings*, Oct. 5–7, 1972, cited in ref. 52.
52. Ouellette, E. M. (1974): The child who convulses with fever. *Pediatr. Clin. North. Am.*, 21:467–481.
53. Ounsted, C. (1951): Significance of convulsions in children with purulent meningitis. *Lancet*, 1:1245–1248.
54. Ounsted, C. (1952): The factor of inheritance in convulsive disorders in childhood. *Proc. R. Soc. Med.*, 45:865–868.
55. Ounsted, C. (1955): Genetic and social aspects of the epilepsies of childhood. *Eugen. Rev.*, 47:33–49.
56. Ounsted, C. (1955): Hyperkinetic syndrome in epileptic children. *Lancet*, 1:303–311.
57. Ounsted, C. (1969): Aggression and epilepsy: Rage in children with temporal lobe epilepsy. *J. Psychosom. Res.*, 13:237–242.
58. Ounsted, C., Lindsay, J., and Norman, R. (1966): *Biological Factors in Temporal Lobe Epilepsy*. Heinemann, London.

59. Patrick, H. T., and Levy, D. M. (1924): Early convulsions in epileptics and others. *JAMA*, 82:375–381.
60. Portnov, V. A., and Kantor, M. G. (1972): Hereditary aspects of childhood epilepsy. *Genetica (Leningrad)*, 8:142–147 (Russian).
61. Praud, E. (1971): Convulsions due to hyperpyrexia in children. *Rev. Prat.*, 21:4499–4512.
62. Roger, J. (1975): Personal communication.
63. Rose, S. W., Penry, J. K., Markush, R. E., Radloff, L. A., and Putnam, P. L. (1973): Prevalence of epilepsy in children. *Epilepsia*, 14:133–152.
64. Scanabissi, E. (1974): Terapia dell'accesso convulsivo febrile. *Clin. Pediatr.*, 56:399–410.
65. Schiøttz-Christensen, E. (1972): Genetic factors in febrile convulsions. *Acta Neurol. Scand.*, 48:538–546.
66. Schiøttz-Christensen, E. (1973): Rate of birth history in the aetiology and course of febrile convulsions: A twin study. *Neuropaediatrie*, 4:238–244.
67. Schiøttz-Christensen, E. (1973): Neurological findings in twins discordant for febrile convulsions. *Acta Neurol. Scand.*, 49:368–378.
68. Schiøttz-Christensen, E., and Bruhn, P. (1973): Intelligence, behaviour and scholastic achievement subsequent to febrile convulsions: An analysis of discordant twin-pairs. *Dev. Med. Child. Neurol.*, 15:565–575.
69. Schuman, S. H., and Miller, L. J. (1966): Febrile convulsions in families: Findings in an epidemiologic survey. *Clin. Pediatr. (Phila.)*, 5:604–608.
70. Scott, D. F., and Swash, M. (1972): Febrile convulsions in early childhood. *Br. Med. J.*, 3:415–416.
71. Smith, B. T., and Masotti, R. E. (1971): Intravenous diazepam in the treatment of prolonged seizure activity in neonates and infants. *Dev. Med. Child. Neurol.*, 13:630–634.
72. Svensmark, O., and Buchthal, F. (1963): Dosage of phenytoin and phenobarbital in children. *Dan. Med. Bull.*, 10:234–235.
73. Svensmark, O., and Buchthal, F. (1964): Diphenylhydantoin and phenobarbital: Serum levels in children. *Am. J. Dis. Child.*, 108:82–87.
74. Taylor, D. C., and Ounsted, C. (1971): Biological mechanisms influencing the outcome of seizures in response to fever. *Epilepsia*, 12:33–45.
75. Thorn, I. (1975): A controlled study of prophylactic long-term treatment of febrile convulsions with phenobarbital. *Acta Neurol. Scand. (Suppl.)*, 60:67–73.
76. Tibbles, J. A. R. (1973): Febrile convulsions in children. *Nova Scotia Med. Bull.*, 52:162–163.
77. Trojaborg, W. (1969): Personal communication, cited in ref. 43.
78. Van den Berg, B. J. (1974): Studies on convulsive disorders in young children. III. Recurrence of febrile convulsions. *Epilepsia*, 15:177–190.
79. Van den Berg, B. J. (1974): Studies on convulsive disorders in young children. IV. Incidence of convulsions among siblings. *Dev. Med. Child. Neurol.*, 16:457–464.
80. Van den Berg, B. J., and Yerushalmy, J. (1969): Studies on convulsive seizures in young children. I. Incidence of febrile and nonfebrile convulsions by age and other factors. *Pediatr. Res.*, 3:298–304.
81. Van den Berg, B. J., and Yerushalmy, J. (1971): Studies on convulsive disorders in young children. II. Intermittent phenobarbital prophylaxis and recurrence of febrile convulsions. *J. Pediatr.*, 78:1004–1012.
82. Vestermark, S. (1972): Fits in children. *Manedsskr. Prakt. Laegegern.*, 50:552–563 (Danish).
83. Vogel, F., and Krüger, J. (1967): Multifactorial determination of genetic affections. In: *Proceedings of the Third International Congress of Human Genetics*, edited by J. F. Crow and J. V. Niel, pp. 437–445. Johns Hopkins Press, Baltimore.
84. Wallace, S. J. (1972): Aetiological aspects of febrile convulsions: Pregnancy and perinatal factors. *Arch. Dis. Child.*, 47:171–178.
85. Wallace, S. J. (1974): Recurrence of febrile convulsions. *Arch. Dis. Child.*, 49:763–765.
86. Wallace, S. J. (1975): Continuous prophylactic anticonvulsants in selected children with febrile convulsions. *Acta Neurol. Scand. [Suppl.]*, 60:62–65.
87. Wallace, S. J. (1976): Neurological and intellectual deficits: Convulsions with fever viewed as acute indications of life-long developmental defects. *This volume.*
88. Weinberg, W. (1972): Epilepsy: a study of a school population. In: *The Epidemiology of Epilepsy: A Workshop*, pp. 57–58. NINDS Monograph No. 14.

89. Willis, T. (1685): *The London Practise of Physick or the Whole Practical Part of Physick.* George and Crooke, London.
90. Wiygul, F. M., Jr. (1972): Epilepsy in high risk groups. In: *The Epidemiology of Epilepsy: A Workshop.* pp. 59–61. NINDS Monograph No. 14.
91. Yssing, M. (1975): Personal communication.

AUTHOR INDEX

Author Index

Abel-Latif, A. A., 49(1)*
Abrahams, S. J., 35(27)
Adair, E. R., 70(4)
Adinolfi, A. M., 169(24), 172(24)
Adler, R. D., 141(1), 144(1)
Agid, Y., 26(22), 33(22)
Aguiar, A. J., 61(36)
Aicardi, J., 214(1), 218(1, 2), 219(1,2), 247 (3), 251(1), 253(2), 254(1), 255(3)
Ajmone-Marsan, C., 189(1,44,45), 190(45), 220(45)
Alberici, M., 219(9)
Alderdice, M. T., 141(9)
Allen, I. V., 89(1), 120(1)
Allison, M., 141(2)
Altman, J., 26(17), 31(16), 163(1)
Amin, A. N., 77(1), 78(2)
Amsile, J., 247(3), 255(3)
Anden, N-E., 41(2)
Andersson, B., 81(3)
Änggård, E., 60(2), 62(1)
Aprison, M. H., 29(20)
Arias, L. P., 218(3)
Athar, S., 183(21)
Atkins, E., 107(1), 117(21), 120(2-9, 15,16,24,25,33,34), 122(7,8,17,18,28), 123(21), 141(2)
Atkins, L., 90(23)
Avery, D. D., 80(4,5), 89(2,3), 101(3), 102(3)
Avery, D. L., 167(26,30), 168(2,26,30), 169(26)

Axelrod, J., 26(10–12), 27(10–12), 28(10), 31(10)
Ayala, G. F., 190(4,46), 191(2), 197(3), 204(3), 207(3)

Baird, J. A., 156(11)
Bak, I. J., 26(1), 31(1)
Baker, M. A., 179(12), 180(12,13), 181(12), 182(12,13), 183(12, 13), 184(12,13)
Baker, P. C., 48(3)
Baldwin, M., 219(10)
Baldy-Moulinier, M., 218(3)
Baraton, J., 214(1), 218(1), 219(1), 251(1), 254(1)
Barbour, H. G., 141(3,4), 179(1)
Barker, J. L., 190(5), 195(5)
Barstad, J. A. B., 194(6)
Bartholini, G., 34(30), 41(34,51)
Beaujouan, J. C., 26(22), 33(22), 34(21), 41(21), 48(21)
Becker, C. G., 27(46)
Beckman, A. L., 89(4,5), 102(5)
Bedard, P., 41(2)
Beere, A., 41(23), 48(23), 49(23)
Beeson, J. P., 144(5)
Beeson, P. B., 107(2,3), 122(10)
Behrman, H. R., 147(46)
Beleslin, D. B., 81(64),

102(37)
Bennett, I. L., Jr., 107(3), 122(10)
Bennett, J. W., 156(11)
Bergstrom, S., 64(3)
Berlin, R. D., 120(11), 144(6)
Bernard, C., 75(8)
Bernardi, G., 169(14), 170(14,15), 174(14)
Bernhard, C. G., 199(7)
Bernheimer, H., 25(2)
Bertilsson, L. M., 49(4)
Bertin, R., 76(9)
Bhargava, A. K., 90(48), 98(49), 99(49)
Bhargava, K. P., 90(48), 98(49), 99(49)
Biggio, G., 42(5)
Bird, E. D., 25(3)
Birkmayer, W., 25(2)
Bishai, I., 60(4)
Bishop, E. J., 199(8)
Bito, L., 60(5,6)
Blatteis, C. M., 155(1)
Bligh, J., 69(3), 72(2), 77(11), 78(12), 79(12), 80(11,12), 81(10,12), 99(6), 101(6), 102(6), 130(1), 146(7), 156(3), 157(2,4), 158(4)
Bloom, F. E., 26(42), 27(42), 29(28), 41(22), 63(7,52)
Bodel, P., 107(1), 117(21), 120(8,13,15,16), 121(19,22), 122(8, 14,17,18,20,22,28), 123(12,13,21)
Bogdanski, D. F., 102(7)

---

*Numbers in parentheses represent reference numbers.

SUBJECT INDEX

Subject Index